*Recent Advances in*
# OPHTHALMOLOGY-16

# Recent Advances in
# OPHTHALMOLOGY-16

*Editor*

**Nitin Nema**  MS DNB
Professor
Department of Ophthalmology
Sri Aurobindo Medical College and
Postgraduate Institute of Medical Sciences
Indore, Madhya Pradesh, India

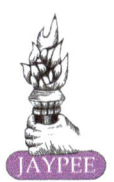

**JAYPEE BROTHERS MEDICAL PUBLISHERS**
*The Health Sciences Publisher*
**New Delhi | London**

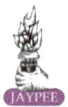 **Jaypee Brothers Medical Publishers (P) Ltd**

**Headquarters**
Jaypee Brothers Medical Publishers (P) Ltd
EMCA House, 23/23-B, Ansari Road, Daryaganj
New Delhi 110 002, India
Landline: +91-11-23272143, +91-11-23272703
+91-11-23282021, +91-11-23245672
Email: jaypee@jaypeebrothers.com

**Corporate Office**
Jaypee Brothers Medical Publishers (P) Ltd
4838/24, Ansari Road, Daryaganj
New Delhi 110 002, India
Phone: +91-11-43574357
Fax: +91-11-43574314
Email: jaypee@jaypeebrothers.com

**Overseas Office**
JP Medical Ltd
83 Victoria Street, London
SW1H 0HW (UK)
Phone: +44 20 3170 8910
Fax: +44 (0)20 3008 6180
Email: info@jpmedpub.com

Website: www.jaypeebrothers.com
Website: www.jaypeedigital.com

© 2023, Jaypee Brothers Medical Publishers

The views and opinions expressed in this book are solely those of the original contributor(s)/author(s) and do not necessarily represent those of editor(s) or publisher of the book.

All rights reserved. No part of this publication may be reproduced, stored or transmitted in any form or by any means, electronic, mechanical, photocopying, recording or otherwise, without the prior permission in writing of the publishers.

All brand names and product names used in this book are trade names, service marks, trademarks or registered trademarks of their respective owners. The publisher is not associated with any product or vendor mentioned in this book.

Medical knowledge and practice change constantly. This book is designed to provide accurate, authoritative information about the subject matter in question. However, readers are advised to check the most current information available on procedures included and check information from the manufacturer of each product to be administered, to verify the recommended dose, formula, method and duration of administration, adverse effects and contraindications. It is the responsibility of the practitioner to take all appropriate safety precautions. Neither the publisher nor the author(s)/editor(s) assume any liability for any injury and/or damage to persons or property arising from or related to use of material in this book.

This book is sold on the understanding that the publisher is not engaged in providing professional medical services. If such advice or services are required, the services of a competent medical professional should be sought.

Every effort has been made where necessary to contact holders of copyright to obtain permission to reproduce copyright material. If any have been inadvertently overlooked, the publisher will be pleased to make the necessary arrangements at the first opportunity.

Inquiries for bulk sales may be solicited at: jaypee@jaypeebrothers.com

*Recent Advances in Ophthalmology-16*

*First Edition*: **2023**

ISBN: 978-93-5696-196-8

**Dedicated to**
*My father, Dr Hari Vallabh Nema,
with immense love and regards*

# Contributors

**Aishwarya Joshi** MBBS DNB
Fellow
Vitreoretina Services
Narayana Nethralaya
Bengaluru, Karnataka, India

**Anand Vinekar** DNB FRCS FPVR PhD
Senior Consultant
Narayana Nethralaya
Bengaluru, Karnataka, India

**Anthony Vipin Das** FRCS
Network Associate Director
Department of eyeSmart EMR and
AEye and Indian Health Outcomes
Public Health and Economics
Research Center
LV Prasad Eye Institute
Hyderabad, Telangana, India

**Arjun Bamel** DOMS DNB
Vitreoretinal Fellow
Sankara Nethralaya
Medical Research Foundation
Chennai, Tamil Nadu, India

**Arthi Mohankumar**
MS MRCS (Ed) FICO FAICO (Retina)
Vitreoretinal Consultant
Rajan Eye Care Hospital
Chennai, Tamil Nadu, India

**Arup Chakrabarti** MS
Cataract and Glaucoma Consultant
Chakrabarti Eye Care Centre
Thiruvananthapuram, Kerala, India

**Brughanya Subramanian**
M Optom
Research Optometrist
Shri Bhagwan Mahavir Vitreoretinal
Services
Sankara Nethralaya
Chennai, Tamil Nadu, India

**Chaitra Jayadev** MBBS DOMS FVR PhD
Head
Vitreoretina Services
Narayana Nethralaya
Bengaluru, Karnataka, India

**Chitralekha S Devishamani**
M Optom
Research Optometrist
Shri Bhagwan Mahavir Vitreoretinal
Services
Sankara Nethralaya
Chennai, Tamil Nadu, India

**Dinesh Visva Gunasekeran**
MBBS
Senior Instructor and Faculty Advisor
Medical Innovation
National University of Singapore
Singapore

**Dipankar Das** MBBS MS
Head and Senior Consultant
Uveitis-Ocular Pathology Services
Department of Ocular Pathology
Uveitis and Neuro-ophthalmology
Sri Sankaradeva Nethralaya
Guwahati, Assam, India

## Contributors

**Divyansh Kailashchandra Mishra**
DO DNB FVRS FGO FICO FAICO
Consultant
Department of Vitreoretina and
Ocular Oncology
Sankara Eye Hospital
Bengaluru, Karnataka, India

**Gangadhara Sundar** DO FRCS (Ed) FAMS
Diplomate, The American Board of
Ophthalmology
Head, Orbit and Oculofacial Surgery
Department of Ophthalmology
National University Hospital
National University of Singapore
Singapore

**Giridhar Anantharaman** MS
Senior Consultant
Vitreoretinal Services
Giridhar Eye Institute
Kochi, Kerala, India

**Gitansha Sachdev** MS FICO
Senior Consultant
Cataract, Refractive Surgery
The Eye Foundation
Coimbatore, Tamil Nadu, India

**Gopal R** DO DNB
Senior Consultant
Cataract, Glaucoma and
Refractive Surgery
The Eye Foundation
Kochi, Kerala, India

**Hima Pendharkar**
DNB (Radiodiagnosis) DM (Neuroimaging and
Interventional Neuroradiology)
Professor
Department of Nuroimaging and
Interventional Radiology
National Institute of Mental Health and
Neurosciences
Bengaluru, Karnataka, India

**Kalpita Das** MS DNB
Associate Consultant
Vitreoretina and Ocular
Oncology Services
Kamalnayan Bajaj Sankara Nethralaya
Kolkata, West Bengal, India

**Kiran Chandran** MS
Associate Consultant Medical Retina
Vitreoretinal Services
Giridhar Eye Institute
Kochi, Kerala, India

**Lingam Gopal**
MS FRCS DNB MSC (Epidemiology)
Senior Consultant
Sankara Nethralaya
Medical Research Foundation
Chennai, Tamil Nadu, India
National University Hospital
Singapore

**Madhusmita Mahapatra** MBBS
Sri Sankaradeva Nethralaya
Guwahati, Assam, India

**Mahesh Shanmugam Palanivelu**
DO FRCS (Ed) PhD
Head
Department of Vitreoretina and
Ocular Oncology
Sankara Eye Hospital
Bengaluru, Karnataka, India

**Meena Chakrabarti** MS
Vitreoretinal Consultant
Chakrabarti Eye Care Centre
Thiruvananthapuram, Kerala, India

**Mohan Rajan**
DO DNB FMRF MCh FIAMS FACS FRCS PhD DSc
Chairman and Medical Director
Rajan Eye Care Hospital
Chennai, Tamil Nadu, India

## Contributors

**Mohana Sinnasamy** MBBS DO
Consultant
Swamy Eye Clinic
Chennai, Tamil Nadu, India

**Murali Ariga** MS DNB FAICO (Glaucoma)
Head
Department of Ophthalmology
Sundaram Medical Foundation
Chennai, Tamil Nadu, India

**Ng Yu Ci Faye**
Medical Student
Yong Loo Lin School of Medicine
National University of Singapore
Singapore

**Nishanth Murali** MBBS FEM
Medical Officer
Swamy Eye Clinic
Chennai, Tamil Nadu, India

**Obaidur Rehman** MS
Fellow
Ophthalmic Plastic and Reconstructive
Surgery and Facial Aesthetics
Department of Oculoplasty
Sri Sankaradeva Nethralaya
Guwahati, Assam, India

**Parul Ichhpujani** MS MBA (HA)
Professor
Department of Ophthalmology
Government Medical College and
Hospital
Chandigarh, India

**Parveen Sen** MS
Senior Retina Consultant
Shri Bhagwan Mahavir Vitreoretinal
Services
Sankara Nethralaya
Chennai, Tamil Nadu, India

**Pawan Garde** MS
Senior Resident
M & J Western Regional Institute
of Ophthalmology
Ahmedabad, Gujarat, India

**Payal Naresh Shah** DNB FVRS
Consultant and Research Associate
Department of Vitreoretina and
Ocular Oncology
Sankara Eye Hospital
Bengaluru, Karnataka, India

**Purvi Bhagat** MS DO FAIMER
Professor and Head
M & J Western Regional Institute of
Ophthalmology
Ahmedabad, Gujarat, India

**Raghulnadhan Ramanadhane** MS
Clinical Fellow Vitreoretinal Services
Kamalnayan Bajaj Sankara Nethralaya
Kolkata, West Bengal, India

**Rajesh Sinha** MD DNB FIACLE FRCS
Professor
Dr Rajendra Prasad Centre for
Ophthalmic Sciences
All India Institute of Medical Sciences
New Delhi, India

**Rajiv Raman** MS DNB FRCS (Ed) Hon DSc
Senior Retina Consultant
Shri Bhagwan Mahavir Vitreoretinal
Services
Sankara Nethralaya
Chennai, Tamil Nadu, India

**Rakesh K** MS
Vitreoretinal Fellow
Rajan Eye Care Hospital
Chennai, Tamil Nadu, India

**Ramamurthy D** MD DNB
Chairman
The Eye Foundation Group of Hospitals
Coimbatore, Tamil Nadu, India

**Rishabh Rathi** MS
Senior Resident
Department of Ophthalmology
Sri Aurobindo Medical College and
Postgraduate Institute of
Medical Sciences
Indore, Madhya Pradesh, India

## Contributors

**Rupesh Agrawal**
DNB FRCS (G) MMed (Ophth) MD (Research)
Senior Consultant
Department of Ophthalmology
Tan Tock Seng Hospital
Associate Professor
Lee Kong Chian School of Medicine
Singapore

**Sakshi Mishra** MBBS
Sri Sankaradeva Nethralaya
Guwahati, Assam, India

**Shahnaz Anjum** MD
Registrar
Dr Rajendra Prasad Centre for
Ophthalmic Sciences
All India Institute of Medical Sciences
New Delhi, India

**Shreesha Kumar Kodavoor**
MS DNB MNAMS
Senior Consultant
Cornea, Cataract, and Refractive
Surgery
The Eye Foundation
Coimbatore, Tamil Nadu, India

**Sushmita Kaushik** MS FAICO
Professor Glaucoma Services
Advanced Eye Center
Postgraduate Institute of Medical
Education and Research
Chandigarh, India

**Yashas Goyal** MS
VST Centre for Glaucoma Care
LV Prasad Eye Institute
Hyderabad, Telangana, India

# Preface

The main theme of *"Recent Advances in Ophthalmology-16"* is *Artificial Intelligence in Ophthalmology* as envisaged by late Dr Hari Vallabh Nema. Artificial intelligence (AI) technology utilizes computational methods to mimic human behavior and thought process. Its application includes assisting a medical practitioner to understand the disease in a better way and take correct decisions. Moreover, it is a sophisticated and reliable diagnostic tool that can be used to detect an ophthalmic disease and monitor the treatment response.

Anthony Vipin Das et al. have lucidly described in Chapter 1 about the medical data, its generation and collection, and development of algorithms to train neural networks for the purpose of AI. High-quality ophthalmic imaging has enabled image-based deep learning to become an integral part of eyecare to diagnose ocular diseases. However, despite the increasing application of AI in ophthalmic practice, there exist some limitations—data safety, the patient's privacy, and ethical concerns.

One of the leading causes of visual impairment is uncorrected refractive errors. Fundus photographs, optical coherence tomography (OCT) images, and eccentric photorefraction techniques are utilized to predict refractive errors by AI.

Artificial intelligence algorithms have been developed to diagnose corneal ectasias, especially keratoconus and forme fruste keratoconus. Rajesh Sinha and colleagues have given a detailed description of the application of machine learning technology in detection and management of keratoconus.

Patients undergoing refractive surgery have extremely high expectations for excellent unaided visual acuity. The refractive surgeons, therefore, must remain updated with the newer refractive procedures, surgical skills, and technological advancements. This has been described vividly in Chapter 4 by Shreesha Kumar Kodavoor et al.

Optical coherence tomography is increasingly being used in the pre-perimetric glaucoma diagnosis. The OCT machines have inbuilt dedicated glaucoma software and algorithms to detect early glaucomatous damage and disease progression. Sushmita Kaushik and coauthors have presented a detailed account of the use of OCT in the diagnosis of glaucoma.

Images derived from multiple imaging modalities used in the diagnosis of glaucoma can be deployed to develop machine learning algorithms. However, a number of challenges, such as data validation, black-box phenomenon, data privacy, and acceptability of patients, must be addressed before AI can be effectively used to diagnose and predict progression of glaucoma.

Preoperative estimation of intraocular lens power in patients of postvitrectomy cataract or with existing posterior segment pathology is of paramount importance in giving satisfactory postoperative visual results to them. Arup Chakrabarti et al. have emphasized the need to measure the axial length correctly and choose an appropriate IOL power in these cases to achieve the desired goal.

Management of complicated uveitic cataract is elaborately reviewed by Mohan Rajan and colleagues. They have suggested that a surgeon should plan cataract surgery only after aggressive ocular inflammation control. Careful surgical maneuvers and management of concurrent ocular pathologies result in excellent postoperative visual gains in these eyes.

Automated image analysis by deep learning finds enormous scope and application in disorders of posterior segment of the eye. AI algorithms are clinically employed in the screening and management of diseases such as diabetic retinopathy, retinopathy of prematurity, retinal detachment, and age-related macular degeneration. This volume of *Recent Advances in Ophthalmology-16* contains separate dedicated chapters on these conditions.

Color fundus photography, near-infrared reflectance, OCT, fundus fluorescein angiography, indocyanine angiography, and optical coherence tomography angiography are frequently used in diagnosing and managing macular pathologies. Giridhar et al. have beautifully described the utility of multimodal imaging in macular diseases.

A detailed account of diagnosis and treatment of commonly encountered optic nerve tumors is presented by Dipankar Das and coauthors. Moreover, the book includes a chapter on choroidal metastasis—one of the most common intraocular malignancies of adults.

Neuro-ophthalmic evaluation not only facilitates detecting underlying systemic diseases but is also considered both life saver and sight saver for the patient. Technological advances have been applied in neuro-ophthalmology too with the application of AI and machine learning algorithms to diagnose and monitor papilledema, anterior ischemic optic neuropathy, optic neuritis, intracranial tumors, and other disorders. Hima Pendharkar et al. have given a classy description of utility of AI in neuro-ophthalmology.

The chapter "Updates in Artificial Intelligence in Ophthalmology" is covered by Gangadhara Sundar and colleagues wherein they have reviewed the various applications of AI technology, the future opportunities, and practical challenges in its use in the field of ophthalmology.

Ophthalmology has witnessed tremendous advancements in the past few years. Introduction of newer technology to diagnose, manage, and monitor ocular diseases has resulted in better patient care. However, it is not possible to include all advances in Ophthalmology in one volume and, therefore, only selected topics are chosen. It is presumed that postgraduate students, fellows in ophthalmology, and practicing ophthalmologists will find this book useful and informative.

**Nitin Nema**

# Acknowledgments

I find no words to express my gratitude of thanks and appreciation for all contributors of *Recent Advances in Ophthalmology-16*. Their commitment, dedication, and hard work were exemplary throughout.

I am highly indebted to Dr Lingam Gopal, Senior Consultant, Sankara Nethralaya, Medical Research Foundation, Chennai, and National University Hospital, Singapore; Dr Sushmita Kaushik, Professor, Glaucoma Services, Advanced Eye Center, Postgraduate Institute of Medical Education and Research, Chandigarh; Dr Anthony Vipin Das, Network Associate Director, Department of eyeSmart EMR and AEye and Indian Health Outcomes, Public Health and Economics Research Center, LV Prasad Eye Institute, Hyderabad; Dr Rajiv Raman, Senior Retina Consultant, Shri Bhagwan Mahavir Vitreoretinal Services, Sankara Nethralaya, Chennai; and Dr Hima Pendharkar, Professor, Department of Neuroimaging and Interventional Radiology, National Institute of Mental Health and Neurosciences, Bengaluru, for agreeing to contribute their chapters on a short notice as well as for their extraordinary support and cooperation.

A very special thanks to my students Dr Rishabh Rathi, Senior Resident, Department of Ophthalmology, Sri Aurobindo Medical College and Postgraduate Institute of Medical Sciences, Indore, Madhya Pradesh, India, and Dr Yashas Goyal, VST Centre for Glaucoma Care, LV Prasad Eye Institute, Hyderabad, Telangana, India, for helping me in my endeavor.

I am grateful to Shri Jitendar P Vij (Group Chairman) and Mr Ankit Vij (Managing Director) who have shown their continued interest in publication of *Recent Advances in Ophthalmology volumes*. The work and devotion of Ms Nikita Chauhan (Senior Development Editor) and other staff of Jaypee Brothers Medical Publishers (P) Ltd are praiseworthy.

Finally, I acknowledge the endless support and encouragement rendered to me by my wife and children.

# Contents

1. **Clinical Application, Limitations, and Future of Artificial Intelligence in Ophthalmology** ......................................................... 1
   *Anthony Vipin Das, Yashas Goyal*

2. **Artificial Intelligence in Refractive Errors** ..................................... 20
   *Purvi Bhagat, Pawan Garde*

3. **Artificial Intelligence in Keratoconus** ............................................. 33
   *Shahnaz Anjum, Rajesh Sinha*

4. **Advances in Refractive Surgery** ...................................................... 43
   *Shreesha Kumar Kodavoor, Gitansha Sachdev, Gopal R, Ramamurthy D*

5. **Optical Coherence Tomography in the Diagnosis of Glaucoma** ............................................................................... 80
   *Parul Ichhpujani, Obaidur Rehman, Sushmita Kaushik*

6. **Pitfalls in the Diagnosis of Glaucoma by Artificial Intelligence** ................................................................... 97
   *Mohana Sinnasamy, Murali Ariga, Nishanth Murali*

7. **Optimizing Intraocular Lens Power Calculation in Eyes with Posterior Segment Diseases and Following Posterior Segment Surgery** .......................................... 107
   *Meena Chakrabarti, Arup Chakrabarti*

8. **Management of Uveitic Cataract** ................................................... 118
   *Mohan Rajan, Arthi Mohankumar, Rakesh K*

9. **Artificial Intelligence in Diabetic Retinopathy** ........................... 132
   *Payal Naresh Shah, Divyansh Kailashchandra Mishra, Mahesh Shanmugam Palanivelu*

10. **Artificial Intelligence in Retinopathy of Prematurity** ................ 151
    *Lingam Gopal, Arjun Bamel, Anand Vinekar*

11. **Diagnosis of Retinal Detachment by Artificial Intelligence** ...... 174
    *Chaitra Jayadev, Aishwarya Joshi*

12. **Artificial Intelligence in Age-related Macular Degeneration** .... 182
    *Brughanya Subramanian, Chitralekha S Devishamani, Parveen Sen, Rajiv Raman*

13. **Multimodal Imaging in Macular Diseases** .................................................. 193
    *Giridhar Anantharaman, Kiran Chandran*

14. **Recent Advances in Optic Nerve Tumors** .................................................. 223
    *Dipankar Das, Obaidur Rehman, Sakshi Mishra,*
    *Madhusmita Mahapatra*

15. **Choroidal Metastasis** .................................................................................... 244
    *Kalpita Das, Raghulnadhan Ramanadhane*

16. **Artificial Intelligence in Neuro-ophthalmology** ........................................ 253
    *Hima Pendharkar, Rishabh Rathi*

17. **Updates in Artificial Intelligence in Ophthalmology** ................................ 272
    *Ng Yu Ci Faye, Dinesh Visva Gunasekeran, Rupesh Agrawal,*
    *Gangadhara Sundar*

*Index* .................................................................................................................... 289

# CHAPTER 1

# Clinical Application, Limitations, and Future of Artificial Intelligence in Ophthalmology

*Anthony Vipin Das, Yashas Goyal*

## ABSTRACT

Data defines our lives today! Ophthalmology is one of the most data-friendly specialties in medicine with a great potential and promise to redefine patient care. The ability to quantify outcomes and the diverse spectrum of images enables the application of various algorithms to the data to generate newer insights. There is a need for eyecare organizations to embark on their digital journeys to generate quality data for meaningful applications of data science. We must also be careful of the cycle of the innovation trigger that leads to the peak of inflated expectations before the slope of enlightenment sets in. There are exciting developments around the world to automate ocular diagnosis, predict patient outcomes, and understand disease progression using the large datasets generated in ophthalmology. There is no better time such as this to harness the true potential of big data and use this technology to impact eyecare services globally, so that all may see.

***Keywords:*** Electronic medical records; big data; machine learning; artificial intelligence; India.

## ■ INTRODUCTION

Big data and artificial intelligence (AI) have the potential to revolutionize ophthalmology practice. Big data helps to identify patterns in large datasets that may not be obvious to conventional analysis, leading to insights that would otherwise remain undetected. Further, it allows doctors to have a better understanding of their patients' medical history and improve accuracy and precision when providing treatment for vision impairment. AI can be used to analyze trends in patient outcomes which helps to inform future decisions about treatment options. Moreover, it aids in diagnostics, provides better patient monitoring, and enhances surgical precision. AI-based systems can quickly detect, analyze, and classify images of the eye, detect early signs of glaucoma, diabetic retinopathy, and age-related macular degeneration. With massive amounts of data and growing computing power, AI is showing promise in transforming the field of ophthalmology. Another significant impact of big data in ophthalmology is the ability to identify population-level trends in eye disease prevalence and incidence. Analysis of large datasets assists researchers to identify risk factors of eye diseases and develop targeted intervention strategies to prevent their occurrence in at-risk populations. Additionally, big data facilitates the development of teleophthalmology, which is a telemedicine approach that enables remote diagnosis and management of eye diseases using digital technologies. These advances are already being used for screening of diabetic retinopathy and retinopathy of prematurity in rural and semi-urban areas. By leveraging big data, ophthalmologists can provide high-quality care to patients in remote areas, improving access to eye care services and reducing burden on healthcare systems.

## ■ WHAT IS DATA AND ITS CHARACTERISTICS?

The staggering explosion of the generation of data from us all has defined the past two decades. It is estimated that in 2021, people created 2.5 quintillion bytes of data every day. By 2022, 70% of the globe's gross domestic product (GDP) will have undergone digitization.[1] The sheer magnitude of the data points generated in a single second has exponentially increased to an extent that >90% of the data of the world has been generated over the last 2 years. The volume of data/information created, captured, copied, and consumed worldwide has increased from 2 zettabytes in 2010 to >97 zettabytes in 2020, with a projected forecast of 181 zettabytes in 2025 **(Fig. 1)**.[2] *Big data* is a term that describes a large volume of data that may be analyzed computationally to reveal trends, associations, and patterns in the area of interest. There are specific attributes to big data that are more popularly known as the 5 "V"s

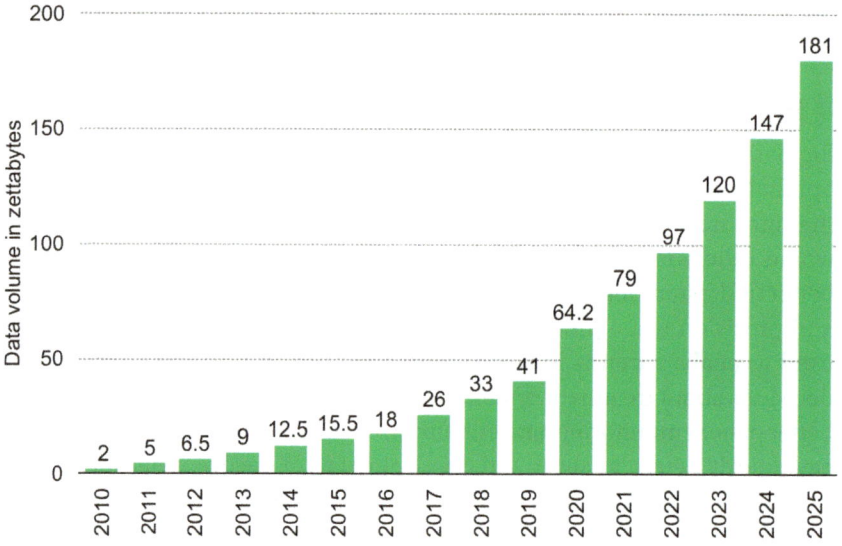

**Fig. 1:** Volume of data/information created, captured, copied, and consumed worldwide from 2010 to 2020, with forecasts from 2021 to 2025 (in zettabytes).

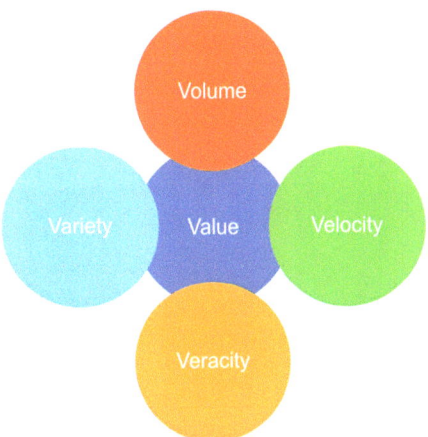

**Fig. 2:** 5 "V"s of big data.

and are defined as volume, velocity, veracity, variety, and value **(Fig. 2)**.[3] Volume is characterized by the sheer number of records or transactions being generated with time. Velocity is characterized by the real-time creation or streaming of data at a constant rate. Veracity is characterized by the trustworthiness and authenticity of the data being generated. Variety is characterized by structured, unstructured, and multimodal datasets. Value is finally dependent on all of the above attributes and provides insights to drive growth and impact. Healthcare data is unique in its diversity across various populations and geographies. While the challenges of standardization of the delivery of care are compounded by the partial digitization of its capture across the world, there is a great opportunity to work on the generation of quality healthcare data to realize the vision of value-based care. While various other sectors including social data, machine data, and transactional data have progressed into billion, trillion to quintillion bytes of data, structured healthcare data that can be mined is lagging behind on the scale.

## ■ WHERE IS DATA GENERATED?

Healthcare data is growing with the increasing integration of technology into the delivery of care around the world. Today, the healthcare industry generates approximately 30% of the world's data by volume.[4] By 2025, the compound annual growth rate of data for healthcare will reach 36%. This growth rate is 6% faster than manufacturing, 10% faster than financial services, and 11% faster than media and entertainment **(Fig. 3)**. The various sources that generate big data in the healthcare industry include hospital records, medical records of patients, results of medical examinations, biomedical research, and devices that are a part of internet of things (IoT). A healthcare data point is created with the first interaction of the patient

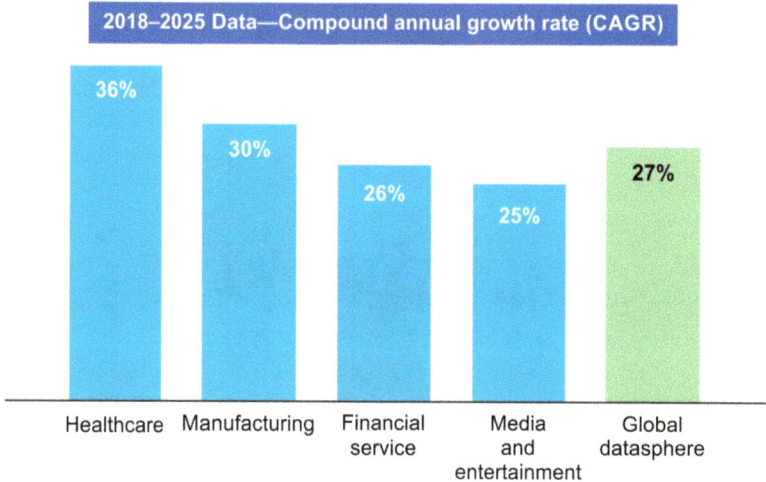

**Fig. 3:** Compound annual growth rate (CAGR) of healthcare data. *Source:* Coughlin et al. (2018).

with the care provider through patient registration that captures the most important aspect of the sociodemographic information of the patient. Age, gender, socioeconomic status, and geographic location form one of the most crucial signals that guide the identification of vulnerable cohorts to suffer from a particular disease. The clinical history and symptoms elicited from the patient and the documentation of the signs from the examination further add to the deduction of the diagnosis that determines the next steps of medical or surgical care. The data generated from investigations form the bulk of the data in healthcare that ranges from various media such as clinical imaging [X-ray, computed tomography (CT) scan, magnetic resonance imaging (MRI)], clinical photographs, audio, and video. There has been a rise in the use of personalized IoT devices globally. From the smartphone device in our hand to the wearable device on our wrist, there is a vast amount of digital health information being captured from the users. It is expected that our digital device interactions will increase from 1,400 interactions per person per day by the end of 2020 to 4,909 interactions per person per day by 2025. There are large healthcare datasets that exist across different regions, notably the National Health Service (NHS) digital,[5] Intelligent Research in Sight (IRIS) Registry,[6] European Health Data Space,[7] Global Health Observatory Data Repository,[8] and eyeSmart electronic medical record (EMR).[9] Big data allows us to look at patterns in the presentation of disease, treatment outcomes, and the possibility to offer personalized templates to deliver care for the patients. There has been an evolution of the size of the patient sample from hundreds and thousands to million and beyond[10] over the past decades **(Fig. 4)**, and there is an increasingly evolving debate on the insights that are derived at

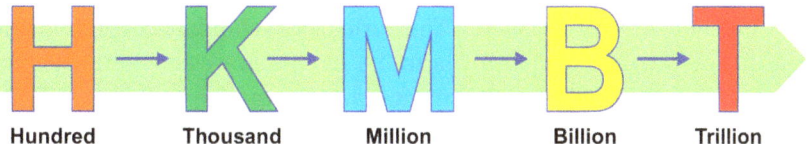

**Fig. 4:** Evolution of the sample size in healthcare research.

each stage.[11] About 80% of all of the healthcare data is unstructured leading to various challenges. There is a growing constraint of the lack of structured healthcare data from the hospitals in different geographies around the world. There is a need to be cautious with algorithms built on smaller datasets[12] that might not be representative of the population and also the synthetic datasets[13] that are not a substitute for real-world data (RWD). RWD and real-world evidence (RWE) play an increasing role in healthcare decisions. The US Food and Drug Administration (FDA) uses RWD and RWE to monitor postmarket safety and adverse events and to make regulatory decisions. The healthcare community use these data to support coverage decisions and to develop guidelines and decision support tools for use in clinical practice. Medical product developers use RWD and RWE to support clinical trial designs (e.g., large simple trials, pragmatic clinical trials) and observational studies to generate innovative, new treatment approaches. RWD can come from a number of sources such as EMRs, claims and billing activities, product and disease registries, patient-generated data including in-home-use settings and data gathered from other sources that can inform on health status, such as mobile devices and wearables. RWE is the clinical evidence regarding the usage and potential benefits or risks of a medical product derived from the analysis of RWD and represents a more realistic picture of the health outcomes.

## ■ HOW IS DATA GENERATED?

There has been an increasing debate on the ownership of patient data over the past few years. Healthcare providers must ensure a culture of trust and transparency in the delivery of care to patients in accordance with data privacy and legal regulations. There has been a paradigm shift in the way personal data is being perceived in the hands of service providers across various domains. The United Nations Conference on Trade and Development (UNCTAD) reports that 137 out of 194 countries had put in place legislation to secure the protection of data and privacy: 71% of the countries have legislation in place, 9% of the countries have draft legislation, 15% of the countries do not have any legislation, and 5% of the countries have no data.[14] The Health

Insurance and Portability and Accountability Act (HIPAA) enacted in 1996 in the United States determines the data privacy and security requirements of Protected Health Information (PHI) and all stakeholders handling these data must ensure compliance.[15] The various stakeholders covered include healthcare providers, health planners, healthcare clearinghouses, and business associates. Most of the privacy laws around the world have defined precise geolocation data, ethnic origin, genetic data, biometric information for purposes of identification, and health information as sensitive personal information. In the hospital life cycle of a patient, data is generated at multiple points clinically, surgically, and financially. The first touchpoint for the patient involves providing sociodemographic details such as national identity, age, gender, location, socioeconomic status, and ethnicity among others. Then the healthcare provider (clinical or paraclinical) elicits the symptoms for which the patient has presented to the clinic. The healthcare provider with the consent of the patient then proceeds to elicit signs and correlates them with the symptoms mentioned by the patient. The next course of action can involve ordering a set of diagnostic tests (invasive or noninvasive) to gather additional information. Once this data is in place, a combination of self-reported information by the patient coupled with the examination and expertise of the healthcare provider is analyzed to arrive at a diagnosis. Hence, the argument here is that the data is *co-created*. It is not only the patient but also the healthcare provider who participates together to generate this PHI. The notion that the entire PHI belongs to the patient alone merits debate. The perspective that patients own their entire healthcare data and they decide whom to share with different healthcare providers and still maintain continuity of care has not really taken off at scale. Collaborative creation of data ensures that both parties have equal access to the data they have co-created. It is the accountability of the healthcare provider to ensure the privacy of the healthcare data that they have created with the patient according to the legal regulations. Informed consent is a key component in medicine, and it is the explicit documented approval given by the patient to receive the medical intervention after having reflected on the pros and cons of the same.[16] Making informed consent an informed choice in the language known to the patient is of utmost importance to prevent the misuse of information collected by the healthcare provider. In most of the low- and middle-income countries (LMICs), general practitioners do not maintain a standard consent form. It is either implied or risks being coercive and is usually collected during registration or prior to any intervention.[17] Broad blanket consents collected by the industry are to be discouraged that may run the risk of misuse of the healthcare data, but on the other hand, may prevent the realization of the true potential of the application of machine learning (ML) or artificial intelligence (AI) algorithms on large datasets gathered from the population.

## ■ WHO IS COLLECTING THE DATA?

A very important aspect to understand is the drive behind the collection of data. There are many stakeholders in the ecosystem and the final value that is generated depends significantly on the comprehensive definition of the data points that are being collected. From the perspective of the clinicians, the data must be comprehensive in the sociodemographics to understand the distribution of the diseases. The medical and surgical documentation at the presenting visit helps to understand the severity of the disease at presentation. The temporal trends also help to quantify the treatment outcomes for the patients. From a healthcare organization perspective, the operational efficiency and costs of the delivery of healthcare services and the reimbursements from the public and private sectors are some of the most important key performance indicators (KPIs) that need to be tracked at regular intervals. The insurance industry mandates the collection of basic information for claims verification and reimbursements, but it lacks the granularity of the clinical documentation including outcomes that will help define value-based healthcare services. Patient engagement groups would want to collect the quality of life data, patient apprehensions, confidence, and trust levels in the system. Public health researchers collect sample population data and basic scientists collect the genome data, which are stored in disparate databases that do not interact with each other. Nongovernmental organizations (NGOs) collect data from the field for the evaluation of government schemes and to understand the social determinants of health. The government collects large amounts of data from the population because of the sheer magnitude of its presence across the population, but it does have the inherent limitation of not being granular enough. We need to evolve into a value-based approach where the collection of healthcare data points aid in the understanding of the efficiency of the care being provided. This is possible through a holistic approach that combines a piece of everyone. The point of interaction with the patient where this framework is most conducive to being collected is in the hospital. We must encourage our healthcare organizations on their digital transformation journeys and contribute to the value-based healthcare pool of information. We need to be cautious of the inclusivity of the data being collected as well. The Vision and Eye Health Surveillance System (VEHSS) report on the IRIS Registry in the United States highlighted certain limitations such as lack of patient-level data that prevent tracking outcomes at a granular level, not considered representative of the general population due to its current nature, does not include all the ophthalmology practices, cannot identify the payer-specific procedures, and that the eye examination rates are not reported due to the lack of a suitable denominator.[18] The ability to collate nationwide data is a great opportunity to understand the nature of services being provided to the population, but we also need to complete the circle by quantifying the value delivered through the outcomes. This will enable us to prioritize the patients in need and also to create a positive reinforcing mechanism for the healthcare providers to focus on quality rather than the quantity of the care being provided to those in need.

## ELECTRONIC MEDICAL RECORDS: BOON OR BANE

There is an increasing trend over a couple of decades among nations around the world to digitize healthcare processes to improve the quality of delivery and optimize the costs.[19] The global health observatory data reported steady growth in the adoption of EMR over the past 15 years and a 46% global increase in the past 5 years. More than 50% of the upper-middle- and high-income countries have adopted national EMR systems. The adoption of EMR is lower in the lower-middle (35%) and low-income (15%) countries. The most frequently cited barriers to going digital were lack of infrastructure, capacity, funding, and legal frameworks.[20] There is reasonable progress among 56% of the World Health Organization member countries in implementing legislation governing the EMR systems; however, a large proportion of countries lack appropriate legislation. At the end of 2016, the Healthcare Information and Management Systems Society, Asia-Pacific analysis adoption model of EMR reported that only 2.6% of hospitals achieved a level 6 certification in India, which required physician documentation (templates), full clinical decision support system (CDSS), and a closed-loop medication administration. Approximately 1.5% of the hospitals in India are measured at level and of functioning, which involves complete EMR and data analytics to improve care at the end of 2020. Currently, a larger proportion of hospitals (31%) are measured at level 3 certification, which include nursing/clinical documentation, CDSS (error checking), and picture archiving and communication system (PACS) available outside radiology.[21] In April 2013, the Ministry of Health and Family Welfare, Government of India, had launched their recommendations of EMR standards in India and updated them in 2016.[22] The activities in EMR adoption include the creation of the basic information and communication technology infrastructure, following the prescribed standards for the development to ensure interoperability and adhering to the national policy and regulations.

## AEYE PIPELINE

The application of data science to big datasets in ophthalmology can be summarized in *The AEye Pipeline*.[23] The pipeline comprehensively describes seven steps in the application of technology on clinical data sets for the generation of newer insights to the care providers. The steps are detailed in **Figure 5**. Step 1 details the *digitization of data through EMR*, which is the primary step for any kind of research based on big datasets. The IRIS

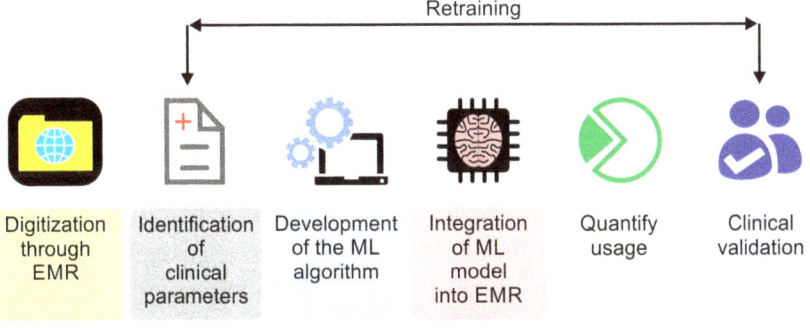

**Fig. 5:** AEye pipeline. (EMR: electronic medical record; ML: machine learning)

registry is the largest national clinical specialty data registry with nearly 50 million patient visits and 14 million unique patients in the United States.[24] The Système national d'information inter-régime de l'assurance maladie (SNIIR-AM) database covers nearly 65 million people and consists of medical and administrative data from 1,546 French private or public healthcare facilities catering to the general population.[25] The National Ophthalmology Database from the United Kingdom was initiated by the Royal College of Ophthalmologists to collate anonymized clinical data from contributing hospitals from the NHS.[26] The United Kingdom Diabetic Retinopathy Electronic Medical Record (UK DR EMR) Users Group has published their comprehensive experience of analyzing big data in patients with diabetic retinopathy (DR) from 20 UK hospital eye services on the real-world prevalence and progression data,[27] impact of cataract surgery on diabetic macular edema,[28] progression of DR,[29] and impact of deprivation on the presentation of diabetic eye disease at hospital services.[30] The eyeSmart EMR database implemented in a multitier ophthalmology network in India has reported an 8-year experience describing 4.7 million patient visits and 2.2 million unique patients seen on EMR.[9] The Ophthatome™ system is an integrated knowledge base of ophthalmic disease and has collected data of 0.5 million unique patients in India.[31] The implementation of EMR systems in large ophthalmology institutions[32] and the use of big data to understand endophthalmitis prophylaxis have been described in India.[33] It is evident that the digitization of clinical data helps generate large datasets for further analysis. Step 2 details the *identification of the clinical parameters* and the benefits of structured datasets and the challenges of unstructured ones. It is important to structure the input of clinical information in a standardized format as far as possible to ensure uniformity of the data for analysis. The use of drop-down menus, multiple selections, and standard forms enables the user to input the data in a repeatable manner. The use of free textboxes in

EMR contributes to unstructured data and missing information that will lead to challenges during analysis.[34] The use of deep learning (DL) techniques in natural language processing (NLP)[35] and finite state modeling to extract information from unstructured data entered in free text boxes[36] can lead to increased information integrity. Step 3 is the *development of ML algorithms* and the application of data science techniques on big data sets. Research using ML models such as linear regression, logistic regression, support vector machine, classification and regression trees, ensemble methods, and artificial neural network has the potential to improve ocular disease diagnosis, disease progression, and risk assessment.[37] The DL algorithm focuses on three major aspects of classification, segmentation, and prediction using the static images generated from an ocular diagnostic device such as fundus photography, optical coherence tomography, visual fields, and others.[38] Step 4 details the *integration of the ML model into the EMR* to complete the loop at the point of care. While a significant amount of research is advanced in the development of algorithms, it is important to integrate the insight into the EMR for efficient care of the patient. The entire purpose is to enhance the provision of care by providing the edge for superior clinical decision-making by the care provider, which otherwise would not have been possible.[39,40] Step 5 details *quantification of the usage* of the insights provided by the machine. This is a crucial dynamic at the intersection of man and machine that evolves with time. How will a clinician with decades of experience trust an AI insight? How can trust in the AI system be optimized to improve decision-making? Interpersonal trust is a human belief based on three main dimensions: Benevolence, integrity, and ability.[41] The reputation of the system, the integrity of the insight, and the user perception of the ability of the AI all influence the reliance of a clinician on the technology.[42] Step 6 is *clinical validation* of the algorithm or the software as a medical device (SaMD) in a real-world setting. Outcomes in healthcare are influenced by many patient-related factors that can or cannot be quantifiable. Hence, tracking the performance of the algorithm over a period of time is important to build trust among clinicians using this technology. Clinical evaluation can either be a *valid clinical association* that generates evidence to demonstrate the association between SaMD output and SaMD-targeted clinical condition, or an *analytical validation* that generated evidence that the SaMD correctly processes input data to generate accurate, reliable, and precise output data, or *clinical validation* that generates evidence that the SaMD's accurate, reliable, and precise data output achieves its intended purpose in its target population in the context of clinical care.[43] There is a need for assurance of the safety and effectiveness of any SaMD by ensuring high-quality data for training, algorithm correctness (verification), performance testing (validation), generalizability (addressing bias), and reliable interpretability. Step and completes the cycle by incorporating *retraining* or continuous learning in real time. The SaMD must be capable of capturing real-world performance data to understand the user interactions with the SaMD and must be able to monitor its technical and analytical performance to evolve into a more efficient and reliable tool for the clinicians. This continuous feedback will connect back to step 2 to include or exclude relevant parameters as input into the ML model to further refine the SaMD. We need to avoid any unintended consequences to the patient due to a wrong insight that can be precipitated due to a break in any of the above seven steps of the AEye pipeline. The key to improving healthcare delivery is digitization through EMR, implementing SaMD and continuous learning.

## ■ ALGORITHMS OVERVIEW

Artificial intelligence is being hailed as one of the key components of the fourth industrial revolution.[44] Nearly all systems for the production, management, and control of goods and services are being transformed by disruptive technologies such as AI and DL. AI, defined simply, is a set of algorithms designed to simulate human behavior. The recent explosion in potential applications of AI can be attributed to three factors: (1) The development of algorithms to train neural networks, (2) flood of available data, and (3) increase in computing capabilities. In its early phase, AI applications were designed to perform tasks that required simulation for intelligent human behavior. These were based on linear regression models which are one of the simplest supervised learning algorithms.[45] Now, AI is evolving to accomplish tasks that simulate intuitive human behavior. DL, a component of ML, is enabled by artificial neural networks and allows AI to learn from experience and understand in terms of the hierarchy of concepts, with each concept defined through its relation to simpler concepts.[46] Convolutional neural networks (CNN) are specifically designed to deal with imaging data. In our daily lives, we are surrounded by AI that works on integrated neural networks: Text recognition, voice recognition, image recognition, language translation, and self-driving.

The technological advancements and digital revolution have enabled AI to become a part of ophthalmology, unlike any other specialty. This accomplishment is attributable to the generation of large amounts of precise data, high-resolution imaging, and EMRs. AI algorithms could be used to modernize and transform clinical care, but current applications are limited to image-based DL.[47] DR, glaucoma, age-related macular degeneration, and retinopathy of prematurity (ROP) are some of the diseases where AI is already being clinically employed. Its applications are also being reviewed for retinal vascular occlusion, corneal ectasias, cataract, refractive errors, retinal detachment, strabismus, and ocular tumors.[48]

Artificial intelligence is increasingly making forays in cataract detection and referral. Early diagnosis and therapeutic intervention help to avoid complications and lead to a better outcome. AI screening allows for a higher population coverage within a short span of time and reduces pressure on tertiary referral centers. Zhang et al. developed a model for cataract severity grading based on fundus image evaluation. As the lenticular opacity increases, the fundus image becomes blurred. They reported an accuracy of 92.66% with this model.[49] A computer-aided diagnosis (CAD) program based on support vector machine regression model developed by Kumar et al. showed high sensitivity (97%), specificity (99%), and predictive accuracy (96.96%) in cataract diagnosis.[50]

Retinopathy of prematurity is a leading cause of preventable childhood blindness. Its impact is even more severe in developing countries where there is an obvious disparity in access to healthcare between urban and rural communities. Also, the incidence of ROP is increasing as a result of better critical care facilities. In a study by Coyner et al., an AI-derived vascular severity score (VSS) was obtained from images from the first examination of newborns after 30 weeks' postmenstrual age from three countries. The model had a sensitivity and specificity, respectively, for each of the datasets as follows: India, 100 and 63.3%; Nepal, 100 and 77.8%; and Mongolia, 100 and 45.8%.[51]

Diabetic retinopathy is a microangiopathy of retinal vasculature, and its incidence is increasing with the aging population. Delayed identification of referable DR leads to significant visual loss and increased financial costs; thus, the requirement of mass screening tools at the primary health level to differentiate between nonreferable and referable DR is the need of the hour.[52] AI tools in DR are one of the most promising avenues for screening and staging in ophthalmology. For DR screening, two AI-based DR screening tools have already received clearance from FDA: IDx-DR and EyeArt. Ting et al. studied a deep learning system (DLS) to identify DR from retina images of 14,880 patients which recorded a sensitivity of 90.5% and specificity of 91.6%.[53,54] Krause et al. demonstrated comparable results of an AI system with three retina specialists and three US board-certified ophthalmologists when validating 2,000 fundus images.[55] An AI system employing a CNN-based model demonstrated 97% sensitivity and 92% specificity for the detection of referable diabetic macular edema in a study by Albahli and Ahmad Hassan Yar that used both fundus and OCT images.[56]

Glaucoma is the leading cause of irreversible blindness worldwide. As screening tools are not ubiquitously available, there is an increasing need for simple tools that can be employed at the primary healthcare level to screen patients for glaucoma. AI algorithms are already in clinical use for glaucoma diagnosis from visual field analysis and optic disk photographs, but no clinically validated algorithm is available for the prediction of progression. The Sensimed Triggerfish contact lens sensor (CLS) has been developed to monitor intraocular pressure (IOP) changes over a 24-hour period. The AI system of the CLS does so by monitoring the changes in corneal strain.[57,58] Al-Aswad et al. tested a DLS named Pegasus to evaluate optic disks for glaucomatous changes in fundus photographs which outperformed five of the six ophthalmologists in diagnostic performance. Pegasus had a sensitivity of 83.7% and a specificity of 88.2%, whereas the ophthalmologists' sensitivity ranged from 61.3 to 81.6% and specificity ranged from 80.0 to 94.1%.[59]

Human communication, as an act of transmitting information to create shared understanding, is an extremely complex task. It requires a range of skills in listening, speaking, questioning, observing, analyzing, and evaluating verbal, emotional, and kinetic actions. Any interaction with the patient in clinical practice is recorded as natural language text which is difficult to analyze by electronic systems because for information to be electronically reproducible and retrievable, it needs to be structured and coded.[60] This unstructured free text in the EMR and patient feedback responses represent a tremendous amount of underutilized data in clinical research and predictive AI. NLP is a type of AI that transforms written text into datasets that ML and statistical models can process, interpret, and analyze.[61] This vast quantity of textual data can be used to develop automated algorithms that process human language. Those algorithms can help with the early identification of critical disorders, better triage, differentiating between referable and nonreferable patients, prediction of disease outcomes, generation of new diagnostic models, and personalizing healthcare to individual needs.[62] As reported by Yang et al., the integration of NLP with clinical care in some test models has resulted in better disease screening, risk stratification, and treatment monitoring.[63] Such models can be employed in routine clinical practice, but the biggest challenges in the development of NLP systems are the amount of training dataset and parameters required for ML, huge computational costs to manage that data, and manpower to train the systems.[59] AI-powered health chatbots are the next avenue in NLP. The goal of these chatbots would be to simulate human conversation and would achieve the same through natural language understanding (NLU) and natural language generation (NLG) algorithms.[64]

An overview of the algorithms used in medicine is summarized in **Table 1**.

## ■ FUTURE DIRECTION

The uniform adoption of these AI-powered technologies will transform healthcare. A key problem with the current AI-based systems is the singularity in disease identification. An IDx-DR system when shown a photograph of central retinal vein occlusion would try to classify it as DR. We need an integrated AI system that is capable of detecting multiple ophthalmic pathologies. AI screening applications currently undergoing validation testing are singular in their approach while most patients present

**TABLE 1:** An overview of algorithms used in data science on medical datasets.

| | |
|---|---|
| Classification model | • Supervised learning algorithm<br>• Used when the output variable is categorical |
| Linear regression | • Simplest supervised learning algorithm<br>• Primary building block for neural networks<br>• Used to predict the value of continuous data variable |
| Logistic regression | • Supervised learning algorithm<br>• Used to calculate the probability of an event when the dependent variable is dichotomous |
| Feed-forward neural network | • Nonlinear regression and classification model<br>• Regression with a two-neuron hidden layer |
| Convolutional neural network | • Deep learning architecture<br>• Inspired by natural visual perception mechanism of humans<br>• Used to perform image-driven pattern recognition tasks<br>• Contains at least a three-layered neural network<br>• Designed to learn spatial hierarchies automatically and adaptively<br>• Highly efficient |
| Recurrent neural network | • Output from the previous step is fed as input to the next step<br>• Network has a hidden layer that has memory of all calculated parameters<br>• Reduces complexity in the calculation of parameters<br>• Also known as long short-term memory (LSTM)<br>• Difficult to train<br>• Cannot process very long sequences |
| Support vector machine | • Supervised learning algorithm<br>• Classification and regression model<br>• Both linear and nonlinear applications<br>• Robust prediction capabilities |
| Decision tree | • Nonlinear supervised learning algorithm<br>• Encode input–output variables in a tree-like structure<br>• Easy interpretation of data |
| Transformer | • Works on mechanism of self-attention<br>• Differentially weighs the significance of each part of input data<br>• Primarily used in natural language processing |
| Random forest | • Supervised learning algorithm<br>• Operates by constructing a multitude of decision trees<br>• Used as "black-box" models |

with multicategorical disorders. We are witnessing a changing demographic trend worldwide. As the percentage share of the aging population is increasing, so are ophthalmic disorders, which have become a matter of public health concern.[65] Recognizing ocular disorders at an early stage and their appropriate management is important to reduce morbidity associated with vision loss and to improve quality of life. We are also witnessing a shift from hospital-centered healthcare practices to home-based healthcare and telemedicine. AI-powered systems are thus uniquely positioned to help improve all avenues of healthcare.[66] One of the most significant problems that the developing countries face, apart from the lack of universal healthcare, is the widening gap between healthcare spending and disease outcomes, and AI-powered algorithms can help to reduce the same. This gap has been analyzed to be caused by inadequate management of research insights, unsatisfactory use of the available evidence, and deficiencies in the recording of patient care experience, all of which resulted in missed opportunities, wasted resources, and potential harm to the patient. The development of a continuous learning healthcare system could help bridge the gap by creating a loop between the research, operational, and feedback arms of healthcare, so that data could be used efficiently and effectively.[67] Applications of AI can significantly improve the ability to support patients in peripheral locations by sharing specialized knowledge and scarce resources. NLP applications would most likely become a part of routine clinical practice in the future. Although effective communication with patients and doctor–patient interactions continue to be the hallmarks of medicine, NLP may be able to improve knowledge transfer and support clinical workflows in places with limited resources.[47] One of the challenges in the implementation/adoption of AI solutions is the lack of diversity in datasets. Healthcare needs vary with geography and ethnicity and need to be catered to accordingly. AI does not intend to replace the role of a clinician but to bridge the gap between the patient and healthcare provider. The role of AI will be to augment patient care by improving diagnostic efficacy and predicting outcomes. The required number of healthcare providers in LMICs is disproportionately lower than the demand for services. AI can help with screening, staging, and treatment planning, thus allowing for greater population coverage.

## ■ CONCLUSION

Data is the new oil, but oil is of no use if it is not processed appropriately. We have to focus on generating good-quality data points that in turn will enable the application of algorithms to unlock newer insights in patient care. The potential of the use of data science in ophthalmology holds great promise due to the availability of structured datasets and images. We need to complete the circle by integrating these insights gained by the algorithms into the point of care for the benefit of the patient. We must ensure that there is an adequate representation in the datasets used for training and must encourage the development of ethical and trustworthy AI. We must embark on this digital journey as healthcare providers and contribute to the understanding of various diseases, understanding progression, and predicting outcomes of various treatment options. The exciting era of data-driven decisions in ophthalmology has begun!

## REFERENCES

1. Bulao J. How much data is created every day in 2023? [online] Available from: https://techjury.net/blog/how-much-data-is-created-every-day/#gref. [Last accessed February, 2023].
2. Taylor P. Amount of data created, consumed, and stored 2010-2020, with forecasts to 2025. [online] Available from: https://www.statista.com/statistics/871513/worldwide-data-created/. [Last accessed February, 2023].
3. Ishwarappa, Anuradha J. A brief introduction on big data 5Vs characteristics and Hadoop technology. Procedia Comput Sci. 2015;48:319-24.
4. Coughlin S, Roberts D, O'Neill K, Brooks P. Looking to tomorrow's healthcare today: a participatory health perspective. Intern Med J. 2018;48(1):92-6.
5. National Health Services, NHS Digital, Data and information. Data sets. [online] Available from: https://digital.nhs.uk/data-and-information/data-collections-and-data-sets/data-sets. [Last accessed February, 2023].
6. IRIS® Registry (Intelligent Research in Sight). About the IRIS® Registry. [online] Available from: https://www.aao.org/iris-registry/about. [Last accessed February, 2023].
7. European Commission eHealth. Digital health and care, EU Health Data Space. [online] Available from: https://health.ec.europa.eu/ehealth-digital-health-and-care/european-health-data-space_en. [Last accessed February, 2023].
8. World Health Organization. The Global Health Observatory data repository. WHO's gateway to health-related statistics. [online] Available from: https://apps.who.int/gho/data/node.home. [Last accessed February, 2023].
9. Das AV, Kammari P, Vadapalli R, Basu S. Big data and the eye-Smart electronic medical record system—an 8-year experience from a three-tier eye care network in India. Indian J Ophthalmol. 2020;68:427-32.
10. Das AV. People to policy: the promise and challenges of big data for India. Indian J Ophthalmol. 2021;69(11):3052-7.
11. Gumpili SP, Das AV. Sample size and its evolution in research. IHOPE J Ophthalmol. 2022;1:9-13.
12. Kaggle. Dealing with very small datasets. Available from: https://www.kaggle.com/code/rafjaa/dealing-with-very-small-datasets/notebook. [Last accessed February, 2023].
13. Kimmel R, Tai XC (Eds). Processing, Analyzing and Learning of Images, Shapes, and Forms: Part 1, Volume 19. Amsterdam: North-Holland Publishing Co.; 2018. pp. 1-145.
14. United Nations Conference on Trade and Development. Data protection and privacy legislation worldwide. [online] Available from: https://unctad.org/page/data-protection-and-privacy-legislation-worldwide. [Last accessed February, 2023].
15. Centers for Disease Control and Prevention. Public Health Professionals Gateway, Public Health Law. [online] Available from: https://www.cdc.gov/phlp/publications/topic/hipaa.html. [Last accessed February, 2023].
16. Agency for Healthcare Research and Quality. Department of Health & Human Services, USA. AHRQ's making informed consent an informed choice: training modules for health care leaders and professionals. [online] Available from: https://www.ahrq.gov/health-literacy/professional-training/informed-choice.html. [Last accessed February, 2023].
17. Saksena N, Matthan R, Bhan A, Balsari S. Rebooting consent in the digital age: a governance framework for health data exchange. BMJ Global Health. 2021;6:005057.

18. CDC. Vision Health Initiative, VEHSS initiative, Information on Data Sources, Electronic Health Records and Registries. IRIS® Registry. [online] Available from: https://www.cdc.gov/visionhealth/vehss/data/ehr-registries/iris.html. [Last accessed February, 2023].
19. Health Information and Management Systems Society. Electronic Health Records: A Global Perspective, 2nd edition. Chicago, IL: Healthcare Information and Management Systems Society; 2010. [online] Available from: https://www.himss.org. [Last accessed February, 2023].
20. World Health Organization. (2016). Global diffusion of eHealth: making universal health coverage achievable: report of the third global survey on eHealth. [online] Available from: https://apps.who.int/iris/handle/10665/252529. [Last accessed February, 2023].
21. Sharma M, Aggarwal H. EHR adoption in India: potential and the challenges. Indian J Sci Technol. 2016;9(34):1-7.
22. National Health Portal. Electronic health record standards for India. [online] Available from: https://www.nhp.gov.in/ehr_standards_mtl_mtl. [Last accessed February, 2023].
23. Verkicharla PK, Das AV. Technology and myopia. Community Eye Health. 2019;32(105):S9-10.
24. Parke II DW, Lum F, Rich WL. The IRIS® Registry: purpose and perspectives. Ophthalmologe. 2017;114(Suppl. 1):1-6.
25. Daien V, Korobelnik JF, Delcourt C, Cougnard-Gregoire A, Delyfer MN, Bron AM, et al. French medical-administrative database for epidemiology and safety in ophthalmology (EPISAFE): The EPISAFE collaboration program in cataract surgery. Ophthalmic Res. 2017;58:67-73.
26. Jackson TL, Donachie PH, Sparrow JM, Johnston RL. United Kingdom National Ophthalmology Database Study of Vitreoretinal Surgery: report 1; case mix, complications, and cataract. Eye (Lond). 2013;27(5):644-51.
27. Egan CA, Lee A, Zhu H, Crabb D, Tufail A, Johnston R, et al. UK DR EMR Users Group: report 1—real world prevalence and progression data for diabetic retinopathy for 56 211 patients from 20 United Kingdom hospital eye services. Invest Ophthalmol Vis Sci. 2015;56(7):1448.
28. Denniston AK, Chakravarthy U, Zhu H, Lee AY, Crabb DP, Tufail A, et al. The UK Diabetic Retinopathy Electronic Medical Record (UK DR EMR) Users Group: report 2: real-world data for the impact of cataract surgery on diabetic macular oedema. Br J Ophthalmol. 2017;101(12):1673-8.
29. Lee CS, Lee AY, Baughman D, Sim D, Akelere T, Brand C, et al. The United Kingdom Diabetic Retinopathy Electronic Medical Record Users Group: report 3: baseline retinopathy and clinical features predict progression of diabetic retinopathy. Am J Ophthalmol. 2017;180:64-71.
30. Denniston AK, Lee AY, Lee CS, Crabb DP, Bailey C, Lip PL, et al. United Kingdom Diabetic Retinopathy Electronic Medical Record (UK DR EMR) Users Group: report 4, real-world data on the impact of deprivation on the presentation of diabetic eye disease at hospital services. Br J Ophthalmol. 2019;103(6):837-43.
31. Raj P, Tejwani S, Sudha D, Narayanan BM, Thangapandi C, Das S, et al. Ophthatome™: an integrated knowledgebase of ophthalmic diseases for translating vision research into the clinic. BMC Ophthalmol. 2020;20:442.
32. Scholl J, Syed-Abdul S, Ahmed LA. A case study of an EMR system at a large hospital in India: challenges and strategies for successful adoption. J Biomed Inform. 2011;44(6):958-67.

33. Haripriya A, Chang DF, Ravindran RD. Endophthalmitis reduction with intracameral moxifloxacin prophylaxis: analysis of 600 000 surgeries. Ophthalmology. 2017;124(6):768-75.
34. Bowman S. Impact of electronic health record systems on information integrity: quality and safety implications. Perspect Health Inf Manag. 2013;10:1c.
35. Ting DSW, Peng L, Varadarajan AV, Keane PA, Burlina PM, Chiang MF, et al. Deep learning in ophthalmology: the technical and clinical considerations. Prog Retin Eye Res. 2019;72:100759.
36. Prashanthi G, Deva A, Vadapalli R, Das AV. Automated categorization of systemic disease and duration from electronic medical record system data using finite-state machine modeling: prospective validation study. JMIR Form Res. 2020;4(12):e24490.
37. Lin W-C, Chen JS, Chiang MF, Hribar MR. Applications of artificial intelligence to electronic health record data in ophthalmology. Trans Vis Sci Tech. 2020;9(2):13.
38. Tong Y, Lu W, Yu Y, Shen Y. Application of machine learning in ophthalmic imaging modalities. Eye Vis (Lond). 2020;7:22.
39. Sagkriotis A, Chakravarthy U, Griner R, Doyle O, Wintermantel T, Clemens A. Application of machine learning methods to bridge the gap between non-interventional studies and randomized controlled trials in ophthalmic patients with neovascular age-related macular degeneration. Contemp Clin Trials. 2021;104:106364.
40. Lin H, Long E, Ding X, Diao H, Chen Z, Liu R, et al. Prediction of myopia development among Chinese school-aged children using refraction data from electronic medical records: a retrospective, multicentre machine learning study. PLoS Med. 2018;15(11):e1002674.
41. Mayer RC, Davis JH, Schoorman FD. An integrative model of organizational trust. Acad Manage Rev. 1995;20(3):709-34.
42. Lee JD, See KA. Trust in automation: designing for appropriate reliance. Hum Factors. 2004;46(1):50-80.
43. Patel B. Digital Health Center of Excellence. Artificial intelligence-machine learning: validation. Available from: https://www.fda.gov/media/143303/download. [Last accessed February, 2023].
44. World Economic Forum. The Fourth Industrial Revolution: what it means and how to respond. World Economic Forum. [online] Available from: https://www.weforum.org/agenda/2016/01/the-fourth-industrial-revolution-what-it-means-and-how-to-respond. [Last accessed February, 2023].
45. Benet D, Pellicer-Valero OJ. Artificial intelligence: the unstoppable revolution in ophthalmology. Surv Ophthalmol. 2022;67(1):252-70.
46. Goodfellow I, Bengio Y, Courville A. Deep Learning. Cambridge, MA: The MIT Press; 2016.
47. Chen JS, Baxter SL. Applications of natural language processing in ophthalmology: present and future. Front Med. 2022;9:906554.
48. Ting DSW, Pasquale LR, Peng L, Campbell JP, Lee AY, Raman R, et al. Artificial intelligence and deep learning in ophthalmology. Br J Ophthalmol. 2019;103(2):167-75.
49. Zhang H, Niu K, Xiong Y, Yang W, He Z, Song H. Automatic cataract grading methods based on deep learning. Comput Methods Programs Biomed. 2019;182:104978.

50. Mahesh Kumar SV, Gunasundari R. Computer-aided diagnosis of anterior segment eye abnormalities using visible wavelength image analysis based machine learning. J Med Syst. 2018;42(7):128.
51. Coyner AS, Oh MA, Shah PK, Singh P, Ostmo S, Valikodath NG, et al. External validation of a retinopathy of prematurity screening model using artificial intelligence in 3 low- and middle-income populations. JAMA Ophthalmol. 2022;140(8):791-8.
52. Ting DSW, Cheung GCM, Wong TY. Diabetic retinopathy: global prevalence, major risk factors, screening practices and public health challenges: a review. Clin Exp Ophthalmol. 2016;44(4):260-77.
53. Ting DSW, Cheung CYL, Lim G, Tan GSW, Quang ND, Gan A, et al. Development and validation of a deep learning system for diabetic retinopathy and related eye diseases using retinal images from multiethnic populations with diabetes. JAMA. 2017;318(22):2211-23.
54. Arsalan M, Owais M, Mahmood T, Cho SW, Park KR. Aiding the diagnosis of diabetic and hypertensive retinopathy using artificial intelligence-based semantic segmentation. J Clin Med. 2019;8(9):1446.
55. Ruamviboonsuk P, Krause J, Chotcomwongse P, Sayres R, Raman R, Widner K, et al. Deep learning versus human graders for classifying diabetic retinopathy severity in a nationwide screening program. NPJ Digit Med. 2019;2:25.
56. Albahli S, Ahmad Hassan Yar GN. Automated detection of diabetic retinopathy using custom convolutional neural network. J Xray Sci Technol. 2022;30(2):275-91.
57. Dunbar GE, Shen BY, Aref AA. The Sensimed Triggerfish contact lens sensor: efficacy, safety, and patient perspectives. Clin Ophthalmol. 2017;11:875-82.
58. Sharma R, Ong ZZ. Sensimed Triggerfish® contact lens sensor for 24-hour intraocular pressure profile-safety and validity. Invest Ophthalmol Vis Sci. 2021;62(8):2564.
59. Al-Aswad LA, Kapoor R, Chu CK, Walters S, Gong D, Garg A, et al. Evaluation of a deep learning system for identifying glaucomatous optic neuropathy based on color fundus photographs. J Glaucoma. 2019;28(12):1029-34.
60. Friedman C, Hripcsak G. Natural language processing and its future in medicine. Acad Med J Assoc Am Med Coll. 1999;74(8):890-5.
61. Harrison CJ, Sidey-Gibbons CJ. Machine learning in medicine: a practical introduction to natural language processing. BMC Med Res Methodol. 2021; 21(1):158.
62. Locke S, Bashall A, Al-Adely S, Moore J, Wilson A, Kitchen GB. Natural language processing in medicine: a review. Trends Anaesth Crit Care. 2021;38:4-9.
63. Yang LWY, Ng WY, Foo LL, Liu Y, Yan M, Lei X, et al. Deep learning-based natural language processing in ophthalmology: applications, challenges and future directions. Curr Opin Ophthalmol. 2021;32(5):397-405.
64. Khadija A, Zahra FF, Naceur A. AI-powered health chatbots: toward a general architecture. Procedia Comput Sci. 2021;191:355-60.
65. Swenor BK, Ehrlich JR. Ageing and vision loss: looking to the future. Lancet Glob Health. 2021;9(4):e385-6.
66. Lu W, Tong Y, Yu Y, Xing Y, Chen C, Shen Y. Applications of artificial intelligence in ophthalmology: general overview. J Ophthalmol. 2018;2018:5278196.
67. Lee CH, Yoon HJ. Medical big data: promise and challenges. Kidney Res Clin Pract. 2017;36(1):3-11.

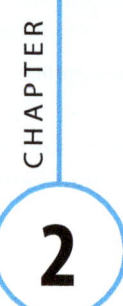

# Artificial Intelligence in Refractive Errors

*Purvi Bhagat, Pawan Garde*

## ABSTRACT

Worldwide, the most common cause of visual impairment is uncorrected refractive errors. With increase in population, the incidence of refractive errors is on the rise as well, particularly myopic errors in Western and Asian populations. We can diagnose refractive errors using objective and subjective refraction. Objective refraction includes retinoscopy, autorefractometry, photorefraction, and electrophysiological methods.

Subjective refraction includes monocular subjective refraction, binocular balancing, and correction for near vision. Artificial intelligence (AI), the science of making intelligent machines, is now being increasingly utilized in all healthcare fields, including ophthalmology. It is widely used for the accurate diagnosis and interpretation of medical imaging and is a branch of engineering that implements novel concepts and solutions to resolve complex challenges. A type of AI called "deep learning" enables systems to learn predictive features from the images of certain labeled data. In this chapter, we shall discuss the use of AI in prediction of refractive errors and the various AI methods, including their merits and demerits.

***Keywords:*** Refraction; refractive error; artificial intelligence; deep learning; refractive error detection network (REDNet).

## ■ WHAT IS ARTIFICIAL INTELLIGENCE?

Artificial intelligence (AI) is the use of a computer to model intelligent behavior with minimal human intervention. It is a branch of engineering that implements novel concepts and novel solutions to resolve complex challenges. Application of AI in medicine has two main branches:[1]
1. Virtual
2. Physical.

Virtual component includes machine learning and deep learning (DL). These use mathematical algorithms and improve learning through experience. Currently, three types of machine learning algorithms are in vogue:
1. *Unsupervised:* Here, the machine uses its ability to find patterns.

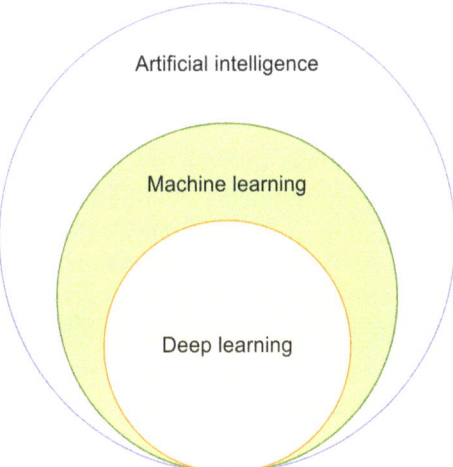

**Fig. 1:** Artificial intelligence and its subsets.

2. *Supervised:* Classification and prediction algorithms are developed based on previous examples.
3. *Reinforcement learning:* Sequences of rewards and punishment are designed to form a strategy for operation in specific problem space.

The physical component of AI includes objects, medical devices, and sophisticated robots known as carebots.

Machine learning is computer learning from data making use of algorithms in order to perform a task without being explicitly programmed. DL uses a complex structure of algorithms modeled on the human brain and is a subset of machine learning **(Fig. 1)**. This enables the processing of unstructured data such as documents, images, and text.

Deep learning uses representation-learning methods with multiple levels of abstraction to process input data without the need for manual feature engineering, automatically recognizing the intricate structures in high-dimensional data through projection onto a lower-dimensional manifold.[2] Compared with conventional techniques, DL has been shown to achieve significantly higher accuracies in many domains, including natural language processing, computer vision,[3-6] and voice recognition.[6] In healthcare, DL has been primarily applied to medical imaging analysis showing robust diagnostic performance in detecting various medical conditions. DL has similarly been applied to ocular imaging, principally fundus photographs and optical coherence tomography (OCT). Major ophthalmic diseases which DL techniques have been used for are as follows:

- Diabetic retinopathy (DR)[7-11]
- Glaucoma[7,12]
- Age-related macular degeneration (AMD)[7,13,14]

- Retinopathy of prematurity (ROP)[15]
- Refractive errors.

## ARTIFICIAL INTELLIGENCE IN REFRACTION

Deep learning methods have been developed to use AI for creating automated, time-efficient, and accurate refraction methods. Different methods use different data for the training and testing of algorithm, but the basic concept remains the same.

*Step 1:* Create an algorithm which can predict a certain entity (diopter power in case of refraction).

*Step 2:* Train the algorithm with adequate data.

*Step 3:* Algorithm defines specific features that it can use to predict refraction (different methods of feature definition are used, compared, and the best one is selected); for example, long short-term memory (LSTM)[16] algorithm is used in refractive error detection network (REDNet).

*Step 4:* Algorithm used on testing data (indices such as mean absolute errors are calculated)

*Step 5:* Algorithm accurately predicts the refractive error.

In REDNet, a convolutional neural network (CNN) extracts features from multiple directions of images and then obtains a feature sequence. Recurrent neural network (RNN) processes feature sequence and fuses features. A fully connected neural network gives spherical power, cylindrical power, and spherical equivalent (SE). At the end, another layer of CNN is added which calculates the average of multiple feature maps. This helps in making the algorithm feature fusion efficient.

The feature fusion extractor CNN was designed based on the Xception network structure with sufficient features and fewer parameters.

The refractive errors can be determined by using the following methods:[16]
- *Fundus images:* Wide field fundus photography, color fundus images
- Posterior segment OCT
- Eccentric photorefraction.

## PREDICTING REFRACTIVE ERRORS WITH RETINAL FUNDUS IMAGES

Refractive errors can be predicted from fundus images using a DL model that can be trained using multiple datasets.[17] Fundus changes are typical of refractive errors, especially axial ametropia. These characteristic changes which happen in the retina due to the associated changes in ocular size and shape can be used to identify the specific refractive error. The term

**Flowchart 1:** Attention model.

```
Algorithm
   ↓
Predict favorable outcome
   ↓
Apply attention technique
   ↓
Identify regions which predict the outcome
   ↓
Use the regions in subsequent images to predict accurate outcomes
```

"attention technique" refers to the practice of using visualization and feature detection methods to locate and characterize image characteristics linked to increased predictive accuracy.[17] Using this method, we can decipher the model and learn which retinal landmarks may be causal in the development of ametropia.

## What is an Attention Model?

Attention models or attention mechanisms are input processing techniques for neural networks that allow the network to focus on specific aspects of a complex input, one at a time, until the entire dataset is categorized. The goal is to break down complicated tasks into smaller areas of attention that are processed sequentially **(Flowchart 1)**.

## How to Collect the Different Types of Data?

Patients undergo ophthalmologic examination which includes refractive error checkup using an autorefraction device as well as paired nonmydriatic OCT and retinal fundus imaging. This gives the data that can be used for training as well as testing of the deep neural networks.

Deep neural network is a sequence of multiple mathematical operations which are then applied to various data inputs.[18] When it is used for image segmentation, the data is usually the pixel value of an image, for example, fundus photograph. Through the process of DL, the network is taught correct parameter values. The network then performs a given task. This includes predicting refractive error from pixel values of the retinal fundus photograph. Open-source deep-learning software libraries, such as TensorFlow,[19] Keras, Caffe, Microsoft's Cognitive Toolkit, PyTorch, and Apache MXNet, are used to train the neural network models.[20]

The training data can be either "train" set or "tune" (validation) set. These sets are divided by the subject. It is common practice to generate random values for the neural network's parameters before beginning the training

**Flowchart 2:** Deep neural network architecture—fundus images form the input of a deep neural network consisting of three residual blocks, an attention layer to learn the most predictive eye features and two fully connected layers.

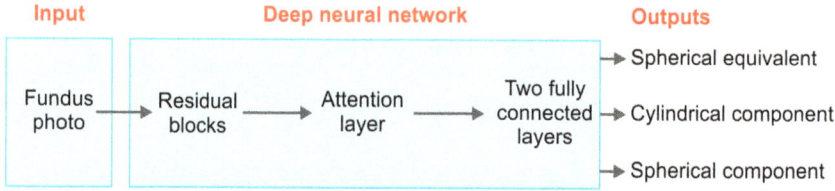

process. Then for each image, the prediction given by the model is compared to the known label from the training set and parameters of the model are then modified slightly to decrease the error on that image. This process, known as stochastic gradient descent, is repeated for every image in the training set until the model "learns" how to accurately compute the label from the pixel intensities of the image for all images in the training set. The tuning dataset is drawn at random from the development dataset; it is not used to hone the model's parameters but rather as a miniature evaluation dataset for fine-tuning the model. The resulting model can be fine-tuned and fed enough information to predict about the labels (such as refractive error) on the new images.

To calculate the degree of a refractive error, one can use a deep neural network model **(Flowchart 2)** that combines a residual network (ResNet)[21] and a soft-attention[22] structure. Layers are used to scale down the input image, three residual blocks are used to learn predictive image features, a soft-attention layer is used to pick the most informative features, and two fully connected layers are used to learn interactions between features.[21,22] Model outputs are SE, cylindrical component, and spherical component.[8]

Thus, the network is made up of:
- ResNet to learn prediction features[21]
- Fully connected layers to learn interactions between selected features
- A soft-attention layer to identify and interpret key aspects of an image.

The fovea in retinal images is an example of an area where soft attention can be used to learn more about which image features are most predictive. The two fully connected layers along with an output layer are used to predict the SE as well as spherical and cylindrical components.

Poor-quality images are filtered out of the training set using an image-quality filtering algorithm. In order to improve model stability, the image-quality algorithm is developed as a CNN trained on 300 manually labeled images to predict the image quality. In order to improve accuracy, the model is calibrated to reject low-quality images (e.g., extremely over or underexposed images). Three different models are developed to make predictions about spherical power, cylindrical power, and SE.

To prevent overfitting, it is helpful to stop training as soon as the model's performance on the tuning dataset stops to show improvement based on an early stopping criterion.[23] Combining the output of multiple neural network models that were trained using the same data (a process known as "ensembling") can further improve accuracy.[24]

Deeper networks are made possible by the residual architecture, which allows them to learn more abstract features and make more accurate predictions.[21] The fovea is clearly the center of attention for all refractive errors, according to both individual and mean attention maps that emphasize features predictive for refractive error. The attention maps' persistent emphasis on the fovea could open up new possibilities for myopia research. Given that fundus images are frequently centered on the fovea, it is possible that this outcome is related to the location of the fovea in relation to other retinal landmarks. It is also conceivable that information concerning refractive error can be gleaned from the way the fovea appears. The fundus may exhibit recognizable clinical signs of pathological myopia that involve the macula.[25] Earlier research using OCT at higher resolutions has shown some data supporting anatomical variation in the thickness or shape of the retina at the fovea in different refractive errors.[26] Although there is some indication that myopic eyes have more widely spaced foveal cone photoreceptors, retinal fundus images alone are not likely to provide solutions.[27] One possibility is that when the fovea is photographed using a fundus camera, there is change in the reflectance or focus due to the variable refractive error. With advancing age or in the presence of macular pathology, the foveal light reflex, as seen with an ophthalmoscope, becomes fainter and less noticeable. However, evidence on the reflex's "brightness" and its connection to refractive errors is still lacking. Another possibility is that the foveal pigment and refractive errors may be related. Nevertheless, Czepita et al. did not discover any such correlation.[28] The density of pigment is often determined through psychophysical methods, although fundus imaging done under blue and green light appears promising enough in assessing the retinal pigment density.[29]

Attention maps also imply that features outside the foveal region, such as diffuse signals from optic nerve head (ONH) and retinal temporal vascular arcades from their exit and as they transit across the fundus, can also help to predict refractive errors, albeit to a lesser extent. Due to contradictory results, the extent of the relationship between the size of the optic disc and refractive errors is still unclear. While a Chinese population-based study indicated that the optic disc size is independent of refractive error within the range of −8 to +4 D, some investigations have found a weakly significant increase in optic disc size with increasing refractive error toward myopia.[30-32] There is no correlation between refractive error and optic disc size, according to Varma et al.[33] Along with disc size, refractive error can also affect how the optic disc looks. The optic discs of axial myopic eyes are known to be tilted.[34] Narrower retinal arterioles and venules, more branching and smaller retinal vascular fractal dimensions have also been linked to myopic refractive errors.[35,36] Additionally, the maps appeared to be quite comparable for images with hypermetropia and myopia, indicating that the neural network makes predictions using the same regions across a range of refractive errors.

While each retinal landmark may individually aid in prediction, the relation between them may also serve as a useful predictor. Numerous studies have been done on the spatial correlations between anatomical characteristics and refractive errors.[37-39] The fovea and ONH being the model's main predictive features, a spatial link between these two as well as other landmarks should be taken into account. Baniasadi et al. discovered a substantial correlation between SE and a number of ONH-related parameters such as the angle between the superior and inferior temporal arteries, ONH tilt and rotation, and location of the central retinal vascular trunk.[40] The ONH and vessels are both prominently emphasized in the averaged attention maps, but it is difficult to gauge the degree of attention paid to these areas because the signals were considerably more diffuse due to the interindividual location differences. Additionally, it is difficult to instantly distinguish between this signal in myopic and hypermetropic eyes. More research should be done on the attention maps and the spatial relations between predictive regions.

## Disadvantages of Retinal Fundus Image Method

- The model predicts spherical power very accurately, however not the cylindrical power probably due to the fact that astigmatism is caused by toricity of the cornea and/or the crystalline lens, information that is unlikely to be contained in retinal fundus images. As previously mentioned, different axial lengths may be related to retinal characteristics linked to different refractive errors. As a result, SE can be predicted with great accuracy in axial ametropia. However, the age-associated increasing lens thickness may influence the camera focus settings and result in image magnification. Spherical power due to lens ametropia is not known to have any specific association with retinal structure. According to Wang et al., presbyopia-related alterations are the main cause of focus and magnification effects beyond 42 years.[39]
- In this model, data is the most essential aspect. Datasets from a wide range of demographics, including those with varying ages, ethnicities, and medical histories, are required. If possible, one should use more than three datasets when training and validating the model. People who have already had eye surgery should be included in a different dataset.
- Data collection is labor- and material-intensive. In order to gather, store, and analyze data, one must have suitable infrastructure. Fundus cameras of sufficient quality and portability are prohibitively expensive.

# PREDICTING REFRACTIVE ERRORS WITH POSTERIOR SEGMENT OPTICAL COHERENCE TOMOGRAPHY IMAGES[41]

Optical coherence tomography-based DL models have also been developed to estimate refractive errors. A regression model based on a pretrained ResNet architecture was trained using horizontal OCT images to predict the SE and the performance of the DL model for detecting high myopia was evaluated, generating a saliency map to visualize the characteristic features.

## Advantages of Posterior Segment Optical Coherence Tomography Method

- Low mean absolute error for SE prediction and, hence, is more accurate.
- Accuracy for detection of high myopia is around 71.4% [95% confidence interval (CI), 65.3–76.9%].[12]
- The inner retinal layers are represented on saliency map.
- Relatively steepened curvatures are highlighted to detect high myopia.

## Disadvantages of Posterior Segment Optical Coherence Tomography Method

- Expensive machine
- Only predicts SE.

# PREDICTING REFRACTIVE ERRORS WITH ECCENTRIC PHOTOREFRACTION[16]

A REDNet is created which uses multiple eccentric photorefraction images. Each image has a different meridian direction. The data is then used to predict the refractive error **(Flowchart 3)**.

**Flowchart 3:** Prediction with eccentric photorefraction.

Convolutional neural network
↓
Extracts features from six eccentric photorefraction images
↓
Fuses feature sequences
↓
Sequence processing
↓
Predicts spherical power, cylindrical power, spherical equivalent

**Flowchart 4:** Visualization in refractive error detection network (REDNet).

```
Gradient weighted class activation mapping[43]
            ⬇
Heat map drawn
            ⬇
Key areas detailed
            ⬇
Meaningful features learnt by neural network
            ⬇
Eccentric photorefraction
            ⬇
Region of eyelashes and Purkinje images avoided
```

## Theory of Photorefraction

Diopters are obtained from grayscale changes in pupil image in different meridian directions. Images are taken from a distance of 1 m. Routinely, this estimation is hampered due to occlusion by eyelashes and disturbance created due to corneal Purkinje images.[42] In REDNet, use of Rectified Linear Unit (ReLU6) helps in excluding the eyelashes and Purkinje images **(Flowchart 4)**.[43] Hence, ReLU6 has an activation function.

## Advantages of Eccentric Photorefraction Method

- Improved prediction of single orientation diopter from single image with smaller number of parameters[16]
- Effectively extracts feature information such as diopter power from eccentric photorefraction images
- Higher accuracy than DL based on fundus photography
- Both eyes can be measured simultaneously
- Can measure spherical power, cylindrical power, and SE simultaneously.

A new neural network has been developed which extracts features of each image, utilizes contextual relationship between images, and predicts cylindrical power as well. It is difficult to measure the contextual relationship as diopter difference in different meridians needs to be calculated.

The method used is a stepwise procedure of data acquisition followed by preprocessing. Thereafter, the data is used and a base model is constructed. Features from six different images for a single pupil are fused. The network is then trained to recognize the most predictive feature. Data acquisition is done in six meridians which are 0, 60, 120, 180, 240, and 300°. A near-infrared (NIR) band-pass filter is used to ignore extra light **(Fig. 2)**.

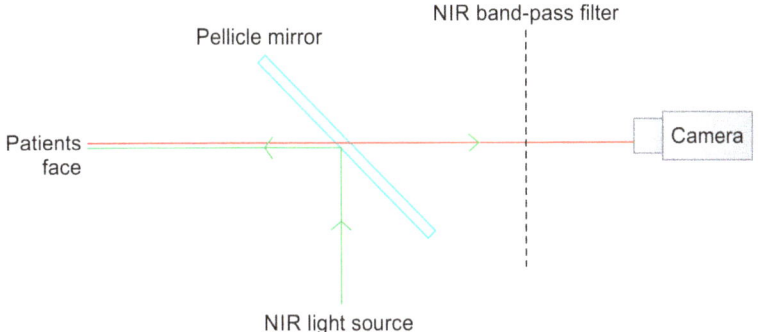

**Fig. 2:** Method of data collection using near-infrared (NIR) band.

The data that is collected contains a lot of details which are not necessary for the final output. Removing this data helps the algorithms to process the remaining data faster and more accurately and come to a conclusion; for example, data such as rest of the face and outside of the pupil are removed. The exposure and brightness of the two pupils are matched for basic diopter prediction. Six images from a single eye are used as they are different in terms of diopter information. A 1,920 × 1,080 pixel size of human face is captured. The position of pupil is located through threshold segmentation and template matching, and the pupil is cropped to 128 × 128 pixels. Diopter is obtained by reflection type and based on the position of eccentric crescent in pupil.

## ■ CONCLUSION

Artificial intelligence represents novel methods for studying the eye and other biological systems. Research utilizing massive retrospective datasets can benefit from the development of medically precise and accurate classification algorithms. The AI algorithms may aid in the study of myopia's epidemiology using large fundus image datasets without refractive error labels. The findings from the attention maps generated may contribute to a better comprehension of the biological and pathophysiological mechanisms underlying myopia. Last but not the least, the processes used to develop the algorithms, such as first utilizing DL to directly predict the outcome or phenotype of interest and then utilizing attention techniques to localize the most predictive features, may be easily transferable. The OCT has the potential to be used as an imaging modality for refractive error estimation, but this use still needs further refinement. **Table 1** gives a quick comparative overview of the three primary AI modalities used to identify refractive errors.

**TABLE 1:** Comparison of the three different major artificial intelligence (AI) modalities used for diagnosis of refractive errors.

| Features | Fundus photo based | OCT based | Eccentric photorefraction based |
| --- | --- | --- | --- |
| Cost | Expensive | Expensive | Relatively cheaper |
| Preprocessing required | Nil | Nil | Extra data such as facial features have to be removed |
| Predicts | Spherical error, spherical equivalent, cylindrical error | Spherical error, spherical equivalent | Spherical error, cylindrical error, spherical equivalent |
| Accuracy | High accuracy for spherical error and spherical equivalents, low accuracy for cylindrical error | Good accuracy for spherical error and spherical equivalent | High accuracy for spherical error, cylindrical error, and spherical equivalents |
| Parameters used for prediction | Large number | Large number | Few |

(OCT: optical coherence tomography)

## ■ REFERENCES

1. Hamet P, Tremblay J. Artificial intelligence in medicine. Metabolism. 2017;69S:S36-40.
2. LeCun Y, Bengio Y, Hinton G. Deep learning. Nature. 2015;521:436-44.
3. Zhang X, Zou J, He K, Sun J. Accelerating very deep convolutional networks for classification and detection. IEEE Trans Pattern Anal Mach Intell. 2016;38(10):1943-55.
4. Shin HC, Roth HR, Gao M, Lu L, Xu Z, Nogues I, et al. Deep convolutional neural networks for computer-aided detection: CNN architectures, dataset characteristics and transfer learning. IEEE Trans Med Imaging. 2016;35:1285-98.
5. Tompson J, Jain A, LeCun Y, Bregler C. Joint training of a convolutional network and a graphical model for human pose estimation. Adv Neural Inf Process Syst. 2014;27:1799-807.
6. Hinton G, Deng L, Yu D, Dahl G, Mohamed AR, Jaitly N, et al. Deep neural networks for acoustic modeling in speech recognition: the shared views of four research groups. IEEE Signal Process Mag. 2012;29:82-97.
7. Ting DSW, Cheung CY, Lim G, Tan GSW, Quang ND, Gan A, et al. Development and validation of a deep learning system for diabetic retinopathy and related eye diseases using retinal images from multiethnic populations with diabetes. JAMA. 2017;318:2211-23.
8. Gulshan V, Peng L, Coram M, Stumpe MC, Wu D, Narayanaswamy A, et al. Development and validation of a deep learning algorithm for detection of diabetic retinopathy in retinal fundus photographs. JAMA. 2016;316:2402-10.
9. Lee CS, Tyring AJ, Deruyter NP, Wu Y, Rokem A, Lee AY. Deep-learning based, automated segmentation of macular edema in optical coherence tomography. Biomed Opt Express. 2017;8:3440-8.

10. Abràmoff MD, Lou Y, Erginay A, Clarida W, Amelon R, Folk JC, et al. Improved automated detection of diabetic retinopathy on a publicly available dataset through integration of deep learning. Invest Ophthalmol Vis Sci. 2016;57:5200-6.
11. Gargeya R, Leng T. Automated identification of diabetic retinopathy using deep learning. Ophthalmology. 2017;124:962-9.
12. Li Z, He Y, Keel S, Meng W, Chang RT, He M. Efficacy of a deep learning system for detecting glaucomatous optic neuropathy based on color fundus photographs. Ophthalmology. 2018;125:1199-206.
13. Burlina PM, Joshi N, Pekala M, Pacheco KD, Freund DE, Bressler NM. Automated grading of age-related macular degeneration from color fundus images using deep convolutional neural networks. JAMA Ophthalmol. 2017;135:1170-6.
14. Grassmann F, Mengelkamp J, Brandl C, Harsch S, Zimmermann ME, Linkohr B, et al. A deep learning algorithm for prediction of age-related eye disease study severity scale for age-related macular degeneration from color fundus photography. Ophthalmology. 2018;125:1410-20.
15. Brown JM, Campbell JP, Beers A, Chang K, Ostmo S, Chan RVP, et al. Automated diagnosis of plus disease in retinopathy of prematurity using deep convolutional neural networks. JAMA Ophthalmol. 2018;136:803-10.
16. Ting DSW, Pasquale LR, Peng L, Campbell JP, Lee AY, Raman R, et al. Artificial intelligence and deep learning in ophthalmology. Br J Ophthalmol. 2019;103(2):167-75.
17. Varadarajan AV, Poplin R, Blumer K, Angermueller C, Ledsam J, Chopra R, et al. Deep learning for predicting refractive error from retinal fundus images. Invest Ophthalmol Vis Sci. 2018;59:2861-8.
18. Angermueller C, Pärnamaa T, Parts L, Stegle O. Deep learning for computational biology. Mol Syst Biol. 2016;12:878.
19. Banoula M. What is Tensorflow? Deep learning libraries and program elements explained. [online] Available from: https://www.simplilearn.com/tutorials/deep-learning-tutorial/what-is-tensorflow. [Last accessed March, 2023].
20. Clark D. Top 16 open source deep learning libraries and platforms. [online] Available from: https://www.kdnuggets.com/2018/04/top-16-open-source-deep-learning-libraries.html. [Last accessed March, 2023].
21. He K, Zhang X, Ren S, Sun J. Identity mappings in deep residual networks. Comput Vis ECCV. 2016;4:630-45.
22. Xu K, Ba J, Kiros R, Cho K, Courville A, Salakhutdinov R, et al. Show, attend and tell: neural image caption generation with visual attention. Proc Int Conf Mach Learn Appl. 2015:2048-57.
23. Caruana R, Lawrence S, Giles L. Overfitting in neural nets: backpropagation, conjugate gradient, and early stopping. In: Leen TK, Dietterich TG, Tresp V (Eds). Advances in Neural Information Processing Systems 13: Proceedings of the 2000 Conference. Cambridge, MA: MIT Press; 2001.
24. Krizhevsky A, Sutskever I, Hinton GE. ImageNet classification with deep convolutional neural networks. Adv Neural Inf Process Syst. 2012:1097-105.
25. Ryan S, Schachat A, Wilkinson C, Hinton D, Sadda S, Wiedemann P. Retina, 5th edition. Amsterdam: Elsevier; 2012.
26. Kitaguchi Y, Bessho K, Yamaguchi T, Nakazawa N, Mihashi T, Fujikado T. In vivo measurements of cone photoreceptor spacing in myopic eyes from images obtained by an adaptive optics fundus camera. Jpn J Ophthalmol. 2007;51:456-61.

27. Newcomb RD, Potter JW. Clinical investigation of the foveal light reflex. Am J Optom Physiol Opt. 1981;58:1110-9.
28. Czepita M, Karczewicz D, Safranow K, Czepita D. Macular pigment optical density and ocular pulse amplitude in subjects with different axial lengths and refractive errors. Med Sci Monit. 2015;21:1716-20.
29. Bour LJ, Koo L, Delori FC, Apkarian P, Fulton AB. Fundus photography for measurement of macular pigment density distribution in children. Invest Ophthalmol Vis Sci. 2002;43:1450-5.
30. Ramrattan RS, Wolfs RC, Jonas JB, Hofman A, de Jong PT. Determinants of optic disc characteristics in a general population: the Rotterdam Study. Ophthalmology. 1999;106:1588-96.
31. Wu RY, Wong TY, Zheng YF, Cheung CY, Perera SA, Saw SM, et al. Influence of refractive error on optic disc topographic parameters: the Singapore Malay Eye Study. Am J Ophthalmol. 2011;152:81-6.
32. Jonas JB. Optic disk size correlated with refractive error. Am J Ophthalmol. 2005;139:346-8.
33. Varma R, Tielsch JM, Quigley HA, Hilton SC, Katz J, Spaeth GL, et al. Race-, age-, gender-, and refractive error-related differences in the normal optic disc. Arch Ophthalmol. 1994;112:1068-76.
34. Vongphanit J, Mitchell P, Wang JJ. Population prevalence of tilted optic disks and the relationship of this sign to refractive error. Am J Ophthalmol. 2002;133:679-85.
35. Lim LS, Cheung CY-L, Lin X, Mitchell P, Wong TY, Mei-Saw S. Influence of refractive error and axial length on retinal vessel geometric characteristics. Invest Ophthalmol Vis Sci. 2011;52:669-78.
36. Li H, Mitchell P, Liew G, Rochtchina E, Kifley A, Wong TY, et al. Lens opacity and refractive influences on the measurement of retinal vascular fractal dimension. Acta Ophthalmol. 2010;88:e234-40.
37. Elze T, Baniasadi N, Jin Q, Wang H, Wang M. Ametropia, retinal anatomy, and OCT abnormality patterns in glaucoma. 1. Impacts of refractive error and interartery angle. J Biomed Opt. 2017;22:1-11.
38. Wang M, Jin Q, Wang H, Li D, Baniasadi N, Elze T. The interrelationship between refractive error, blood vessel anatomy, and glaucomatous visual field loss. Trans Vis Sci Technol. 2018;7(1):4.
39. Wang M, Elze T, Li D, Baniasadi N, Wirkner K, Kirsten T, et al. Age, ocular magnification, and circumpapillary retinal nerve fiber layer thickness. J Biomed Opt. 2017;22:1-19.
40. Baniasadi N, Wang M, Wang H, Mahd M, Elze T. Associations between optic nerve head-related anatomical parameters and refractive error over the full range of glaucoma severity. Trans Vis Sci Technol. 2017;6(4):9.
41. Yoo TK, Ryu IH, Kim JK, Lee IS. Deep learning for predicting uncorrected refractive error using posterior segment optical coherence tomography images. Eye (Lond). 2022;36:1959-65.
42. Crane HD, Steele CM. Generation-V dual-Purkinje-image eyetracker. Appl Opt. 1985;24(4):527-37.
43. Selvaraju RR, Cogswell M, Das A, Vedantam R, Parikh D, Batra D. Grad-CAM: visual explanations from deep networks via gradient-based localization. Proceedings of the IEEE International Conference on Computer Vision. 2017:618-26.

# CHAPTER 3

# Artificial Intelligence in Keratoconus

*Shahnaz Anjum, Rajesh Sinha*

## ABSTRACT

Artificial intelligence (AI) simulates human intelligence processes by a computer or robot. Thus, complex tasks that are commonly done by humans can be achieved easily by these computer systems. AI technology has demonstrated increasing utility in the field of ophthalmology, especially in retinal diseases and glaucoma. Recently, researchers have tried to harness the power of AI to help in diagnosing and treating anterior segment disorders. Common disorders such as keratoconus, infective keratitis, ocular surface disorders, refractive errors, and intraocular lens power calculations are fertile fields for application of AI. We aim to provide an overview of AI in the evaluation and management of keratoconus.

***Keywords:*** Artificial intelligence; deep learning; machine learning; keratoconus.

## ■ INTRODUCTION

Keratoconus (KCN) is one of the most common bilateral corneal non-inflammatory conditions, primarily affecting young adults and children, and characterized by an abnormally steep cornea due to progressive corneal thinning resulting in decreased vision.[1-3] Often in advanced stage, KCN patients require corneal transplant, exposing them to various associated risks.[4,5]

While frank KCN may be diagnosed based on slit-lamp findings and corneal topography, early diagnosis of subclinical or forme fruste KCN remains a challenge, particularly in patients planned for refractive surgery. At present, we primarily rely on imaging modalities such as corneal topography, Scheimpflug imaging, and spectral domain optical coherence tomography (SD-OCT) for screening these patients. Various parameters from these modalities have been employed for timely diagnosis as well as for predicting the development of KCN; the availability of huge amount of data and its complexity for interpretation is a limiting factor.

Artificial intelligence (AI) is a machine's ability to perceive or infer information and to retain it as knowledge to be applied toward adaptive behaviors within an environment or context.[6]

Deep learning (DL), a type of AI, has been previously applied to other ophthalmic fields such as ocular imaging, including fundus photographs and OCT which assisted in the diagnosis and follow-up of diseases such as diabetic retinopathy (DR), glaucoma, age-related macular degeneration (AMD), and retinopathy of prematurity (ROP).[7-11] DL has also been applied to estimate refractive error and cardiovascular risk factors (e.g., age, blood pressure, smoking status, and body mass index).[12,13]

Artificial intelligence algorithms that integrate the data from various diagnostic imaging modalities have shown promise in improving the diagnostic efficiency to differentiate normal eyes from that of subclinical or forme fruste KCN. Furthermore, AI is also used to predict the refractive and topographical outcomes following the implantation of intracorneal ring segments in KCN patients.[14] More recently, AI has been explored in identifying susceptibility genes for KCN.[15]

## ■ TYPE OF ARTIFICIAL INTELLIGENCE ALGORITHMS

The different types of AI algorithms include simple automated detectors, and basic and advanced machine learning (ML) and DL **(Flowchart 1)**.

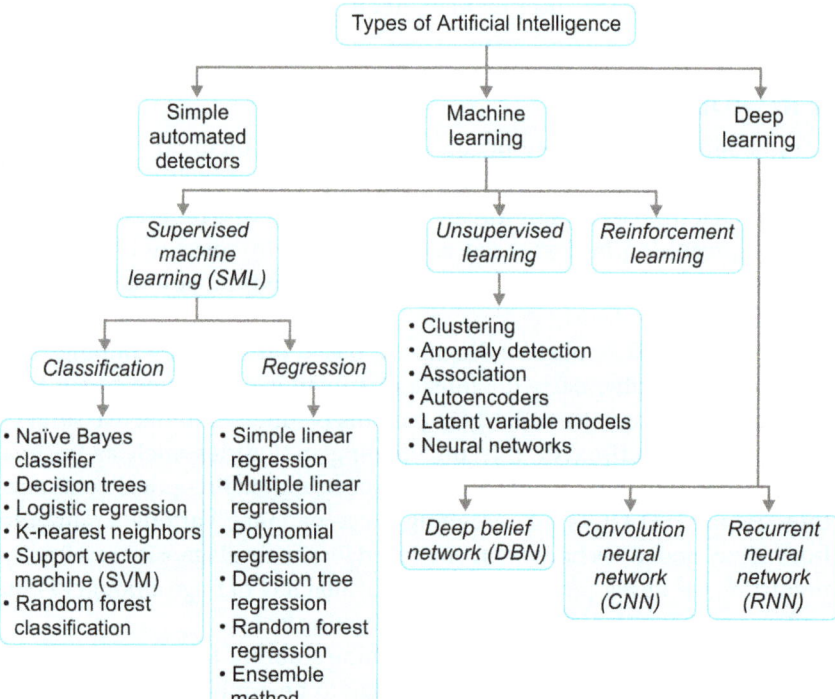

**Flowchart 1:** Types of artificial intelligence algorithms.

## Simple Automated Detectors

These are the simplest form of AI. Programmers give the software a mathematical description of the features to detect.

## Basic and Advanced Machine Learning

Machine learning is a subfield of AI technology that systematically implements algorithms to synthesize the underlying interrelation between data and information. Programmers provide a training set of images from the affected (diseased), eye or unaffected (normal) eye. This algorithm examines the images to learn about the differences. Advanced ML has an algorithm that consists of one or two interconnected layers of small computing units called "neurons." ML can be supervised, semisupervised, or unsupervised learning, making use of deep neural networks which are inspired by the structure and function of the human brain.[16,17]

### *Supervised Machine Learning*

In a supervised learning model, a prelabeled dataset is introduced to the machine to train it to detect a desired response of the new dataset.[18] However, this algorithm is time-consuming and cumbersome as it requires a large amount of dataset to be manually labeled before training the machine. Supervised machine learning (SML) algorithms include classification and regression:
- *Classification:* Based on training data, this algorithm can be used to predict discrete binary values such as yes or no, male or female. Different types of classification algorithms are logistic regression, K-nearest neighbors, naive Bayes classifier, decision trees, support vector machine (SVM), and random forest classification.
- *Regression:* These algorithms are utilized to detect data of continuous values. Various types of regression algorithms are simple linear, multiple linear, polynomial regression, decision tree regression, random forest regression, etc.

*Random forest* is a flexible and easy-to-use ML algorithm that belongs to the supervised learning technique. It is one among the most used algorithms due to its simplicity and variety. Random forests are an ensemble learning method that is used for performing classification, regression, and other tasks through the construction of decision trees and providing the output as a class which is the mode or the mean of the underlying individual trees.[18]

### *Unsupervised Learning*

In this model, unlabeled and uncharacterized datasets are given to the algorithm, and the algorithm learns to detect the expected results based on co-occurrence and underlying patterns on its own. This type of algorithm is similar to human learning by experience, and it helps in detecting useful insights from the dataset. Since an unlabeled dataset is used as input, the results can be less precise. Various types of unsupervised learning are clustering (K-mean clustering, hierarchal clustering), latent variable models, anomaly detection, association, and neural networks.[19]

## Reinforcement Learning

Reinforcement learning is an important type of AI that is based on the reward system. Here, unlabeled datasets are used, and the machine/program makes its own sequence of decisions to give an appropriate result. A reward is given if the results are near to the target and vice versa, thus letting the system to identify the right decision. A huge amount of data is needed for such learning, which constitutes its major drawback.

## Deep Learning

Deep learning usually focuses on data representation rather than task-specific algorithms. It means training multiple interconnected layers which are similar to the thinking process.[17,19] It includes:

- *Deep belief network (DBN):* Convolutional deep belief network (CDBN), conditional restricted Boltzmann machine
- *Convolution neural network (CNN):* AlexNet, GoogleNet, visual geometry group network (VGG), deep residual learning, etc.
- *Recurrent neural network (RNN):* Bidirectional RNN, long short-term memory

Various machines with different AI algorithms are utilized in KCN detection that are described below **(Table 1)**:

- *Videokeratoscope:* In 1994, Maeda et al. were the first to develop an automated ML algorithm to differentiate KCN using computer-assisted videokeratoscope. They used a combination of classification tree with a linear discriminant function derived from discriminant analysis of indices obtained from TMS-1 videokeratoscope data. With a validation set, they showed a sensitivity of 89%, specificity of 99%, and accuracy of 96% to detect KCN.[20] Other videokeratoscope-based algorithms were made and analyzed by Kalin et al. and Rabinowitz et al. using a combination of discriminant analysis and classification tree and linear discriminant analysis, respectively.[21,22]
- *Pentacam:* Most AI algorithms utilize Pentacam readings for detection of early and frank KCN. Different kinds of ML methods have been tested, including logistic regression, neural network,[23-25] SVM,[26] discriminate analysis,[27] random forest,[28] etc. Data from the Pentacam using ML demonstrated a higher pooled sensitivity and specificity in detecting

**TABLE 1:** Different types of machine learning utilizing various corneal imaging systems for keratoconus diagnosis.

| Type of corneal imaging system | Studies done (first author) | AI algorithm used | Detects |
|---|---|---|---|
| Videokeratoscope (TMS1) | Maeda et al.[20] | Discriminant analysis and classification tree | KCN eyes from control eyes |
| | Kalin et al.[21] | Discriminant analysis and classification tree | KCN eyes from control eyes |
| | Rabinowitz et al.[22] | Linear discriminant analysis | KCN eyes from control eyes |
| Pentacam | Chandapura et al.[28] | Logistic regression | KCN eyes from control eyes |
| | Kovács et al.[23] | Neural network | Early KCN and KCN eyes from control eyes |
| | Ruiz Hidalgo et al.[26] | Support vector machine | Early KCN and KCN eyes from control eyes |
| | Issarti et al.[24] | Neural network | Early KCN and KCN eyes from control eyes |
| | Lopes et al.[37] | Multiple methods | Early KCN eyes from control eyes |
| Galilei analyzer | Smadja et al.[31] | Decision tree | Early KCN and KCN eyes from control eyes |
| | Mahmoud et al.[32] | Logistic regression | KCN eyes from control eyes |
| OCT | Dos Santos et al.[38] | Convolutional neural network | KCN eyes from control eyes |
| | Kamiya et al.[33] | Convolutional neural network | KCN eyes from control eyes |
| | Yousefi et al.[39] | Density-based clustering | Detects KCN severity |
| CorVis ST | Koprowski et al.[35] | Decision tree | KCN eyes from control eyes |
| | Leão et al.[36] | Discriminant analysis | KCN eyes from control eyes |
| Combinations: Pentacam + CorVis ST | Ambrósio et al.[40] | Multiple methods | Early KCN and KCN eyes from control eyes |
| Artemis-1 + Pentacam | Silverman et al.[27] | Discriminant analysis | KCN eyes from control eyes |
| Pentacam + OCT | Chandapura et al.[28] (2019) | Random forest | KCN eyes from control eyes |

(AI: artificial intelligence; CorVis ST: corneal visualization Scheimpflug technology; OCT: optical coherence tomography)

KCN from control eyes compared to other imaging machines. This can be attributed to the ability of the Pentacam machine to generate a broad spectrum of data than other systems, including data on the front and back of cornea, corneal pachymetry, and other parts of the anterior segment of eye.[1]

- *Other topography measurement machines*: A few authors have utilized other topography measurement machines such as Orbscan,[29,30] Galilie,[31,32] OCT,[33,34] and corneal visualization (CorVis),[35,36] to test different AI algorithms.

Cao et al. conducted an extensive meta-analysis on AI in KCN. They showed that based on a large amount of datasets from variable corneal topography/tomography machines, ML can give genuine and reliable results in terms of distinguishing KCN from normal eyes (pool sensitivity >0.90). However, ML models did not perform well in differentiating and detecting early KCN from controls (maximum pooled sensitivity of around 0.88). This implies that more sophisticated ML algorithms are needed to detect early KCN in order to give an edge over manual diagnosis for its timely pickup and management.[1]

# LIMITATIONS OF ARTIFICIAL INTELLIGENCE IN KERATOCONUS

## Lack of Interchangeability Among Models

Various ML algorithms were developed using a variety of imaging systems. Models/algorithms themselves are, therefore, not directly interchangeable owing to the different input expectations. This may have a detrimental effect on the clinical translation of these models. For example, Smadja et al. developed an ML model that had a sensitivity of 93.6% and a specificity of 97.2% for discriminating normal eyes from early KCN in their study.[31] This model was constructed using the anterior and posterior asphericity asymmetry index (AAI), opposite sector index (OSI), corneal volume, paracentral mean keratometry, and anterior chamber depth derived from Galilei machine. Parameters such as AAI and OSI are not accessible in other corneal tomography imaging systems, such as Pentacam, suggesting that the generated model cannot be utilized in clinics equipped with the Pentacam system, which is one of the most frequently used corneal tomographic technologies in clinical practice.[25]

## Lack of External Validation

Most of the papers developed newer ML algorithms for KCN detection and did internal validation, and only a few conducted external validation using other data sources.[25,30,32,37] A major concern is that local datasets used for validation are unlikely to be representative of the target population on a global scale. The ML model developed in a cross-ethnic research by Mahmoud et al. performed differently when it was evaluated on datasets collected in the United States and Switzerland.[32] This implies that most of the current identified models cannot be used in a broad clinical setting since their performance may vary and it will most likely be poorer when applied to other external clinics or nations.

## Exclusion of Demographic and Clinical Signs

Various clinical symptoms such as frequent change of glasses, decreased vision, associated symptoms such as itching, and other slit-lamp findings also point toward the development of KCN. No study has been done incorporating all such pertinent data.[34,41] Demographic data such as age and gender, as well as potential risk factors for KCN, such as eye rubbing and family history, may also aid in KCN detection.[1]

## Lack of Integration of Data from Multiple Imaging Modalities

The majority of ML algorithms were trained based on datasets from one type of corneal topography/tomography device. Thus, there is a lack of information on impact and use of combining data from multiple devices on ML models in the detection of KCN. To improve the performance and detection rate of early KCN using ML models, integrating data from multiple devices can be tested.[1]

## Use of Training Data from Local Set of Population

There is a lack of large patient population validation of various ML models using different imaging modalities. Often, ML models were used on a local participant group comprised of individuals of various ethnic backgrounds. Therefore, external model validation needs to be done on a diverse patient population, as well as the generation of variable-independent models that can be generalized through varied corneal imaging systems.

## ■ FUTURE DIRECTIONS

Despite the high level of accuracy of the AI-based ML models in many ophthalmic conditions, the practical universal adoption of these models in day-to-day clinical practice still faces numerous clinical and technical hurdles. These difficulties could appear at various points in both research and therapeutic contexts. First of all, a lot of studies have employed training datasets from generally homogeneous populations. To solve this problem, the dataset's ethnic and image-capture hardware diversity could be increased. The algorithm picks up new information from the input it receives. More evidence on ways of getting high-quality ground-truth labeled datasets is required for different imaging tools.

To improve clinical implications of ML systems, it is important to unravel and explore various newer modes of machine and DL using existing and future methodologies. However, even with existing challenges, ML/DL will find a deep impact and likely change the practice of medicine and ophthalmology in the coming decades.

Integrating ML technologies into clinical practice by incorporating them into advanced imaging modalities in the future will aid widespread implementation of the technology. Despite the challenges, ML has significant potential for continuous advancements and should be further investigated for widespread application in KCN detection and management.

## CONCLUSION

Artificial intelligence helps in the early diagnosis of KCN, especially in young and post-refractive surgery patients, which might be missed by conventional techniques. It is a promising tool for monitoring progression in KCN.

## REFERENCES

1. Cao K, Verspoor K, Sahebjada S, Baird PN. Accuracy of machine learning assisted detection of keratoconus: a systematic review and meta-analysis. J Clin Med. 2022;11(3):478.
2. Buzzonetti L, Bohringer D, Liskova P, Lang S, Valente P. Keratoconus in children: a literature review. Cornea. 2020;39(12):1592-8.
3. Sharif R, Bak-Nielsen S, Hjortdal J, Karamichos D. Pathogenesis of keratoconus: the intriguing therapeutic potential of prolactin-inducible protein. Prog Retin Eye Res. 2018;67:150-67.
4. Rock T, Bartz-Schmidt KU, Rock D. Trends in corneal transplantation at the University Eye Hospital in Tubingen, Germany over the last 12 years: 2004-2015. PLoS One. 2018;13(6):e0198793.
5. Davidson SC, Bohrer G, Gurarie E, LaPoint S, Mahoney PJ, Boelman NT, et al. Ecological insights from three decades of animal movement tracking across a changing Arctic. Science. 2020;370(6517):712-5.
6. Mintz Y, Brodie R. Introduction to artificial intelligence in medicine. Minim Invasive Ther Allied Technol. 2019;28(2):73-81.
7. Ting DSW, Cheung CY, Lim G, Tan GSW, Quang ND, Gan A, et al. Development and validation of a deep learning system for diabetic retinopathy and related eye diseases using retinal images from multiethnic populations with diabetes. JAMA. 2017;318(22):2211-23.
8. Lee CS, Tyring AJ, Deruyter NP, Wu Y, Rokem A, Lee AY. Deep-learning based, automated segmentation of macular edema in optical coherence tomography. Biomed Opt Express. 2017;8(7):3440-8.
9. Li M, Wan C. The use of deep learning technology for the detection of optic neuropathy. Quant Imaging Med Surg. 2022;12(3):2129-43.

10. Dong L, Yang Q, Zhang RH, Wei WB. Artificial intelligence for the detection of age-related macular degeneration in color fundus photographs: a systematic review and meta-analysis. EClinicalMedicine. 2021;35:100875.
11. Yildiz VM, Tian P, Yildiz I, Brown JM, Kalpathy-Cramer J, Dy J, et al. Plus disease in retinopathy of prematurity: convolutional neural network performance using a combined neural network and feature extraction approach. Transl Vis Sci Technol. 2020;9(2):10.
12. Varadarajan AV, Poplin R, Blumer K, Angermueller C, Ledsam J, Chopra R, et al. Deep learning for predicting refractive error from retinal fundus images. Invest Ophthalmol Vis Sci. 2018;59(7):2861-8.
13. Poplin R, Varadarajan AV, Blumer K, Liu Y, McConnell MV, Corrado GS, et al. Prediction of cardiovascular risk factors from retinal fundus photographs via deep learning. Nat Biomed Eng. 2018;2(3):158-64.
14. Valdés-Mas MA, Martín-Guerrero JD, Rupérez MJ, Pastor F, Dualde C, Monserrat C, et al. A new approach based on machine learning for predicting corneal curvature (K1) and astigmatism in patients with keratoconus after intracorneal ring implantation. Comput Methods Programs Biomed. 2014;116(1):39-47.
15. Hosoda Y, Miyake M, Meguro A, Tabara Y, Iwai S, Ueda-Arakawa N, et al. Keratoconus-susceptibility gene identification by corneal thickness genome-wide association study and artificial intelligence IBM Watson. Commun Biol. 2020;3(1):410.
16. LeCun Y, Bengio Y, Hinton G. Deep learning. Nature. 2015;521(7553):436-44.
17. Schmidhuber J. Deep learning in neural networks: an overview. Neural Netw. 2015;61:85-117.
18. Rigatti SJ. Random forest. J Insur Med. 2017;47(1):31-9.
19. Tong Y, Lu W, Yu Y, Shen Y. Application of machine learning in ophthalmic imaging modalities. Eye Vis (Lond). 2020;7(1):22.
20. Maeda N, Klyce SD, Smolek MK, Thompson HW. Automated keratoconus screening with corneal topography analysis. Invest Ophthalmol Vis Sci. 1994;35(6):2749-57.
21. Kalin NS, Maeda N, Klyce SD, Hargrave S, Wilson SE. Automated topographic screening for keratoconus in refractive surgery candidates. CLAO J. 1996;22(3):164-7.
22. Rabinowitz YS, Rasheed K, Yang H, Elashoff J. Accuracy of ultrasonic pachymetry and videokeratography in detecting keratoconus. J Cataract Refract Surg. 1998;24(2):196-201.
23. Kovács I, Miháltz K, Kránitz K, Juhász É, Takács Á, Dienes L, et al. Accuracy of machine learning classifiers using bilateral data from a Scheimpflug camera for identifying eyes with preclinical signs of keratoconus. J Cataract Refract Surg. 2016;42(2):275-83.
24. Issarti I, Consejo A, Jiménez-García M, Hershko S, Koppen C, Rozema JJ. Computer aided diagnosis for suspect keratoconus detection. Comput Biol Med. 2019;109:33-42.
25. Issarti I, Consejo A, Jiménez-García M, Kreps EO, Koppen C, Rozema JJ. Logistic index for keratoconus detection and severity scoring (Logik). Comput Biol Med. 2020;122:103809.
26. Ruiz Hidalgo I, Rodriguez P, Rozema JJ, Ní Dhubhghaill S, Zakaria N, Tassignon MJ, et al. Evaluation of a machine-learning classifier for keratoconus detection based on Scheimpflug tomography. Cornea. 2016;35(6):827-32.

27. Silverman RH, Urs R, Roychoudhury A, Archer TJ, Gobbe M, Reinstein DZ. Epithelial remodeling as basis for machine-based identification of keratoconus. Invest Ophthalmol Vis Sci. 2014;55(3):1580-7.
28. Chandapura R, Salomão MQ, Ambrósio Jr R, Swarup R, Shetty R, Sinha Roy A. Bowman's topography for improved detection of early ectasia. J Biophotonics. 2019;12(10):e201900126.
29. Bessho K, Maeda N, Kuroda T, Fujikado T, Tano Y, Oshika T. Automated keratoconus detection using height data of anterior and posterior corneal surfaces. Jpn J Ophthalmol. 2006;50(5):409-16.
30. Saad A, Gatinel D. Topographic and tomographic properties of forme fruste keratoconus corneas. Invest Ophthalmol Vis Sci. 2010;51(11):5546-55.
31. Smadja D, Touboul D, Cohen A, Doveh E, Santhiago MR, Mello GR, et al. Detection of subclinical keratoconus using an automated decision tree classification. Am J Ophthalmol. 2013;156(2):237-46.e1.
32. Mahmoud AM, Nuñez MX, Blanco C, Koch DD, Wang L, Weikert MP, et al. Expanding the cone location and magnitude index to include corneal thickness and posterior surface information for the detection of keratoconus. Am J Ophthalmol. 2013;156(6):1102-11.
33. Kamiya K, Ayatsuka Y, Kato Y, Fujimura F, Takahashi M, Shoji N, et al. Keratoconus detection using deep learning of colour-coded maps with anterior segment optical coherence tomography: a diagnostic accuracy study. BMJ Open. 2019;9(9):e031313.
34. Lavric A, Popa V, Takahashi H, Yousefi S. Detecting keratoconus from corneal imaging data using machine learning. IEEE Access. 2020;8:149113-21.
35. Koprowski R, Ambrósio R. Quantitative assessment of corneal vibrations during intraocular pressure measurement with the air-puff method in patients with keratoconus. Comput Biol Med. 2015;66:170-8.
36. Leão E, Ing Ren T, Lyra JM, Machado A, Koprowski R, Lopes B, et al. Corneal deformation amplitude analysis for keratoconus detection through compensation for intraocular pressure and integration with horizontal thickness profile. Comput Biol Med. 2019;109:263-71.
37. Lopes BT, Ramos IC, Salomão MQ, Guerra FP, Schallhorn SC, Schallhorn JM, et al. Enhanced tomographic assessment to detect corneal ectasia based on artificial intelligence. Am J Ophthalmol. 2018;195:223-32.
38. Dos Santos VA, Schmetterer L, Stegmann H, Pfister M, Messner A, Schmidinger G, et al. CorneaNet: fast segmentation of cornea OCT scans of healthy and keratoconic eyes using deep learning. Biomed Opt Express. 2019;10(2):622-41.
39. Yousefi S, Yousefi E, Takahashi H, Hayashi T, Tampo H, Inoda S, et al. Keratoconus severity identification using unsupervised machine learning. PLoS One. 2018;13(11):e0205998.
40. Ambrósio Jr R, Lopes BT, Faria-Correia F, Salomão MQ, Bühren J, Roberts CJ, et al. Integration of Scheimpflug-based corneal tomography and biomechanical assessments for enhancing ectasia detection. J Refract Surg. 2017;33(7):434-43.
41. Maeda N, Klyce SD, Smolek MK. Comparison of methods for detecting keratoconus using videokeratography. Arch Ophthalmol. 1995;113(7):870-4.

CHAPTER 4

# Advances in Refractive Surgery

*Shreesha Kumar Kodavoor, Gitansha Sachdev,
Gopal R, Ramamurthy D*

## ABSTRACT

Refractive surgery remains an exciting and rapidly evolving field within ophthalmology. Extensive research has provided advancements and invaluable refinements in laser technology and diagnostic methods and tools to develop a safe and predictable treatment option for the entire gamut of refractive disorders.

Though laser in situ keratomileusis (LASIK) is the mainstay in refractive surgery and can be used in its various forms of laser vision surgeries or even combined with cataract surgery, presbyopic correction, and phakic intraocular lenses (IOLs), the refractive surgery has evolved beyond the traditional LASIK to advanced procedures such as small incision lenticule extraction (SMILE), Contoura vision, intracorneal implants and segments, phakic IOLs, and laser refractive cataract surgery with refractive lens exchange with advanced optics that provide more options in carefully selected patients.

We have techniques and technologies to suit practically all individual patients today. Possibilities with refractive surgery are mind-boggling. Selecting a particular type of procedure to suit a particular eye becomes the responsibility of a refractive surgeon and failure to do so can result in catastrophe.

***Keywords:*** LASIK; Contoura vision; SMILE; phakic intraocular lens; Pentacam; excimer laser; femtosecond laser; microkeratome; bioptics.

## ■ INTRODUCTION

Today, refractive surgery has evolved beyond the traditional laser refractive surgery termed laser in situ keratomileusis (LASIK) to advanced procedures such as small incision lenticule extraction (SMILE), Contoura vision, intracorneal implants, and phakic intraocular implants. Laser refractive cataract surgery with refractive lens exchange with advanced optics provides more options in carefully selected patients. The advent of the femtosecond (FS) laser provides unparalleled safety, precision, and predictability. An intensive evaluation is mandatory to assess the ocular status and determine the ideal surgical procedure. Additionally, complications must be managed with utmost caution and care to prevent loss of corrected visual acuity.

## ■ EXCIMER LASER

The excimer laser system was first developed in 1970 and more than a decade later used in the human eye to perform corneal photoablation.[1]

### Principle

The excimer laser system works on the principle of ablative photodecomposition using argon fluoride (ArF) as the essential gas mixture. When electric energy is applied, the argon molecule is stimulated to form an "excited dimer" or "excimer." This unstable dimer reverts quickly to its original state, emitting a charged photon. The charged photon has high energy, enabling breakdown of collagen bonds or "photoablation." It is a class IV laser with a near X-ray wavelength of 193 nm. This affords low tissue penetration, thereby allowing the laser to work only directly on the intended surface, unlike the FS laser. Thus, the excimer laser requires removal of the epithelium in photorefractive keratectomy (PRK) or creation of a flap in LASIK to gain direct access to the underlying stromal surface.

For myopic correction, greater ablation is carried out in the center of the cornea to flatten it, whereas in hyperopia, a doughnut-shaped mid-peripheral ablation is required, allowing incoming light to be refracted strongly when meeting the steeper flanks of the dome. Astigmatic correction is along one particular meridian. The ablation protocol is determined specifically for each individual's refractive error and calculated by a software program in the laser system. The depth of tissue ablation is calculated by Munnerlyn equation which in a simplified way states that:

$$\text{Ablation depth } (\mu m) = \frac{\text{Optic zone}^2 \times \text{Dioptric correction required}}{3}$$

Hence, the extent of stromal tissue ablation is dependent on the refractive error corrected and the optic zone diameter.

All laser systems come with their recommended list of safety precautions. Odors and fumes interfere with laser function and should not be allowed inside the laser room. The gas cylinders used in the laser have fluorine, argon, helium, and neon. Fluorine is a highly toxic gas with a sharp odor that causes irritation to nose, eyes, and throat at extremely low concentrations. Excimer lasers use <0.25% concentration of fluorine. Argon, helium, and neon are inert nontoxic gases with no color, odor, or taste.

Strict environmental conditions need to be maintained in the laser suite for proper functioning of the laser system. Temperature range should not fluctuate beyond 60–80°F and relative humidity should be between 35 and 65%.

Advances in Refractive Surgery

**BOX 1:** Types of excimer laser.

- *Broad beam laser:*
  - Large diameter ~ 7 mm
  - High-energy per pulse
  - Lesser pulses required
  - Lower repetition rate
  - Correction may be limited as central islands of cornea may be subtotally treated, secondary to plume of ejected particles shadowing the underlying tissue
- *Flying spot laser* **(Fig. 1)**:
  - Smaller diameter ~ 0.5–2 mm
  - Higher repetition rate
  - Higher frequency
  - *Smoother stromal bed:* Since the laser shots are distributed in placement, it allows adequate time for plume dissipation before the next laser shot is fired on the same area
- Slit scanning laser

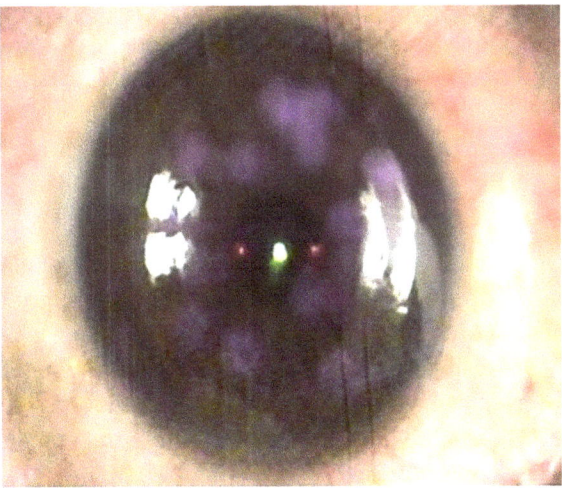

**Fig. 1:** Flying spot placement of an excimer laser.

## Types of Excimer Laser

Types of excimer laser are given in **Box 1**.

## Types of Ablation Profiles

Refractive corrections are engineered on the anterior corneal surface as the cornea is responsible for two-thirds of the refractive power of the eye. Additionally, the air-tear film anterior cornea demonstrates the greatest change in refractive index; therefore, any treatment administered here

gives maximum refractive results. Types of ablation profiles can be broadly classified into the following:
- *Conventional ablation:* It entails the correction of lower-order aberrations (defocus or sphere and astigmatism or cylinder). However, this induces spherical aberrations secondary to peripheral loss of fluence. As the laser beam spot peripherally is more oblique as compared to circular in the center, a resultant loss of laser energy causes reduced effect in the periphery. This induces greater flattening centrally, making the corneal shape oblate, thereby inducing spherical aberrations.
- *Wavefront-guided* (*WFG*) *ablation:* This combines the conventional ablation (treatment of lower-order aberrations) with treatment of preexisting higher-order aberrations (HOAs) (coma, trefoil, and spherical aberrations). However, it does not compensate for the treatment-induced spherical aberrations.
- *Wavefront-optimized* (*WFO*) *ablation:* This compensates for loss of fluence by increasing the number of peripheral pulses. This reduces the treatment-induced spherical aberrations, which provides higher quality of vision especially in mesopic conditions. WFO ablation additionally treats preoperative lower-order aberrations but does not treat preexisting HOAs.
- *Topo-guided ablation profile:* It is a combination of WFO ablation along with treatment of preexisting corneal HOAs.

## Eye Tracking in Excimer Laser

With the advent of excimer laser treatments, accurate ocular alignments are important to optimize refractive results. The pupillary center serves as the anatomical landmark for the centration of the laser ablation. Any misalignment of the ablation profile due to shifting of the pupillary center or cyclotorsion can result in undercorrection of existing aberrations or induction of newer ones. Hence, the need for an efficient eye tracking to optimize the placement of laser pulses arises.[2]

The tracking system is based on iris registration and includes both passive and active tracking. The system includes an active x-y and a passive z tracker in addition to a rotational eye tracker. The assessment is based on the difference in the position of the iris landmarks between the preoperative and intraoperative images. These images are compared using infrared cameras.

## Iris Registration

An infrared camera captures the characteristic iris landmarks in the sitting position during the preoperative measurement. Prior to laser ablation, another infrared image is acquired in supine position. The difference between the two images determines the extent of cyclotorsion and pupil centroid shift, realigning the treatment plan accordingly. Iris registration is a static process and does not actively track eye movements during the excimer ablation.

## Active Tracking

The incorporation of iris registration allows static eye movement compensation. However, active cyclotorsion and eye movements have been noted during laser ablation. Active tracking utilizes an image of the iris taken prior to ablation and measures subsequent changes to determine the intraoperative eye movement rather than using the preoperative image. Dynamic trackers reduce enhancement rates. The eye tracker locks onto the patient's iris just before the treatment and monitors the pattern throughout the procedure. The direction of the laser pulses is automatically adjusted, based on the rotation of the iris pattern. Newer advances in eye-tracking systems enable the compensation of subtler movements such as pupil centroid shift and cyclotorsion.

## Cyclotorsion Compensation

While the preoperative wavefront and topographic data are collected in the sitting position, the laser ablation is delivered in the supine position. The intraoperative cyclotorsion can serve as a potential source of error during the laser treatment, especially in errors that are not radially symmetrical such as astigmatism, coma, and trefoil.[3] Intraoperative cyclotorsion can result due to a variety of factors including rotation of the head and body, distortion of globe due to placement of the eyelid speculum, unmasking of cyclophoria, and dynamic eye movements. The extent of cyclorotation is typically between 2° and 7°. Theoretically, a 5° misalignment results in 17% less effect in astigmatic reduction and a misalignment of 15° can result in an under-correction of up to 50% of astigmatism.[2]

Cyclotorsion is divided into two components: (1) Static which comprises the difference between the supine and prone position; (2) Dynamic which comprises further rotational movements during ablation treatment.

## Pupil Centroid Shift

An important consideration for the centration of the laser ablation is the position of the pupil centroid. The preoperative wavefront data is captured under dim illumination, while the illumination increases during laser ablation.[4] As the lighting conditions vary, the diameter of the pupil fluctuates with a corresponding pupil centroid shift **(Fig. 2)**. Since the laser ablation is centered around the pupil centroid, any shift can lead to a decentered ablation with subsequent visual symptoms such as glare, haloes, and starbursts. Decentrations as small as 0.2 mm significantly increase the HOAs after LASIK. Theoretically, if the ablation is completed without correction

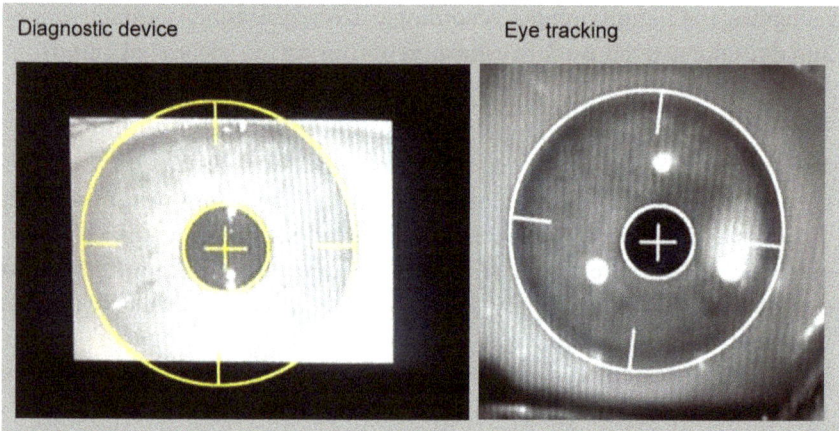

**Fig. 2:** Registration of iris landmarks to determine the extent of cyclotorsion and pupil centroid shift (WaveLight® Ex500 Excimer Laser, Alcon). Note a nasal shift of the pupil centroid and a cyclotorsion of –6°.

of pupil centroid shift, >40% of the patients would present with increased postoperative HOAs and reduced quality of vision.[5]

# PHOTOREFRACTIVE KERATECTOMY OR SURFACE ABLATION

Photorefractive keratectomy or surface ablation entails the removal of the corneal epithelium followed by excimer laser stromal ablation to offer a refractive correction.

Various techniques may be employed for the removal of corneal epithelium including laser in transepithelial PRK **(Figs. 3A to D)**, alcohol in laser epithelial keratomileusis (LASEK), microkeratome in epi-LASIK **(Figs. 4A to D)**, and mechanical debridement in surface ablation.

Several methods have been postulated for epithelial removal in surface ablation corrections. No differences in refractive outcomes and haze have been demonstrated between various techniques including LASEK, epi-LASIK, and transepithelial PRK in myopia. However, faster re-epithelization and lower pain may be associated with the transepithelial PRK approach.[6]

## Advantages of Photorefractive Keratectomy

- *Flapless procedure:* Flap-associated complications including flap striae and epithelial ingrowth are not associated with this procedure.
- *Biomechanical superiority:* PRK offers biomechanical superiority over SMILE and LASIK. This is secondary to two factors: Variable strength of the collagen lamellae and impact of penetrating cuts. The cohesive tensile strength of the cornea decreases from anterior to posterior cornea within

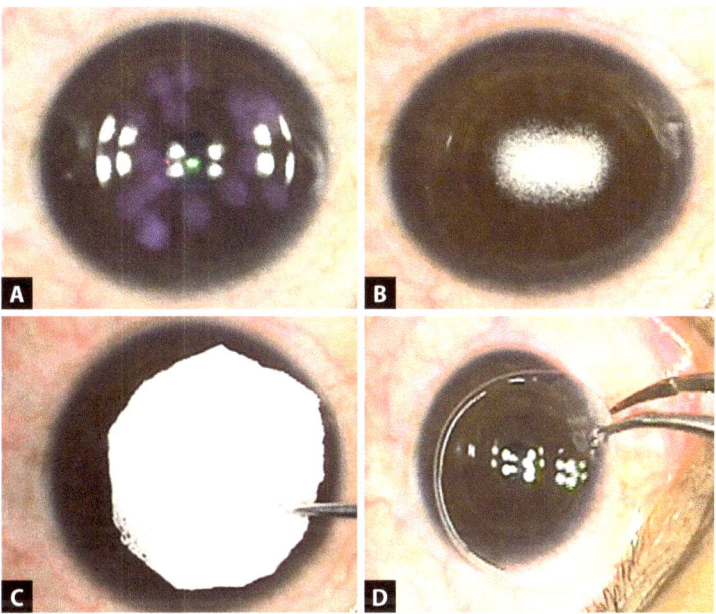

**Figs. 3A to D:** Steps of transepithelial photorefractive keratectomy (PRK): (A) Epithelial removed using phototherapeutic keratectomy (PTK) mode; (B) Excimer laser ablation is performed on the stromal bed; (C) Mitomycin C (MMC) 0.02% placed for 30 seconds; (D) Bandage contact lens placed after thorough saline wash.

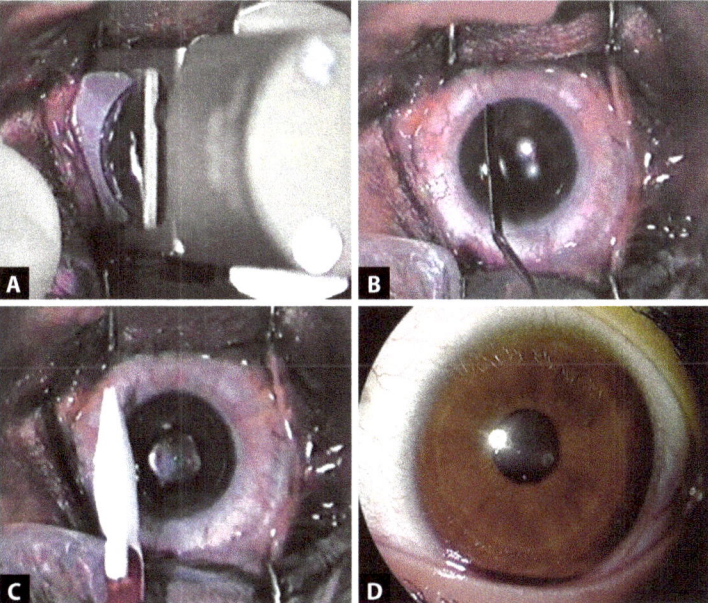

**Figs. 4A to D:** Steps of Epi-LASIK: (A) Epikeratome creates an epithelial flap; (B) Flap is subsequently reflected; (C) Excimer laser ablation is performed on the stromal bed and epithelial flap is reposited; (D) Postoperative image with bandage contact lens in situ.

the central region. As there is a greater change in the anterior corneal stroma in LASIK vis-à-vis PRK, the biomechanical strength of collagen fibers following PRK is greater.

The vertical cuts have a greater biomechanical effect in comparison to stromal ablation for refractive correction. As PRK does not involve any cuts, unlike the flap cut and corneal side cut, it induces lower biomechanical weakness in comparison to LASIK and SMILE.

- *Thinner corneas:* PRK allows treatment in thinner corneas between 475 and 490 μm. However, the final corneal thickness post-ablation should not be reduced beyond 400 μm.
- *Topo-guided approach for keratoconic eyes:* Topography-guided transepithelial PRK in combination with corneal collagen cross-linking is used in mild-to-moderate cases of keratoconus will well-centered cones.[7]

## ■ TOPOGRAPHY-GUIDED TREATMENT FOR KERATOCONUS

Keratoconus is a corneal ectasia characterized by progressive steepening and thinning of corneal tissue. The ectasia can lead to refractive error and degradation of visual quality. Corneal cross-linking (CXL) is recommended for stopping the progression of keratoconus.[8] The efficacy of CXL for arresting disease progression in keratectasia, both idiopathic and iatrogenic, is well established.[9] While cross-linking achieves disease stability, corneal surface irregularities and aberrations remain untreated requiring rigid gas permeable (RGP) contact lens postoperatively. RGP also brings with it the unique challenges including reduced patient comfort, poor fit in case of increased flattening, or haze caused by cross-linking.[10] The advent of topography-guided excimer laser ablation with concomitant CXL allows the reduction of corneal anterior surface irregularities along with disease stability. Kanellopoulos and Binder first described the novel application of topography-guided ablation in a cross-linked eye to improve visual acuity. Following this, a report of two cases exhibiting stability for over a period of 30 months was published.[11]

The same author then subsequently went on to describe the stability and anterior surface normalization in a larger cohort of 232 eyes. These results were then replicated by other groups as well, demonstrating the safety and efficacy of the treatment over a 2-year follow-up period.[12] The subsequent discussion entails a comprehensive overview of the preoperative requisites, treatment parameters, and visual outcomes of this technique. Keratometric flattening is seen in most corneas undergoing CXL. However, conventional uniform intensity CXL does not reduce HOAs significantly. In contrast, topography-guided ablation of keratoconus improves the visual acuity and reduces the HOAs by regularizing the anterior corneal surface.[13] The ablation is calculated using either the anterior corneal surface features (topography-guided treatment) or the total ocular wavefront (WFG). The superiority of visual outcomes of corneal aberration-guided ablation compared to CXL is known from multiple studies.[14]

The conventional topography-guided PRK (TGPRK) ablation profile is centered at the geometric center of the cornea and treats an optical diameter ranging from 5.5 to 6.5 mm. A significant amount of tissue is removed at and around the region of steepest anterior curvature (the cone). As a rule of thumb, the maximum stromal ablation depth is limited to 50 μm. Further, the location of the cone relative to the geometric center can impact the visual acuity outcomes after TGPRK.[15] A centered transepithelial phototherapeutic keratectomy (PTK) can also deliver patient-specific regularization of the corneal surface.[16] However, a centered PTK also causes unnecessary laser ablation of potentially normal regions of the keratoconic cornea. In this study, 1-year outcomes of a tissue-conserving customized ablation approach were analyzed. This approach, named the topography-assisted removal of epithelium, was performed at the region of the "cone." A decentered elliptical shape "single-step" PTK [topography-assisted phototherapeutic keratectomy (TPTK)], centered at the steepest tangential curvature point, was performed. This was followed by manual removal of the epithelium up to a diameter of 8 mm and accelerated CXL of the entire deepithelialized zone.[17] The outcomes of TPTK were comparable with the outcomes of patients who underwent TGPRK and accelerated CXL.

## ■ LASER IN SITU KERATOMILEUSIS

Laser in situ keratomileusis or LASIK was originally conceived by Dr José I Barraquer in 1949 where he created a free cornea flap, froze it, sculpted the undersurface on a cryolathe, and sutured it back to the cornea. Then came the advent of automated lamellar keratoplasty, which entailed the creation of a flap followed by a disc of stromal tissue excision using a microkeratome. Burrato and Pallikaris were the first to combine the microkeratome flap with subsequent excimer laser ablation. Subsequent modification in this technique led to the current form of LASIK, wherein a microkeratome blade is used to create a hinged corneal flap. This is subsequently raised, the stroma ablated with excimer laser, and the flap is then reposited back.

Laser in situ keratomileusis has become increasingly popular since 1995 and is now one of the most commonly performed refractive procedures to correct myopia, hyperopia, and astigmatism. It is also a modality of treatment for residual refractive errors after radial keratotomy and cataract surgery.

The basic instruments required for LASIK procedure include a microkeratome or FS laser for flap creation and excimer laser unit for stromal bed ablation. The details regarding excimer laser have already been covered in depth under PRK.

## Microkeratome Laser In Situ Keratomileusis

A microkeratome consists of a fine oscillating blade which can cut through the cornea at predetermined depths to form a smooth flap. The adjustable parameters allow the surgeon to decide the depth of the corneal flap with an accuracy of 10 μm. The assembly, operation, and maintenance of the microkeratome system are crucial to ensure accurate and predictable resections of the corneal tissue. The microkeratome head includes a pneumatic suction ring which elevates the intraocular pressure to above 65 mm Hg and allows stable fixation of the globe during flap creation. The surface of the suction ring has dove-tailed grooves over which the microkeratome head is placed. The surgeon-controlled foot-pedal activates the motor allowing the blade to advance forward till the ideal hinge is achieved, after which it is reversed, and the microkeratome head and suction ring removed. The flap is subsequently raised followed by excimer laser ablation of the stromal bed (**Figs. 5A to C**).

## Femtosecond Laser In Situ Keratomileusis

*Principle:* The FS laser is a solid-state neodymium glass laser with pulse duration in the FS range ($10^{-15}$ seconds). The wavelength falls in the

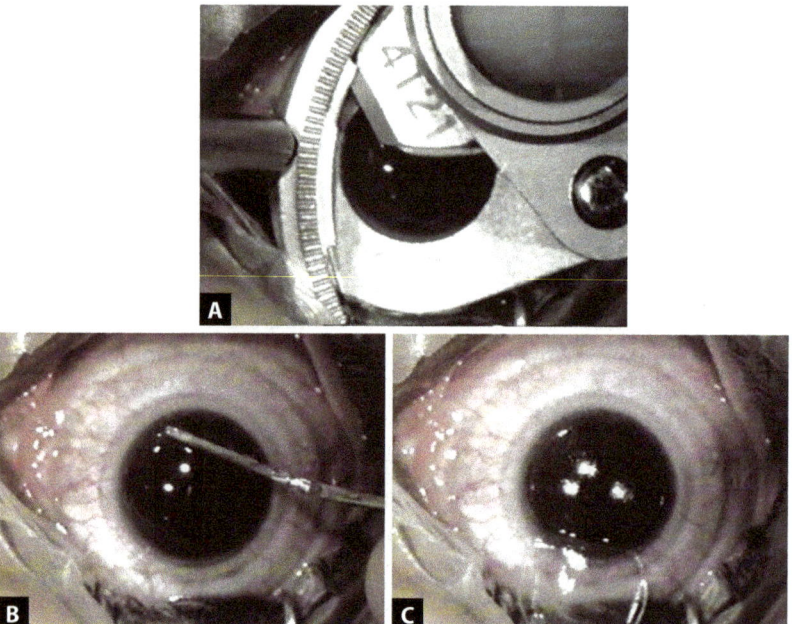

**Figs. 5A to C:** Steps of microkeratome laser in situ keratomileusis (LASIK): (A) Microkeratome head is placed on the suction ring; subsequent forward and reverse movement allows creation of a flap; (B) Flap is subsequently raised; (C) Underlying stroma is treated with excimer laser ablation.

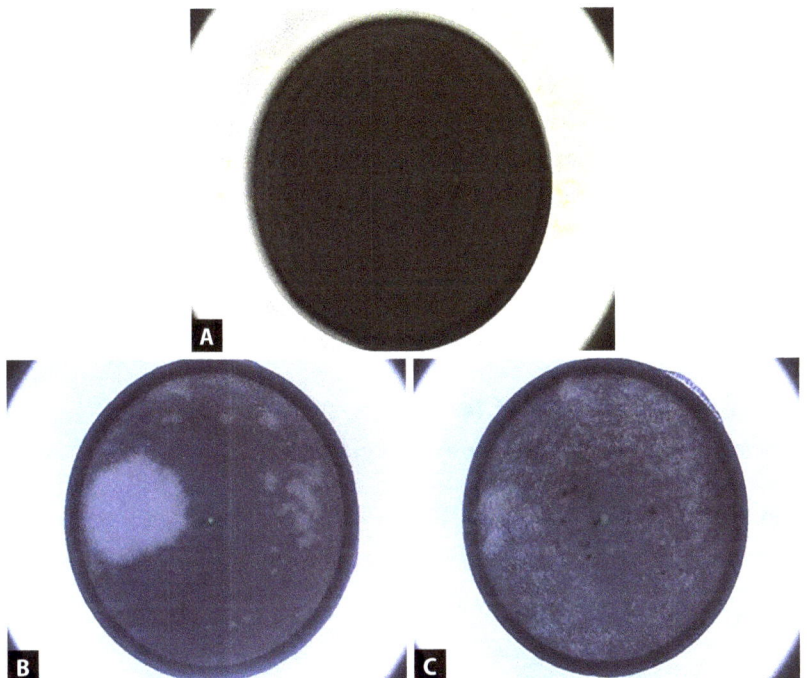

**Figs. 6A to C:** (A) Ideal opaque bubble layer (OBL); (B) High-energy OBL; (C) Low-energy OBL.

near-infrared range (1,053 nm). The FS laser can form precise cuts with minimum collateral damage by a process called *photodisruption*. The process begins with a sequence of laser pulses applied at a specific depth within the cornea in a predetermined pattern. The photon excites bound electrons by transmitting energy as heat, freeing them and initiating a vaporization cascade or microplasma formation. The microplasma expands to form cavitation bubbles, cleaving the tissue plane. Once the expansion stops, the cavitation bubbles collapse, emitting acoustic waves.

The following components of the FS procedure can be used to guide the surgeon in the process of optimization:[18]

*Pattern of opaque bubble layer:* The opaque bubble layer (OBL) is a collection of gas bubbles in the intralamellar spaces of the cornea **(Figs. 6A to C)**. OBL spontaneously clears in around 30–45 minutes. Predisposing factors for increased OBL formation include older patients and smaller and steeper corneas. The nature of the OBL allows determination of the laser energy and subsequent optimization of energy parameters.

In *OBL, secondary to high energy*, higher energy results in the formation of larger cavitation bubbles, wherein the incoming laser pulse will fall within the boundaries of the previously formed pulse (ideally the new pulse should fall adjacent to the previous pulse). Rather than vaporizing tissue, the new pulse will simply transfer heat to the existing cavitation bubble, increasing its size and causing a thicker OBL.

In OBL, secondary to low energy, small microplasma bubbles prevent easy coalescence during expansion, resulting in thick tissue bridges. Instead, the expanding bubbles may force the collagen around them apart, resulting in secondary bubbles.[19]

*Quality of dissection*
*Postoperative findings:* An increased incidence of diffuse lamellar keratitis (DLK) is associated with high-energy settings.

## Laser Settings for Flap Creation

Laser settings for flap creation are given in **Box 2**.

## Procedure

The surgical steps of LASIK are highlighted in **Figures 7A to F**.

Advantages of FS-LASIK over microkeratome LASIK include the following:
- Precise size and depth of corneal flap, independent of corneal curvature, blade sharpness, and speed of microkeratome pass

---

**BOX 2:** Laser settings for flap creation.

- *Pocket parameters:*
  - A pocket prevents dense OBL formation by allowing excessive gas bubbles to exit from the flap. The pocket depth is usually lower than 50% of corneal thickness (220–250 µm) with an ideal width of 250 µm
  - Pocket formation is associated with flat applanation contact interface, wherein the applanation force on the cornea does not allow the OBL to spread out easily. Newer curved contact interface is not associated with pocket formation
- *Hinge parameters:* The hinge angle varies with the planned ablation zone. A large hinge angle reduces the exposed stromal bed, whereas a narrow hinge will provide an inadequate fulcrum for the flap. The hinge position is fashioned nasally or superiorly.
- *Flap bed parameters:* The laser delivery for the formation of the corneal flap cut may occur in one of the following patterns:
  - Raster pattern
  - *Centrifugal spiral:* In-outward
  - *Centripetal spiral:* Out-inward
- *Side cut parameters:* Steeper side cut angle allows easier flap reposition and decreases the incidence of epithelial ingrowth. Optimal laser delivery allows a smooth and even edge creation; inadequate energy results in uncut areas or peripheral tags while excessive energy increases the risk of postoperative DLK

(DLK: diffuse lamellar keratitis; OBL: opaque bubble layer)

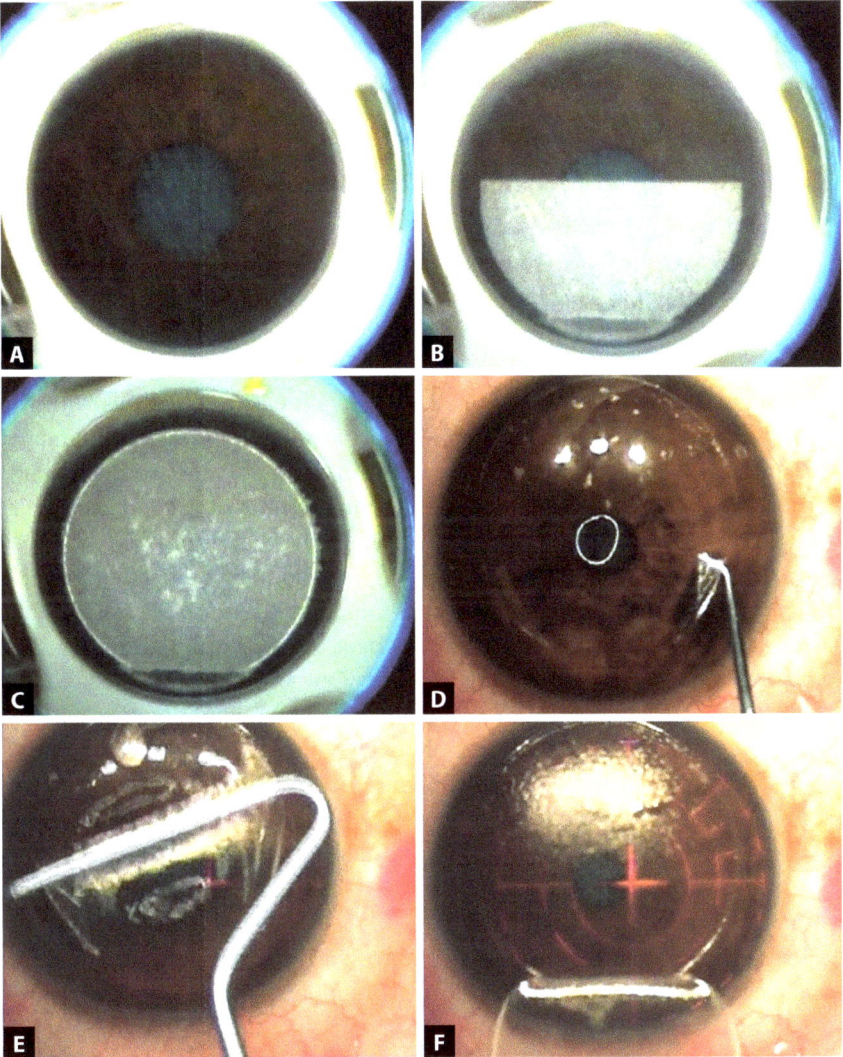

**Figs. 7A to F:** (A) Application of contact interface; (B) Pocket construction followed by flap cut; (C) Completion of flap cut and side cut; (D) Delineation of side cut; (E) Dissection of flap; and (F) Excimer laser stromal ablation.

- Reduced risk of complications such as free flaps, buttonhole formation, and incomplete and decentered flaps[20]
- Creation of a distinctive beveled edge flap which allows for precise repositioning and alignment, with reduced incidence of flap folds and epithelial ingrowth
- Ability to redock the eye and perform a double pass in the same sitting: The precision of the FS laser allows the flap cut to be repeated at the same depth in the event of a suction loss. The newly fired laser pulses percolate

to the same depth as the previously formed cavitation bubbles, which offer a path of least resistance. On the contrary, an incomplete pass with a microkeratome LASIK would require the surgeon to abort the procedure as a repeat pass would risk the formation of a biplanar flap.[21]

## Topography-guided Laser In Situ Keratomileusis

Currently, excimer laser systems designed to perform LASIK can correct astigmatism in different ways. The most basic method is to treat the measured refractive astigmatism based on the manifest refraction. A more advanced alternative is to use a WFG ablation that requires measuring the ocular wavefront of the entire eye and designing a specific ablation pattern to reduce or eliminate the ocular aberrations measured. Results with this approach appear only modestly better than treating the measured refractive astigmatism.[22] It is possible that the ability to accurately measure the ocular wavefront is still insufficient to provide a consistent beneficial effect. A third alternative is topography-guided LASIK **(Fig. 8)** that attempts to create a more uniform corneal surface to reduce aberrations while also correcting the refractive error. This technology was initially reserved to correct irregular astigmatism, although recent advances have led to it being used on virgin corneas as well, with promising results.[23] One of the topography-guided LASIK procedures (Contoura Vision, Alcon) has been shown to provide excellent visual outcomes in normal eyes without irregular astigmatism, with 93% of eyes achieving 20/20 or better uncorrected distance visual acuity (UDVA), 65% achieving 20/16 or better UDVA, and 34% achieving 20/12.5 or better UDVA 1-year postoperatively.[24] After Food and Drug Administration (FDA) approval of the topography-guided Contoura algorithm, it became more widely used in clinical settings.

Treatments were performed on eyes with a greater disparity between the manifest and topographic cylinder measurements. The challenge has been determining the best balance between using the topographic information and the refractive formation to provide an optimal correction for each eye. The topography-guided treatment profile is fixed by the Contoura software,

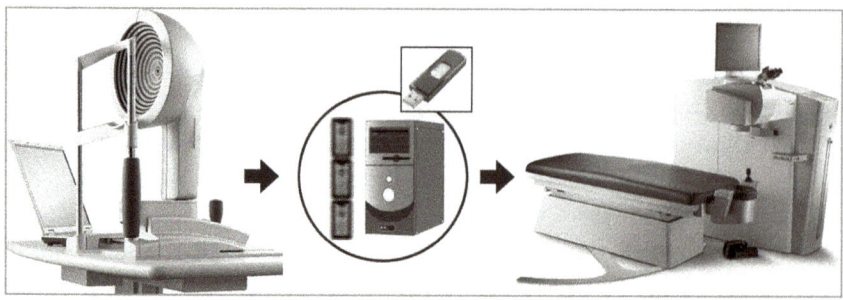

**Fig. 8:** Contoura workstation.

designed to treat all corneal topographic aberrations. However, the sphere and cylinder correction are user-specified; the WaveLight Topolyzer VARIO (Alcon) laser provides the user with the opportunity to select a treatment of sphere and cylinder. Different surgeons have based the sphere and cylinder treatment on the desired clinical outcome, the manifest refraction, the topographic cylinder, and/or other factors. Subjective approaches vary with surgeon, although more objective algorithms for treatment planning, such as that of Kanellopoulos, have been developed.[25] These rely on either treating completely from the measured topographic anterior astigmatic magnitude and axis or systematically combining the elements of both manifest refractive and topographic cylinder measurements. Others have suggested that using the manifest refractive cylinder alone as the basis for topography-guided treatment remains the best option.

A new alternative to the above-noted approaches, the Phorcides Analytic Engine (Phorcides LLC), considers the topography of the cornea in terms of not simply astigmatism but also its varying elevation profile. As such, it is not constrained by using only corneal astigmatism magnitude and axis as an input to the ablation algorithm. It may, therefore, provide an ablation pattern that is more responsive to asymmetry on the cornea. Corneal asymmetry is often the source of HOAs such as coma. A patient's manifest refraction may include a cylinder magnitude that is selected to reduce the blur circle created by coma. If the coma is effectively treated with topography-guided LASIK, the lower-order cylinder correction needed would likely be different.[26] Another consideration is that posterior corneal astigmatism and lenticular astigmatism affect the path of light through the eye. The Phorcides Analytic Engine thus considers the anterior corneal astigmatism, the topographic irregularities that create HOAs, the posterior corneal astigmatism, and the lenticular astigmatism when determining the optimal treatment of an eye with topography-guided LASIK.

Higher-order corneal aberrations such as trefoil, quadrafoil, and coma can create ovalization of the central cornea, which can interact with the ovalization caused by lower-order astigmatism to either induce, cancel out, or modify the manifest refraction. Contoura processing successfully determines the linkage of these interactions resulting in full astigmatism removal. Purely lenticular astigmatism appears to be rare. All aberrations require cerebral compensatory processing and can be removed, supported by the facts that full removal of aberrations and its linkage with lower-order astigmatism with the LYRA (Layer Yolked Reduction of Astigmatism) Protocol does not result in worse or unacceptable vision for any patient. In conclusion, HOAs interacting with lower-order astigmatism is the main reason for the differences between manifest refraction and Contoura-measured astigmatism, and the linkage between these interactions can be successfully treated using Contoura and the LYRA Protocol.[27]

*The LYRA Protocol is as follows:* (1) Enter the manifest/cycloplegic refraction into Contoura during presurgical planning; (2) Zero out the astigmatism and sphere to see an ablation pattern for the aberration correction layer; (3) Enter Contoura-measured astigmatism and axis for the final correction. The ablation map at this point should be similar to the Pentacam anterior elevation map. This will assist in understanding the ablation when there is a significant discrepancy between manifest versus measured astigmatic power and axis; (4) The sphere is now entered after adjustment for the spherical equivalent of the change in astigmatism. Aberration correction is visualized on the treatment. This understanding of how HOAs affect lower-order astigmatism came about as an attempt to understand why the LYRA Protocol using the measured Contoura astigmatism is effective. Different theories were examined, but the underlying fact was that using the LYRA Protocol eliminated astigmatism and resulted in good vision even when the manifest astigmatism/axis differed markedly from the Contoura-measured astigmatism/axis. Over time, examining the HOA pattern of patients in relation to their lower-order astigmatism and the changes from manifest refraction to Contoura measured led to an understanding of how the HOAs were interacting with the lower-order astigmatism. Essentially, this understanding was "reverse-engineered" from the realization that the LYRA Protocol works and creates more uniform corneas.

## ■ SMALL INCISION LENTICULE EXTRACTION

Small incision lenticule extraction entails the creation of four sequential corneal cuts to fashion an intrastromal lenticule using the FS laser. The lenticule is subsequently separated from the surrounding tissue, and refractive lenticule extraction (ReLEx) is done after raising a flap [ReLEx femtosecond lenticule extraction (FLEx)] or via a corneal side cut small incision (ReLEx SMILE).[28] The United States FDA trial provided approval for myopic correction using SMILE in 2016.

Currently, ReLEx SMILE is available as a treatment modality for myopic correction of –10 D and an astigmatic correction of –5 D, with a maximum spherical equivalent correction of –12.5 D. The procedure is currently not commercially available for hyperopic treatment. The preoperative assessment criteria have already been discussed.

Small incision lenticule extraction can be performed using the VisuMax system from Carl Zeiss Meditec AG **(Fig. 9A)**. The FS laser system in the VisuMax remains fixed. A joystick is used to align the patient's eye. Subsequent alignments are done under the integrated microscope for surgical steps. The FS laser is delivered through a contact glass interface attached onto the laser system's optical aperture **(Fig. 9B)**.

Advances in Refractive Surgery

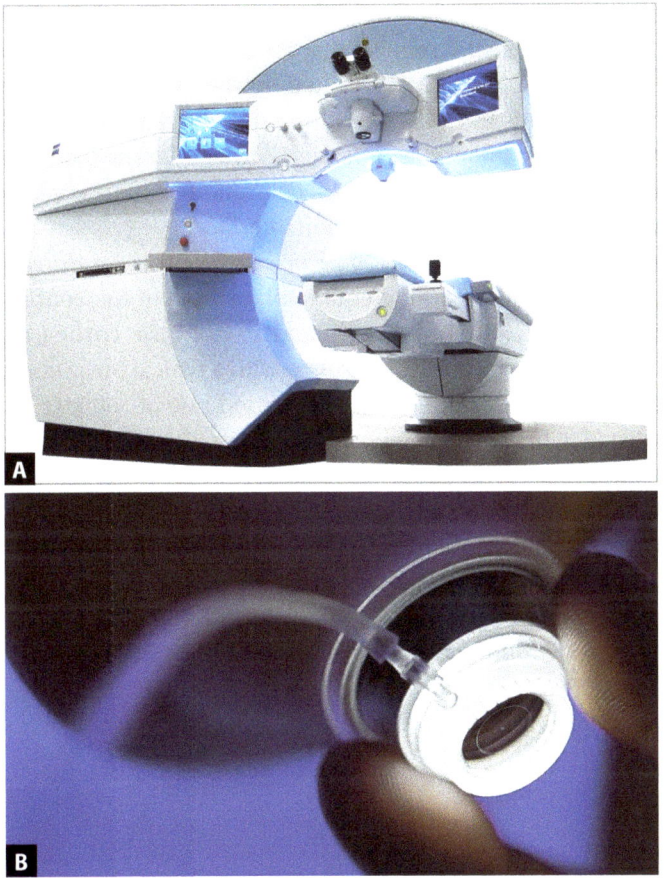

**Figs. 9A and B:** (A) VisuMax femtosecond laser system; (B) Corneal contact interface of the VisuMax femtosecond laser system.

The curved shape of the interface allows maximal surface contact with minimal corneal distortion. Additionally, suction ports afford a peripheral corneal or limbal hold as against a conjunctival suction reducing the incidence of subconjunctival hemorrhage. This allows a low suction force, thereby retaining the normal intraocular circulation and allowing continuous visibility of the fixation light.[29] An infrared illumination mode is incorporated into the system which allows the surgeon to ascertain the pupil centration following initiation of suction.

## Procedure

The procedure is carried out under topical anesthesia. There are three discrete steps involved:
1. *Initial docking with precise centration*: The joystick attached to the movable bed is used to align the patient's eye under the curved

contact glass. A proper head position is achieved by tilting the patient's head medially to avoid nasal contact with the cone of the contact glass interface. The chin must also be tilted upward or downward in a manner that the cornea is in the center of the palpebral fissure and maximum exposure to the contact glass interface is available. The patient is asked to focus on the fixation target. Precise centration should be verified before corneal contact with the applanation interface.

2. *Verification and maintenance of suction during FS laser delivery:* Following proper centration and adequate placement of the contact glass on the patient's eye, suction is initiated to hold the cornea against the contact glass interface. FS laser pulses with a typical pulse energy of 120–170 nJ are delivered with a pulse repetition rate of 500 kHz. The typical spot distance between each pulse is 2–5 µm. The FS laser spots are fired in a spiral track, with either decreasing (posterior lenticule surface) or increasing (anterior lenticule surface) spirals. The entire laser procedure takes around 23 seconds, irrespective of the refractive error to be corrected.

The four tissue disruption planes created by the FS laser in SMILE are shown in **Figure 10** and **Box 3**.

3. *Performing manual lenticule extraction:* Following completion of the FS laser (treatment mode), the suction automatically turns off. The patient's eye is repositioned under the microscope (observation mode).

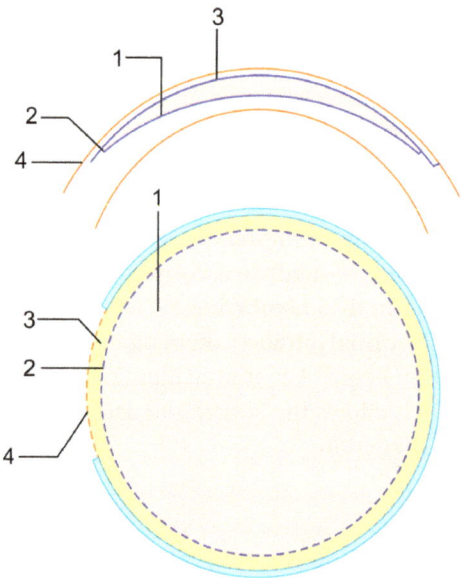

**Fig. 10:** Cross-section of the various cleavage planes created during small incision lenticule extraction (SMILE): (1) Posterior lenticule cut; (2) Lenticule side cut; (3) Anterior lenticule cut; (4) Corneal side cut.

**BOX 3:** Four tissue disruption planes created by a femtosecond laser in small incision lenticule extraction (SMILE).

1. Posterior lenticule surface (from periphery to center) followed by transition zone at the edge of the refractive zone (for spherocylindrical correction). The optical zone selected determines the diameter of the posterior lenticule surface
2. Vertical edge cut along the perimeter of the lenticule
3. Anterior lenticule surface (from center to periphery), which extends about 0.5–1 mm beyond the posterior lenticule surface
4. Peripheral corneal incision for lenticule access and extraction is generally created superiorly or superotemporally to preserve the nasal and temporal nerve arcades and to provide surgical convenience. The corneal incision varies from 250 to 300° in chord length for FLEx and 30–50° in chord length for SMILE

(FLEx: femtosecond lenticule extraction; SMILE: small incision lenticule extraction)

The lenticule extraction can be done manually by the following two techniques:
1. *FLEx:* A sharp-tipped instrument is used to enter vertically and delineate the flap-cut incision. A blunt spatula is subsequently inserted into the cleavage plane, to dissect the flap from the underlying lenticule. The flap is raised similar to that of FS-LASIK. The lenticule is then separated and peeled off from the residual stromal bed using corneal forceps. The interface is washed using balanced salt solution, and the flap is repositioned.
2. *ReLEx smile:* The corneal side cut is opened using a sharp-tipped instrument. This is followed by the delineation of the lenticular edge from the anterior cap and the posterior stroma. A blunt spatula is then inserted to dissect the lenticule completely from the anterior and posterior surfaces. Once the lenticule is freely separated, microforceps are inserted to grasp the lenticule and extract it out **(Figs. 11A to F)**.

## Advantages of Small Incision Lenticule Extraction

- Photodisruptive mechanism in SMILE, unlike the ablative nature of the excimer laser, is independent of factors such as corneal hydration, temperature, atmospheric humidity, and depth of stromal ablation.
- SMILE offers a distinct biomechanical advantage vis-à-vis LASIK due to two differentiating factors: (1) Variable strength of the collagen lamellae and (2) impact of penetrating cuts. The cohesive tensile strength of the cornea decreases from anterior to posterior cornea within the central region. As the stronger anterior and peripheral collagen fibers are left relatively intact in SMILE, therefore, its biomechanics is superior in comparison to LASIK.

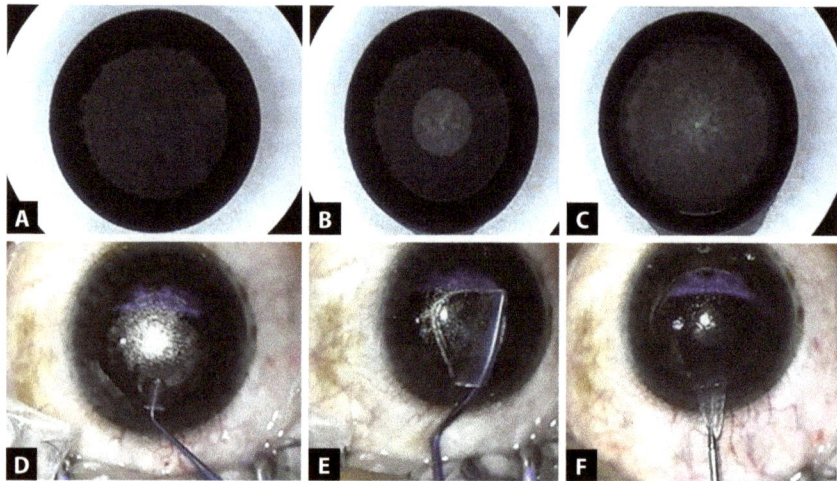

**Figs. 11A to F:** Surgical steps of a femtosecond laser-assisted small incision lenticule extraction (SMILE) procedure: (A) Posterior tissue disruption plane or lenticule cut; (B) Anterior tissue disruption plane or cap cut; (C) Cap side cut incision manual; (D) Delineation of planes; (E) Dissection of planes; (F) Lenticule removal.

The vertical cuts have a greater biomechanical effect in comparison to horizontal cuts, with greater weakening for deeper incisions. As LASIK entails vertical side cuts of a larger area, the corneal strain induced is greater in comparison to SMILE.[30]

- Lower number of corneal nerves are severed due to smaller cap side cut incision, thereby reducing the incidence of postoperative dry eye.[31]
- Lesser induction of HOAs, particularly spherical aberrations:[32] The peripheral loss of fluence in LASIK results in greater induction of spherical aberrations. Moreover, flap creation with subsequent excimer laser ablation induces a greater inflammatory response in comparison to SMILE, with greater wound modulation and induction of aberrations.[33] Additionally, the effective optic zone reduction in LASIK is greater than SMILE, i.e., 77.6 versus 83.4%.[34]
- Significantly, shortened procedural time due to use of a single laser platform instead of the two-platform procedure.

## Retreatment Options Following Small Incision Lenticule Extraction

- Surface ablation
- Thin flap LASIK
- CIRCLE software

A recent adaptation of SMILE software (Circle, Carl Zeiss Meditec AG) enables revision of the previously created cap by remodeling it into a

# Advances in Refractive Surgery

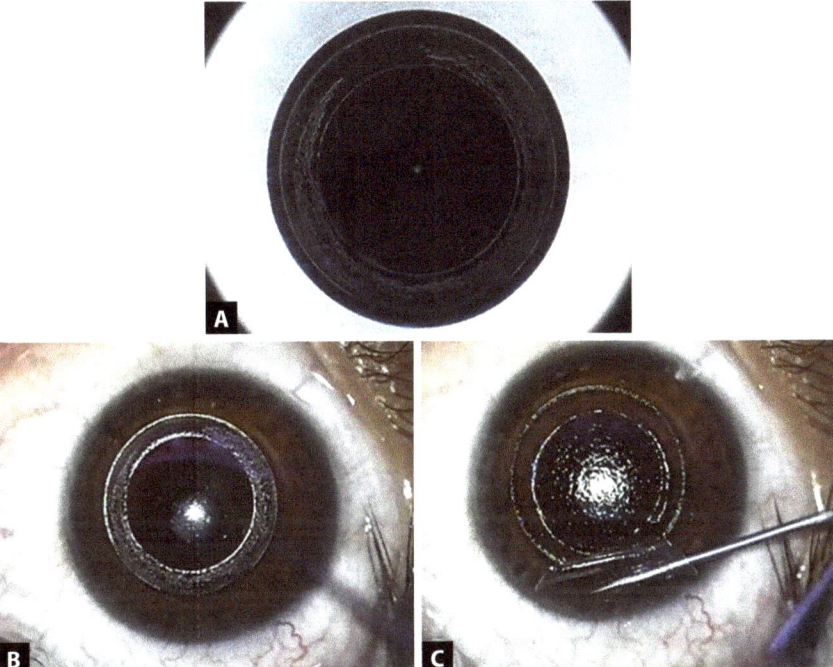

**Figs. 12A to C:** A lamellar ring (A and B) is created at the same depth as the existing small incision lenticule extraction (SMILE) incision allowing the conversion of SMILE cap into a hinged flap; (C) The flap is then raised followed by excimer laser ablation.

larger diameter flap (with hinge) allowing subsequent excimer laser ablation **(Figs. 12A to C)**.

In the CIRCLE procedure, the FS laser is used to create: (1) an incision plane encircling the original "cap" cut as a lamellar ring, (2) a side cut with hinge around the new incision plane, and (3) a "junction cut" which allows the original "cap" and the new incision plane to be part of one larger surface. Riau et al. investigated the use of four different patterns to create the above three cuts in rabbit eyes. They found that the pattern (pattern D) which creates the lamellar ring at the same level as the original "cap" thickness is the easiest to lift, even though all four patterns created a viable flap.[35]

Recently, a new method of lenticule management called "*lenticuloschisis*"[36] **(Fig. 13)**, a no-dissection technique in which the lenticule is gently peeled off the stroma in a rhexis-like pattern without performing actual dissection of the planes using any dissector, is described. The technique may offer better quality of vision immediate postoperative due to minimum manipulation of the tissues compared to the conventional dissection technique as the interface seen on the first postoperative day showed less roughness and irregularity compared to the dissection technique **(Figs. 14A and B)**. However, authors emphasized that the prerequisites such

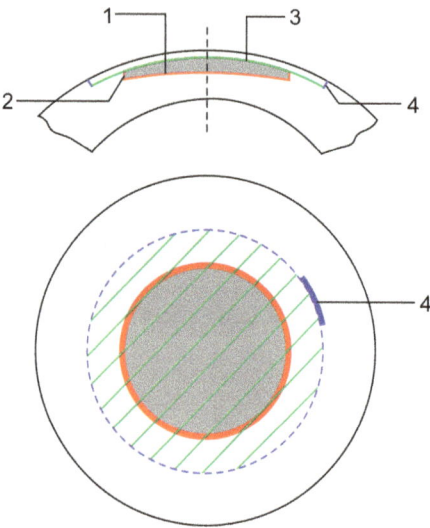

**Fig. 13:** (1) Lenticule cut (underside of lenticule); (2) Lenticule side cut; (3) Cap cut (concurrently the upper side of lenticule); (4) Cap opening incision.

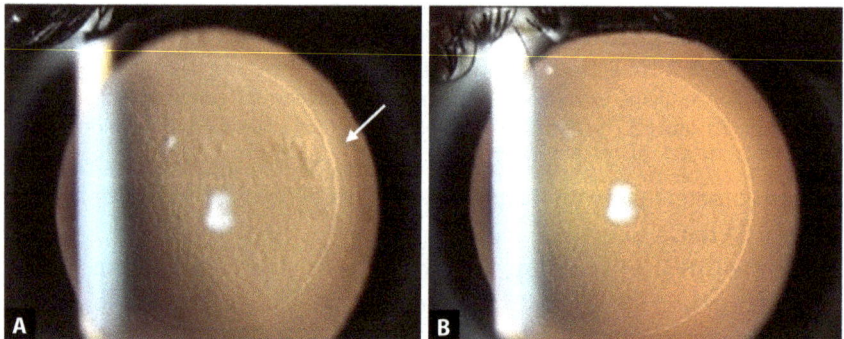

**Figs. 14A and B:** (A) Conventional dissection; (B) Lenticuloschisis.

as optimized energy levels, ideal bubble pattern, myopia >3 D, and good experience in the conventional technique of lenticule dissection must be fulfilled before attempting this technique.

A precursor to modern refractive corneal lenticule extraction (RCLE) was first described in 1996 using a picosecond laser to generate an intrastromal lenticule that was removed manually after lifting a flap in human donor eyes.[37] However, significant manual dissection was required leading to an irregular surface.[38] The switch to FS improved the precision, and studies were performed in rabbit eyes in 1998 and in partially sighted eyes in 2003. Following the introduction of the VisuMax FS (Carl Zeiss Meditec AG, Jena, Germany), in 2007, intrastromal lenticule refractive correction was introduced, in a procedure called FLEx. Ekundo et al. published the 6-month results of the first 10 fully seeing eyes treated in 2008 and a larger series subsequently. The procedure still included the creation of a hinged flap, under which the stromal lenticule was extracted, both cuts by FS laser.

The current SMILE FDA approval is for myopia of −1 to −10 D and astigmatism of −0.75 to −3 D with a maximum spherical equivalent (myopia plus half of the astigmatism) correction of no more than −10 D. The other machines which are recently added to perform the same technique are SCHWIND ATOS FS and FEMTO LDV Z8, both since 2020. The various parameters are given in **Table 1**.

**TABLE 1:** Overview of current femtosecond lasers that offer modern refractive corneal lenticule extraction (RCLE) applications.[38]

| FSL | ATOS SCHWIND | VisuMax Zeiss | Z8 Ziemer |
|---|---|---|---|
| RCLE program | SmartSight | SMILE | CLEAR |
| Possible refractive cuts | Flap/lenticule | Flap/lenticule | Flap/lenticule/arcuate incisions |
| Weight (kg) | <275 kg | 870 | 215 |
| Approval | CE | FDA/CE | CE |
| *Treatment range [diopters (D)]:* | | | |
| Sphere | −0.5 to −12.0 | −0.5 to −10.0 | −0.5 to −10.0 |
| Cylinder | 0 to −6.0 | 0 to −5.0 | 0 to −5.0 |
| SEQ | −0.5 to −14 | −0.5 to −12.5 | −0.5 to −12.5 |
| Repetition rate | Up to 4 MHz | 500 kHz | Up to 20 MHz |
| Energy per pulse (nJ) | 75–135 | 110–150 | <<100 |
| Laser/patient interface | Machine-fixed | Machine-fixed | Handheld |
| Contact glass on suction system | Curved (20 mm) | Curved (22 mm) | Flat |
| iOCT | No | No | Yes |
| Automatic detection of pupil | Yes | No | Yes |
| Pupil central offsetting | Yes | No | Yes |
| Cyclotorsion compensation | Yes | No | Yes |
| Centration | Eye tracking guided (semiautomated) centration | Manual | Eye tracking guided (semiautomated) centration |
| Real-time video recording | Yes | Yes | No—schematic graphic |

*Contd...*

*Contd...*

| FSL | ATOS SCHWIND | VisuMax Zeiss | Z8 Ziemer |
|---|---|---|---|
| Postsuction lenticule adjustment | Lateral electronic adjustment | Nil | Lateral electronic adjustment |
| Laser pattern | Arc segments—centrifugal/centrifugal | Centripetal/centrifugal | Spiral raster |
| Lenticule shape | No side cut | 10 μm side cut | No side cut |
| Number of treatments performed | 700+ | 3.5 million+ | 400+ |
| Incisions (mm) | 1, 2–5 | 1–3, 2–5 | 1–2, 1.5–4 |
| Advantages | Recentering after docking | Established technique | Recentering after docking |
| | Eye tracking with pupil recognition and cyclotorsion compensation | Many treated cases | Eye tracking with pupil recognition and cyclotorsion compensation |
| | Mobile device | Low IOPs during suction | Mobile device |
| | High repetition rate | | Small footprint |
| | Lower pulse energy | | High repetition rate |
| | | | Low pulse energy |
| | | | Guiding incisions and tunnels |
| | | | iOCT |
| | | | Multiuse laser |
| Disadvantages | New procedure lacking clinical experience | No recentering after docking | New procedure lacking clinical experience |
| | | No eye tracking | |

(CLEAR: cornea lenticule extraction for advanced refractive correction; FDA: Food and Drug Administration; FSL: femtosecond laser; iOCT: intraoperative OCT; IOP: intraocular pressure; OCT: optical coherence tomography; SMILE: small incision lenticule extraction; SEQ: spherical equivalent)

## Advantages of Refractive Corneal Lenticule Extraction over LASIK

With laser refractive surgery already achieving excellent clinical visual outcomes, it is often difficult to demonstrate that newer procedures are superior to the established techniques. A recent meta-analysis revealed a similar safety, efficacy, and predictability of SMILE compared to FS-LASIK in the correction of myopia. Similarly, Ang et al. recently published their results of a clinical trial, in 70 patients, performing FS-LASIK in one eye and SMILE in the other.[39] They found excellent, comparable outcomes in terms of refractive predictability, efficacy, and safety for both procedures at 3 months and also after 1 year of follow-up. Vision-related quality of life has also been found to be comparable between SMILE and LASIK. However, potential benefits of RCLE over LASIK are a quicker recovery of dry eye disease (DED), a larger functional optical zone, and no flap-related complications.[31]

## Hyperopic Small Incision Lenticule Extraction

In hyperopic SMILE treatment, the FS laser dissects out a concave lenticule within the corneal stroma which is then extracted by the surgeon, achieving the end result of a steeper central corneal configuration.[40-42] The second option to correct hyperopia is through convex-shaped lenticule reimplantation which has been obtained from a myopic correction of another patient **(Figs. 15A to C)**. The latter has been shown to be efficacious in both human beings and primates.

Previously in the laboratory, the authors have demonstrated the feasibility of reimplantation of refractive lenticules in a rabbit model and nonhuman primate model, with minimal short-term corneal haze and wound healing responses. A special nomogram was used to calculate the geometry and the thickness of the refractive lenticule for the correction of hyperopia.[43] The FS laser parameters used are 120 μm flap thickness, 7.9 mm flap diameter, 170 nJ power, and side cut angles at 90°. The spot distance and tracking spacing will be respectively at 3 and 3 μm for the lenticule, 1 and 1 μm for the lenticule side, 3 and 3 μm for the flap, and 2 and 2 μm for the flap side cut. The diameter of the lenticule will be 7.5 mm, which is equal to the optical zone (5.5 mm) plus the transition zone (1 mm + 1 mm).

Once suction is applied, laser incisions will be made in the following automated sequence:
- A spiral-in pattern on the posterior surface of the lenticule with a 5.5 mm diameter, equating the optical zone
- A spiral-out pattern on the posterior surface of the lenticule, from the edge of the optical zone for 2 mm, corresponding to the transition zone
- A vertical 90° lenticule side cut
- A spiral-out anterior surface of the lenticule cutting 7.9 mm diameter cap
- Followed by a superiorly placed 3 mm wide incision at 120° as previously optimized

After the laser sequence is completed, a Seibel spatula is inserted into the superiorly placed 3 mm incision to gain access to the intrastromal lenticule following which, a SMILE dissector is introduced to dissect microadhesions

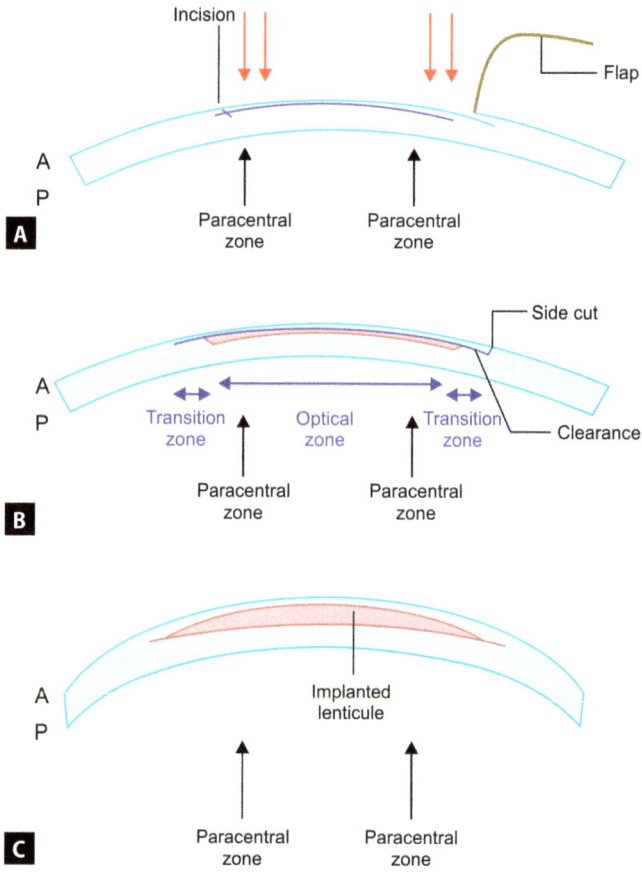

**Figs. 15A to C:** Schematic diagram of hyperopic small incision lenticule extraction (SMILE) treatment.

firstly on the anterior and then the posterior surfaces of the lenticule from the surrounding stroma. Once these planes are separated, the lenticule is extracted using a coaxial Tan Descemet stripping automated endothelial keratoplasty (DSAEK) forceps. The corneal stromal pocket is then irrigated with balanced salt solution with a 25-gauge cannula.

## Characteristics of Different Corneal Lenticule Extraction for Advanced Refractive Correction Systems[44,45]

Cornea lenticule extraction for advanced refractive correction (CLEAR) is a new RCLE procedure for myopic correction of sphere –0.5 to –10 D and cylinder 0 to –5 D. It is an optional software upgrade on the FEMTO LDV Z8 platform. This platform can also be used for cataract surgery, corneal transplantation, pterygium excision, LASIK flap creation, and presbyopic correction (pockets for inlays).[46] The Z8 is based on a low-energy (<100 nJ) and a high-frequency (up to 20 MHz) concept, where the miniaturized scanning optic, integrated into the hand-piece and its high numerical aperture, creates highly focused laser pulses. The advantages of the low-energy concept are the decreased stromal gas generation and a very accurate laser focus. The high-frequency repetition rate leads to overlapping pulses during the procedure. The laser pulses are guided from the laser source through an articulated moveable arm to a handpiece that is adaptable in position and height, with a very close working distance to the eye.

In addition, the FEMTO LDV Z8 offers a wide range of centration options and the options of recentering the treatment area after having performed the docking, including correction of cyclotorsion by adjustment on the touchscreen monitor, without having to release the suction, which is not possible with the current VisuMax Laser System. This ensures accurate centration on the visual axis and adjusted cyclotorsion, which is especially important in patients with cylindrical corrections. In CLEAR, the surgeon can adjust the distance between the incisions and the angle position for greater comfort and can also decide if one or both incisions are created and used. The lenticule has a diameter of 6.5 mm without adding any additional edge thickness.[47] During the cutting of the lenticule, the applied vacuum level to the eye is 700 mbar, the same as used for LASIK flaps with the Z8.

Another ability of the Z8 is the inbuilt intraoperative optical coherence tomography (iOCT). This feature may also be used following lenticule creation. This could be useful in more complicated cases, for example, CLEAR in post-transplant cases. Performing experimental CLEAR on enucleated porcine eyeballs during a medical exhibition in China, Wang et al. found that suction peak pressure, total laser application, and total surgery time in CLEAR takes longer time as compared to SMILE.[48] However, the CLEAR group included OCT scanning and offsetting before performing the laser procedure, which took more time for these crucial steps. The anterior and posterior lenticule surfaces analyzed by scanning electron microscopy were smoother in the FEMTO LDV Z8/CLEAR group compared to the VisuMax/SMILE group. The authors speculated that this might be the reason for easier lenticule separation in CLEAR compared to SMILE.

The atraumatic, smooth cutting of high-frequency low-energy FS has been shown before in rabbit corneas by Riau et al. using the FEMTO LDV Z6 predecessor model by placing laser spots directly adjacent to each other; the Z6 and Z8 are believed to create a smooth stromal interface. Further comparative studies are necessary to evaluate whether these differences in lenticule surface roughness created by different laser platforms could result in different clinical performances with regard to postoperative refraction, optic quality, and tissue response.[49]

## ■ PHAKIC INTRAOCULAR LENS IMPLANTATION

Although the prevalence of high myopia in the general population is exceedingly low, they constitute a significant proportion of the patients presenting for refractive surgery. Moderate and high myopes are 10 and 16 times, respectively, more likely to present for refractive correction in comparison to low myopes.[50]

Regression, ectasia, and compromise in optical quality are some of the limitations of corneal refractive surgery while correcting higher refractive errors. Hence, there is a need for an alternative form of treatment. This is available in the form of phakic intraocular lenses (IOLs) which are implanted between the cornea and the lens. Also termed "pseudophakia" or "artiphakia," the normal crystalline lens is retained, and an additional intraocular lens is placed in front to correct the refractive error.

### Types of Phakic Intraocular Lens

The lens may be fixated in the angle (angle-supported phakic IOLs) or enclavated in the mid-peripheral iris with a claw (iris-supported phakic IOLs). Newer designs entail placement in the posterior chamber (posterior chamber phakic IOLs), and these are the preferred phakic IOLs in today's practice. Posterior chamber phakic IOLs were introduced in the year 1987. Initial models were constituted of silicone with associated complications of cataract, endothelial cell loss, and chronic uveitis. The newer generation IOLs are composed of collamer—a copolymer of hydroxyethyl methacrylate (HEMA) and porcine collagen. The implantable collamer lens (ICL) is now the preferred modality of treatment. It was first developed in the late 1980s in Russia by Dr S Fyodorov, and the first implant was performed in Europe in 1993.[51]

The STAAR® Visian ICL™ is a single-piece, plate haptic lens made from a combination of copolymer and collagen called Collamer.® It is designed to vault anteriorly to the crystalline lens. The Collamer material is biologically inert as the collagen has an affinity for fibronectin. Upon implantation, a layer of fibronectin coats the IOL surface, inhibiting deposition of other proteins and increasing its biocompatibility. It is made up of 60% poly-HEMA, water (36%), benzophenone (3.8%), and collagen (0.2%).

The optic diameter of the myopic ICL ranges from 4.65 to 5.50 mm. The thickness is 50 µm at the center of the optic and 100 µm at the haptic plate. The thickest part of the myopic ICL is optic haptic junction which ranges from 300 to 700 µm. The optic diameter of hyperopic ICL is 5.5 mm for all powers. The lens is thickest at the center. The overall length of the myopic ICL ranges from 11.50 to 13 mm in 0.50 mm increments while that of a hyperopic ICL ranges from 11 to 12.5 mm. Power ranges from -18 to -3 D and +3 to +21.50 D in half-diopter increments. The toric ICL (TICL) has the same overall design as the spherical ICL with the addition of a toric component (+1 to +6 D cylinder). The toricity is manufactured in the plus cylinder axis, within 22° of rotation from the horizontal axis.

The currently available V4 model has a steeper radius of curvature, allowing an additional 0.13–0.21 mm of anterior vaulting in comparison to the earlier model, significantly reducing the incidence of cataract formation. The newer model of Visian ICL with centraFLOW (V4C) has a central artificial hole called the KS-aquaPORT. This improves the aqueous circulation within the eye, improving the lens metabolism and reducing the incidence of cataract formation.[52] Moreover, the need for a peripheral iridotomy is eliminated with reduced risk of complications such as hyphema and inflammation.

## Indications of Phakic Intraocular Lens
- Age of 21 years or greater
- Refractive stability (change in mean refraction in spherical equivalent of not more than –0.25 D over 1 year)
- Internal anterior chamber depth (ACD) (from corneal endothelium to anterior lens capsule) ≥2.8 mm
- Corneal endothelial cell count of >2,500 cells/mm$^2$
- Mesopic pupil size of <6 mm
- Absence of ocular comorbidities including uveitis, glaucoma, and cataract

## Preoperative Measurements

A complete and detailed evaluation of the patient before planning phakic IOL implantation is a must to avoid complications and attain best results.

### Calculation of Power

ICL/TICL calculation and implantation software allows calculation of spherical and cylindrical powers and length and generates the ICL/TICL implantation diagram **(Fig. 16)**.

The calculations are based on preoperative measurements including refraction, ACD, and white-to-white (WTW). Manifest refraction is usually sufficient for myopia. However, in hyperopia, a cycloplegic refraction is recommended to eliminate the possible effect of accommodation. The refraction is carried out for a back-vertex distance at 12 mm. Contact lens over-refraction can be done for high myopes.

### Measurement of WTW Diameter

In the preoperative planning, the critical parameter in sizing the ICL is the WTW measurement which can be measured using a Pentacam **(Fig. 17)**, Orbscan, ultrasound biomicroscopy (UBM), or digital calipers **(Fig. 18)**. WTW measurements with an automated technique offer convenient

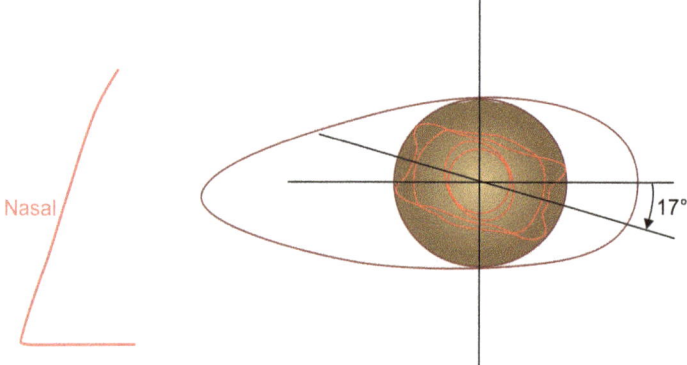

**Fig. 16:** Toric implantable collamer lens (TICL) implantation diagram.

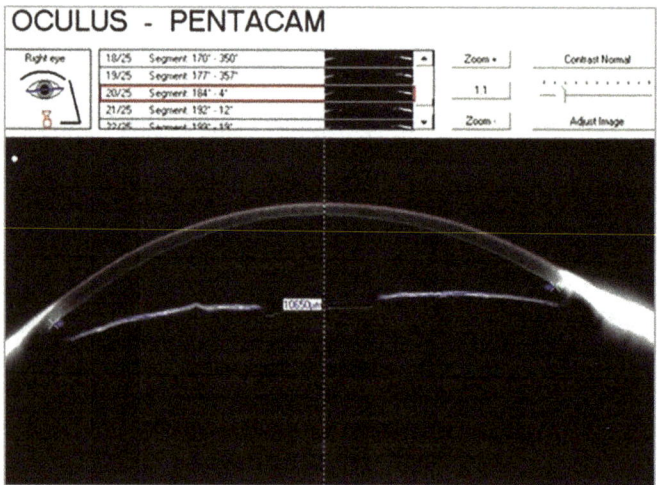

**Fig. 17:** Measurement of white-to-white diameter with Pentacam (Scheimpflug image).

and repeatable measurements. However, measurements with manual calipers afford greater accuracy, especially in eyes with limbal anomalies including a thick arcus, pterygia, and dense pigmentation. In cases of limbal hyperpigmentation, the Orbscan may overestimate the WTW and measurement using digital calipers is preferred. Since the ICL was designed so that its haptic rests horizontally on the ciliary sulcus, the length of the ICL should ideally be equal to the horizontal sulcus diameter. The conventional method for sizing the ICL is an addition of 0.5 mm to the horizontal WTW for an ACD of <3.5 mm and 1 mm for an ACD of >3.5 mm.

If the ICL is too short for the sulcus, the lens vault may be insufficient increasing the risk of anterior subcapsular cataract formation and rotation secondary to unstable fixation. If the implant is oversized, the lens vaults

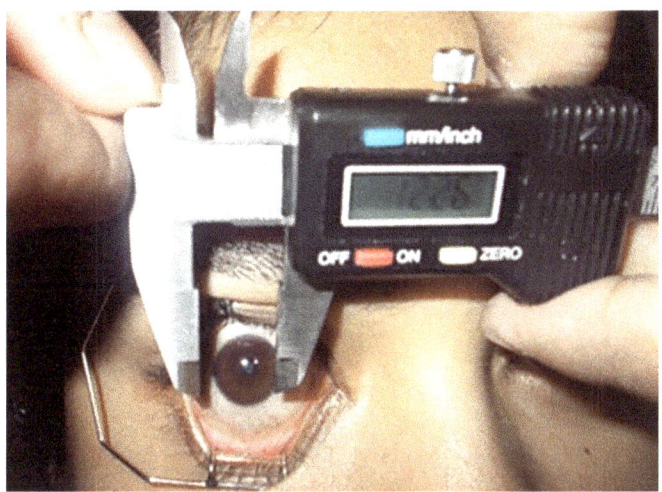

**Fig. 18:** Measurement of horizontal white-to-white using digital calipers.

excessively, crowding the angle and possibly causing secondary angle-closure glaucoma.

Anterior chamber depth can be measured using optical devices including IOLMaster, anterior segment imaging devices such as Orbscan and Pentacam, or A-scan ultrasound. No significant difference was found between most of the devices. However, corneal indentation secondary to contact ultrasound may result in an erroneous ACD measurement.

## Lens Vault

An ideal ICL vault is approximately 250–750 μm, which is roughly half to one and a half corneal thickness **(Fig. 19)**. The vault can be measured using an anterior segment OCT **(Fig. 20)**.

There are concerns about high vault (1,000 μm) leading to angle crowding and resulting in angle closure or synechiae formation. A high vault may also increase iris chaffing and pigment dispersion resulting in pigmentary glaucoma. On the other hand, a low vault (125 μm) may cause ICL contact with the crystalline lens and increase the risk of cataract formation over time.[53]

## Peripheral Iridotomy

A peripheral iridotomy is performed 1–2 weeks before the surgery to provide an outlet for the aqueous flow around the lens. Alternatively, it may be performed intraoperatively after ICL implantation with a Vannas scissors or a vitrectomy cutter. It should be sufficiently wide (at least 500 μm), positioned superiorly (from 11 to 1 o'clock) and well away from the haptics placement.

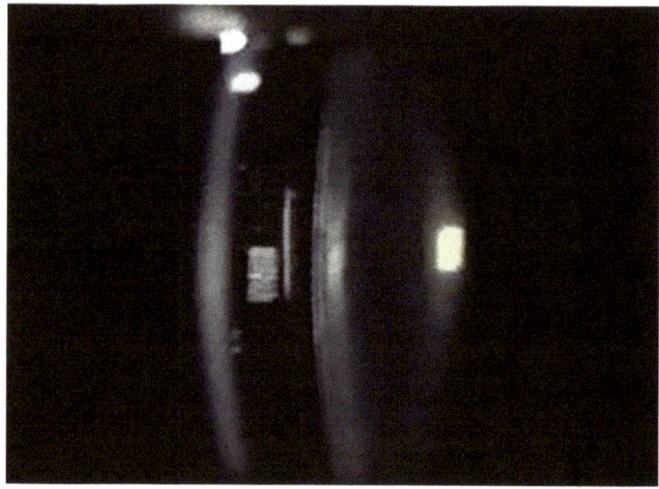

**Fig. 19:** Ideal vaulting of implantable collamer lens (ICL) with vault equal to corneal thickness.

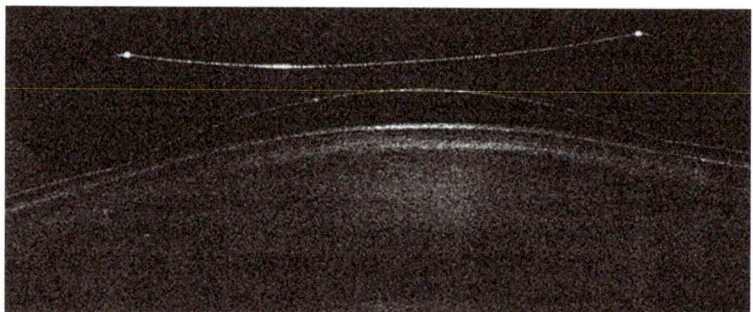

**Fig. 20:** Anterior segment optical coherence tomography (ASOCT) demonstrating phakic intraocular lenses (IOL), crystalline lens, and space between the two (vault).

However, with the advent of the ICL centraFLOW, the need for a peripheral iridotomy is obviated.

## Advantages of Posterior Chamber Phakic Intraocular Lens
- Accommodation is preserved as the crystalline lens is left untouched.
- Preservation of corneal asphericity
- High predictability
- No risk of regression or corneal ectasia
- *Larger effective optic zone:* In corneal ablative procedures, the induced HOAs, particularly the spherical aberrations, deteriorate the visual quality. In high corrections, a large amount of the cornea is ablated in a central 6 mm optic zone diameter. Patients with a mesopic pupil diameter larger than the optic zone diameter might experience night glare and haloes.

Advances in Refractive Surgery

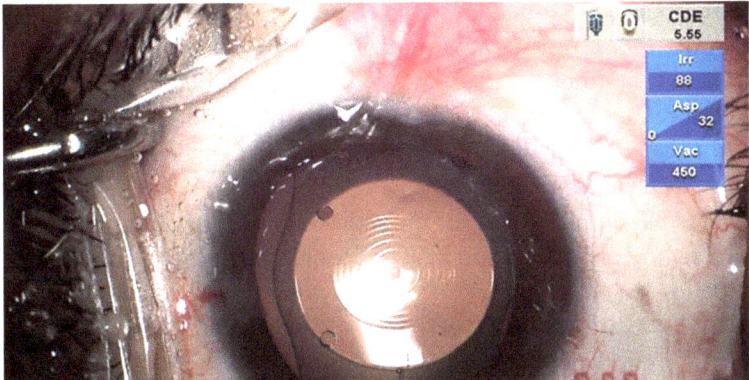

**Fig. 21:** Presbyopic phakic intraocular lenses (IOL) in situ (intraoperative) showing diffractive rings.

Since the ICL is implanted in the posterior chamber, the effective optic diameter at the corneal plane is larger by a factor of 1.25. Thus, the effective optic diameter ranges to a maximum effective diameter of 7.3 mm.

## Presbyopic Phakic Intraocular Lens

Posterior chamber phakic technology (Presbyopic Phakic IOLs, Care Group, India) to correct presbyopia in myopic and myopic astigmatism patients has been introduced with good success. The lens provides near additions ranging from +1.5 to +3.5 D that can be customized to the patient's need and degree of accommodation. This is an interesting lens that can be suggested in myopic or myopic astigmatism patients aged 40–55 years who have not yet developed cataract. It has a diffractive optical zone of 3.5 mm in diameter **(Fig. 21)**, which allows a soft sliding of the iris over the lens and aims at reducing haloes.

## ■ BIOPTICS

The eye offers the surgeon two distinct planes, the lenticular and the corneal, on which to engineer refractive improvements. Sometimes, a correction on one plane is insufficient to achieve emmetropia, hence, the need for bioptics.[54]

Certain examples of bioptics include the following:
- Keratorefractive procedures for correction of residual refractive error following phakic intraocular lens implantation, especially in high ametropia wherein customized IOLs are less economically viable.
- Keratorefractive procedures for residual refractive error following cataract surgery secondary to inaccurate biometry, especially in extremes of IOL powers.

- Keratorefractive procedures for correction of postoperative refractive surprise following cataract surgery in eyes with history of previous LASIK or radial keratotomy surgery.
- Keratorefractive procedures for correction of residual cylindrical power of >0.75 D resulting in a significant decline in the visual quality following multifocal IOL implantation.
- Phakic IOL implantation for refractive correction following intracorneal ring segment implantation in keratoconic eyes: "reverse bioptics."

## Advantages of Laser Vision Correction over Other Modalities of Treatment for Bioptics

- Laser vision correction offers more precise results vis-à-vis arcuate keratotomy/limbal relaxing incision. Additionally, arcuate keratotomies are prone to regression over time.
- Laser vision correction is less invasive, technically less demanding, and safer in comparison to IOL exchange or piggyback IOL.

## CONCLUSION

Refractive surgery has witnessed various advancements both in terms of technology and in terms of understanding of the optical system of the eye, allowing reproducible, precise, and predictable outcomes. Proper planning and selecting an ideal treatment procedure for a particular patient are paramount to success.

## ACKNOWLEDGMENTS

We would like to acknowledge Drs Chitra Ramamurthy, Mahipal Sachdev, and Shreyas Ramamurthy for their contributions in the preparation of this manuscript.

## REFERENCES

1. Trokel SL, Srinivasan R, Braren B. Excimer laser surgery of the cornea. Am J Ophthalmol. 1983;96(6):710-5.
2. Park SH, Kim M, Joo CK. Measurement of pupil centroid shift and cyclotorsional displacement using iris registration. Ophthalmologica. 2009;223(3):166-71.
3. Stevens JD. Astigmatic excimer laser treatment: theoretical effects of axis misalignment. Eur J Implant Refract Surg. 1994;6:310-8.
4. Lawless MA, Hodge C. Wavefront's role in corneal refractive surgery. Clin Experiment Ophthalmol. 2005;33(2):199-209.
5. Schallhorn SC, Kaupp SE, Tanzer DJ, Tidwell J, Laurent J, Bourque LB. Pupil size and quality of vision after LASIK. Ophthalmology. 2003;110(8):1606-14.
6. Zhao LQ, Wei RL, Cheng JW, Li Y, Cai JP, Ma XY. Meta-analysis: clinical outcomes of laser-assisted subepithelial keratectomy and photorefractive keratectomy in myopia. Ophthalmology. 2010;117:1912-22.

7. Kanellopoulos AJ, Asimellis G. Corneal refractive power and symmetry changes following normalization of ectasias treated with partial topography-guided PTK combined with higher-fluence CXL (the Athens protocol). J Refract Surg. 2014;30(5):342-6.
8. Caporossi A, Mazzotta C, Baiocchi S, Caporossi T. Long-term results of riboflavin ultraviolet a corneal collagen cross-linking for keratoconus in Italy: the Siena eye cross study. Am J Ophthalmol. 2010;149(4):585-93.
9. Wollensak G, Spoerl E, Seiler T. Riboflavin/ultraviolet-A-induced collagen crosslinking for the treatment of keratoconus. Am J Ophthalmol. 2003;135:620-7.
10. Kanellopoulos AJ, Binder PS. Collagen cross-linking (CCL) with sequential topography-guided PRK: a temporizing alternative for keratoconus to penetrating keratoplasty. Cornea. 2007;26:891-5.
11. Krueger RR, Kanellopoulos AJ. Stability of simultaneous topography-guided photorefractive keratectomy and riboflavin/UVA cross-linking for progressive keratoconus: case reports. J Refract Surg. 2010;26(10):S827-32.
12. Tuwairqi WS, Sinjab MM. Safety and efficacy of simultaneous corneal collagen cross-linking with topography-guided PRK in managing low-grade keratoconus: 1-year follow-up. J Refract Surg. 2012;28:341-5.
13. Zhu AY, Jun AS, Soiberman US. Combined protocols for corneal collagen cross-linking with photorefractive surgery for refractive management of keratoconus: update on techniques and review of literature. Ophthalmol Ther. 2019;8(Suppl. 1):15-31.
14. Padmanabhan P, Radhakrishnan A, Venkataraman AP, Gupta N, Srinivasan B. Corneal changes following collagen cross-linking and simultaneous topography guided photoablation with collagen cross-linking for keratoconus. Indian J Ophthalmol. 2014;62(2):229-35.
15. Shetty R, Nuijts RM, Nicholson M, Sargod K, Jayadev C, Veluri H, et al. Cone location-dependent outcomes after combined topography-guided photorefractive keratectomy and collagen cross-linking. Am J Ophthalmol. 2015;159(3):419-25.e2.
16. Binder PS. Risk factors for ectasia after LASIK. J Cataract Refract Surg. 2008;34(12):2010-1.
17. Shetty R, Vunnava K, Khamar P, Choudhary U, Sinha Roy A. Topography-based removal of corneal epithelium for keratoconus: a novel and customized technique. Cornea. 2018;37(7):923-5.
18. Faktorovich EG. Femtodynamics: a guide to laser settings and procedure techniques to optimize outcomes with femtosecond lasers. New Jersey: SLACK Incorporated; 2009.
19. Soong HK, Malta JB. Femtosecond lasers in ophthalmology. Am J Ophthalmol. 2009;147:189-97.e2.
20. Montés-Micó R, Rodríguez-Galietero A, Alió JL. Femtosecond laser versus mechanical keratome LASIK for myopia. Ophthalmology. 2007;114(1):62-8.
21. Kymionis GD, Kankariya VP, Plaka AD, Reinstein DZ. Femtosecond laser technology in corneal refractive surgery: a review. J Refract Surg. 2012;28(12):912-20. [Erratum in: J Refract Surg. 2013;29(1):72].
22. Manche E, Roe J. Recent advances in wavefront-guided LASIK. Curr Opin Ophthalmol. 2018;29:286-91.

23. Holland S, Lin DT, Tan JC. Topography-guided laser refractive surgery. Curr Opin Ophthalmol. 2013;24:302-9.
24. Stulting RD, Fant BS, T-CAT Study Group, Bond W, Chotiner B, Durrie D, et al. Results of topography-guided laser in situ keratomileusis custom ablation treatment with a refractive excimer laser. J Cataract Refract Surg. 2016;42:11-8.
25. Kanellopoulos AJ. Topography-modified refraction (TMR): adjustment of treated cylinder amount and axis to the topography versus standard clinical refraction in myopic topography-guided LASIK. Clin Ophthalmol. 2016;10:2213-21.
26. Zhou W, Stojanovic A, Utheim TP. Assessment of refractive astigmatism and simulated therapeutic refractive surgery strategies in coma-like-aberrations-dominant corneal optics. Eye Vis (Lond). 2016;3:13.
27. Motwani M. The use of Wavelight® Contoura to create a uniform cornea: the LYRA Protocol. Part 1: the effect of higher-order corneal aberrations on refractive astigmatism. Clin Ophthalmol. 2017;11:897-905.
28. Sekundo W, Kunert KS, Blum M. Small incision corneal refractive surgery using the small incision lenticule extraction (SMILE) procedure for the correction of myopia and myopic astigmatism: results of a 6 month prospective study. Br J Ophthalmol. 2011;95:335-9.
29. Vetter JM, Faust M, Gericke A, Pfeiffer N, Weingärtner WE, Sekundo W. Intraocular pressure measurements during flap preparation using 2 femtosecond lasers and 1 microkeratome in human donor eyes. J Cataract Refract Surg. 2012;38(11):2011-8.
30. Fernández J, Rodríguez-Vallejo M, Martínez J, Tauste A, Piñero DP. Corneal biomechanics after laser refractive surgery: unmasking differences between techniques. J Cataract Refract Surg. 2018;44(3):390-8.
31. Kobashi H, Kamiya K, Shimizu K. Dry eye after small incision lenticule extraction and femtosecond laser-assisted LASIK: meta-analysis. Cornea. 2017;36:85-91.
32. Chen X, Wang Y, Zhang J, Yang SN, Li X, Zhang L. Comparison of ocular higher-order aberrations after SMILE and wavefront-guided femtosecond LASIK for myopia. BMC Ophthalmol. 2017;17(1):42.
33. Dong Z, Zhou X, Wu J, Zhang Z, Li T, Zhou Z, et al. Small incision lenticule extraction (SMILE) and femtosecond laser LASIK: comparison of corneal wound healing and inflammation. Br J Ophthalmol. 2014;98(2):263-9.
34. Hou J, Wang Y, Lei Y, Zheng X. Comparison of effective optical zone after small-incision lenticule extraction and femtosecond laser-assisted laser in situ keratomileusis for myopia. J Cataract Refract Surg. 2018;44(10):1179-85.
35. Riau AK, Ang HP, Lwin NC, Chaurasia SS, Tan DT, Mehta JS. Comparison of four different VisuMax circle patterns for flap creation after small incision lenticule extraction. J Refract Surg. 2013;29(4):236-44.
36. Ganesh S, Brar S. Lenticuloschisis: a "no dissection" technique for lenticule extraction in small incision lenticule extraction. J Retract Surg. 2017;33:563-6.
37. Ito M, Quantock AJ, Malhan S, Schanzlin DJ, Krueger RR. Picosecond laser in situ keratomileusis with a 1053-nm Nd:YLF laser. J Refract Surg. 1996;12:721-8.
38. Vestergaard A, Ivarsen A, Asp S, Hjortdal JØ. Femtosecond (FS) laser vision correction procedure for moderate to high myopia: a prospective study of ReLEx® flex and comparison with a retrospective study of FS-laser in situ keratomileusis. Acta Ophthalmol. 2013;91:355-62.

39. Ang M, Farook M, Htoon HM, Tan D, Mehta JS. Simulated night vision after small-incision lenticule extraction. J Cataract Refract Surg. 2016;42:1173-80.
40. Sun L, Yao P, Li M, Shen Y, Zhao J, Zhou X. The safety and predictability of implanting autologous lenticule obtained by SMILE for hyperopia. J Refract Surg. 2015;31:374-9.
41. Liu R, Zhao J, Xu Y, Li M, Niu L, Liu H, et al. Femtosecond laser-assisted corneal small incision allogenic intrastromal lenticule implantation in monkeys: a pilot study. Invest Ophthalmol Vis Sci. 2015;56(6):3715-20.
42. Sekundo W, Reinstein DZ, Blum M. Improved lenticule shape for hyperopic femtosecond lenticule extraction (ReLEx FLEx): a pilot study. Lasers Med Sci. 2016;31(4):659-64.
43. Liu YC, Ang HP, Teo EP, Lwin NC, Yam GH, Mehta JS. Wound healing profiles of hyperopic-small incision lenticule extraction (SMILE). Sci Rep. 2016;6:29802.
44. Pajic B, Cvejic Z, Pajic-Eggspuehler B. Cataract surgery performed by high frequency LDV Z8 femtosecond laser: safety, efficacy, and its physical properties. Sensors (Basel). 2017;17:1429.
45. Izquierdo Jr L, Sossa D, Ben-Shaul O, Henriquez MA. Corneal lenticule extraction assisted by a low-energy femtosecond laser. J Cataract Refract Surg. 2020;46:1217-21.
46. Liu YC, Wittwer VV, Yusoff NZM, Lwin CN, Seah XY, Mehta JS, et al. Intraoperative optical coherence tomography-guided femtosecond laser-assisted deep anterior lamellar keratoplasty. Cornea. 2019;38:648-53.
47. Williams GP, Ang HP, George BL, Liu YC, Peh G, Izquierdo L, et al. Comparison of intraocular pressure changes with liquid or flat applanation interfaces in a femtosecond laser platform. Sci Rep. 2015;5:14742.
48. Wang M, Zhang F, Copruz CC, Han L. First experience in small incision lenticule extraction with the femto LDV Z8 and lenticule evaluation using scanning electron microscopy. J Ophthalmol. 2020;2020:6751826.
49. Riau AK, Liu YC, Lwin NC, Ang HP, Tan NY, Yam GH, et al. Comparative study of nJ- and µJ-energy level femtosecond lasers: evaluation of flap adhesion strength, stromal bed quality, and tissue responses. Invest Ophthalmol Vis Sci. 2014;55(5):3186-94.
50. McCarty CA, Livingston PM, Taylor HR. Prevalence of myopia in adults: implications for refractive surgeons. J Refract Surg. 1997;13(3):229-34.
51. Kamiya K, Shimizu K, Igarashi A, Hikita F, Komatsu M. Four-year follow-up of posterior chamber phakic intraocular lens implantation for moderate-to-high myopia. Arch Ophthalmol. 2009;127(7):845-50.
52. Higueras-Esteban A, Ortiz-Gomariz A, Gutiérrez-Ortega R, Villa-Collar C, Abad-Montes JP, Fernandes P, et al. Intraocular pressure after implantation of the Visian implantable Collamer lens with CentraFLOW without iridotomy. Am J Ophthalmol. 2013;156(4):800-5.
53. Gonvers M, Bornet C, Othenin-Girard P. Implantable contact lens for moderate-to-high myopia: relationship of vaulting to cataract formation. J Cataract Refract Surg. 2003;29(5):918-24.
54. Zaldivar R, Oscherow S, Piezzi V. Bioptics in phakic and pseudophakic intraocular lens with the Nidek EC-5000 excimer laser. J Refract Surg. 2002;18:S336-9.

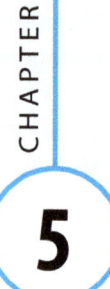

# Optical Coherence Tomography in the Diagnosis of Glaucoma

*Parul Ichhpujani, Obaidur Rehman, Sushmita Kaushik*

## ABSTRACT

Optical coherence tomography (OCT) is a noninvasive imaging modality designed to quantitatively assess the peripapillary retinal nerve fiber layer (pRNFL) and the macular retinal layers in vivo. This chapter gives an outline on leveraging OCT for the management of glaucoma.

***Keywords:*** Optical coherence tomography; glaucoma; ganglion cell layer; retinal nerve fiber layer.

## ■ INTRODUCTION

Optical coherence tomography (OCT) is an imaging modality that provides quantitative information about the various retinal layers, which corresponds to histological tissue sections. It uses low-coherence interferometry to determine the echo time delay and magnitude of backscattered light reflected off the object under consideration.

## ■ OPTICAL COHERENCE TOMOGRAPHY: FROM THEN TO NOW

Optical coherence tomography has a short history within ophthalmology relative to its tremendous impact. The OCT-1, the first time-domain (TD) OCT device, was introduced by Humphrey, which was later acquired by Carl Zeiss in 1991. Its successors, OCT-2 and OCT-3 (Stratus OCT), had better resolution but still had several limitations. The operating principle of TD-OCT was associated with the delay in the reflection time of light. The actual variable in spectral domain (SD)-OCT is the change in the optic frequency.

Now, all OCT devices that are manufactured have SD technology.

Modern SD-OCT devices are characterized by enhanced resolution up to 3 µm, reduced acquisition time, and less operator dependence than TD-OCT.

Hardware and software developments, including three-dimensional (3D) volumetric scanning protocols, have been incorporated in commercially available SD-OCTs, increasing the amount of information available to doctors. It can offset to a great extent the effect of saccades and motion

Optical Coherence Tomography in the Diagnosis of Glaucoma

artifacts. Additionally, software modifications and an expansion in the population-specific normative databases similar to other devices have also been done.

The newer generation of OCT, swept source (SS)-OCT, enhances the visualization of the deep optic nerve head (ONH) and deep parapapillary structures such as the lamina cribrosa (LC) and the choroid. All the above have led to a resultant improvement in repeatability, reproducibility and, hence, reliability for glaucoma diagnostics and monitoring of progression.

## COMMONLY USED SPECTRAL DOMAIN OPTICAL COHERENCE TOMOGRAPHY DEVICES

**Table 1** enlists some of the commonly used SD-OCT devices across the globe. In this chapter, we will touch upon Cirrus high-definition (HD)-OCT (Carl Zeiss Meditec, Inc., Dublin, CA, United States), RTVue-100 (Optovue, Inc., Fremont, CA, United States), and SPECTRALIS SD-OCT (Heidelberg Engineering, Inc., Heidelberg, Germany) at relevant places.

**TABLE 1:** Common spectral domain optical coherence tomography (SD-OCT) devices.

| Model | Carl Zeiss Meditec (Cirrus) | Topcon Medical Systems (3D OCT-2000) | Heidelberg Engineering (SPECTRALIS) | Optovue (RTVue) |
|---|---|---|---|---|
| No. of subjects | 284 | 183 | 201 | 80 |
| Ages (years) | 19–84 | 19–84 | 18–78 | 18–84 |
| Gender F: Female M: Male | 149 F; 133 M | Disk: 92 F/54 M Macula: 112 F/61 M | 90 F; 111 M | N/A |
| Ethnicity | • 43% Caucasian<br>• 24% Asian<br>• 18% African American<br>• 12% Hispanic<br>• 1% Indian<br>• 6% mixed ethnicity | • 64% Caucasian<br>• 21% African American<br>• 15% Hispanic | Caucasian | • 33% Caucasian<br>• 22% Asian<br>• 20% African American<br>• 12% Hispanics<br>• 12% Indian<br>• 1% other |
| Anatomical parameters assessed | • RNFL thickness<br>• ONH parameters<br>• GCL + IPL macular thickness | Optic disk Macula | RNFL thickness | • RNFL thickness<br>• Ganglion cell complex macular thickness |

*Contd...*

*Contd...*

| Model | Carl Zeiss Meditec (Cirrus) | Topcon Medical Systems (3D OCT-2000) | Heidelberg Engineering (SPECTRALIS) | Optovue (RTVue) |
|---|---|---|---|---|
| Refractive error range | −12 to +8 D | −6 to +3 D | −12 to +12 D | −15 to +12 D |
| Maximum signal strength | 10 | 160 | 40 | 100 |
| Minimum signal strength | 6 | 60 | 15 | 30 |
| Speed and resolution | 27,000 A-lines per second 5 μm | 50,000 A-lines per second 5 μm | 40,000 A-lines per second 7 μm | 26,000 A-lines per second 5 μm |

(3D: three-dimensional; GCL: ganglion cell layer; IPL: inner plexiform layer; N/A: not applicable; ONH: optic nerve head; RNFL: retinal nerve fiber layer)

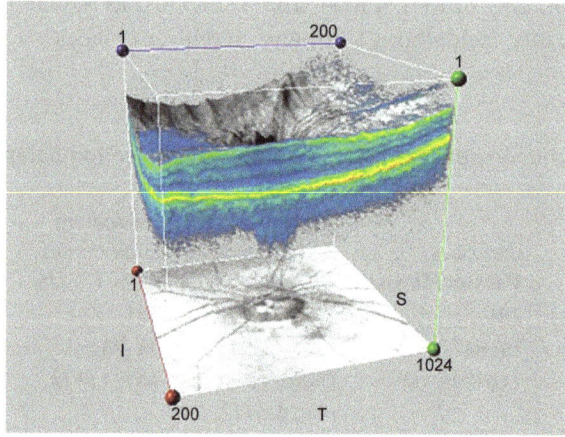

**Fig. 1:** Three-dimensional (3D) image of the optic disk cut at width: 1, 200 height: 1, 200 A-scan: 1, 1024; resultant image is called "*optic disk cube*".

## ■ IMAGING PROTOCOLS

Some common imaging protocols used in SD-OCT are mentioned below.

### Three-dimensional Scan

Three-dimensional scan allows reconstruction in a 3D manner using a series of horizontally or vertically oriented lines. This scan protocol consists of various horizontal line scans in a rectangular box, such as 6 × 6 mm, 7 × 7 mm, and 12 × 9 mm.

The resultant 3D image is referred to as a "cube" **(Fig. 1)**. Optic disk imaging is done using 6 × 6 mm cube consisting of serial B scans that take 30,000–40,000 A-mode scans. A 3.46 mm circle centered at optic disk is identified automatically using 3D software, enabling the analysis of peripapillary retinal nerve fiber layer (pRNFL). The standard OCT acquires

3D images of the ONH region, which enables accurate and reproducible measurements of parameters such as disk and rim area, cup-to-disk ratio (CDR), cup volume, and others.[1] The acquired data is then compared with the normative database of the machine and interpreted in different color codings. Different machines have different color coding schemes to depict the statistical divisions of normative data.

Different machines have different absolute reference values; therefore, the OCT scan taken by one brand of machine cannot be compared with the OCT taken by another brand.

## Radial Scan

Radial scan consists of a 6–12-line scan, wherein the lines are spaced equally around a common axis. For determination of the relationship of a lesion with the fovea, the axis can be focused onto the fovea.[1] **Figure 2** shows a radial scan with focus on the fovea.

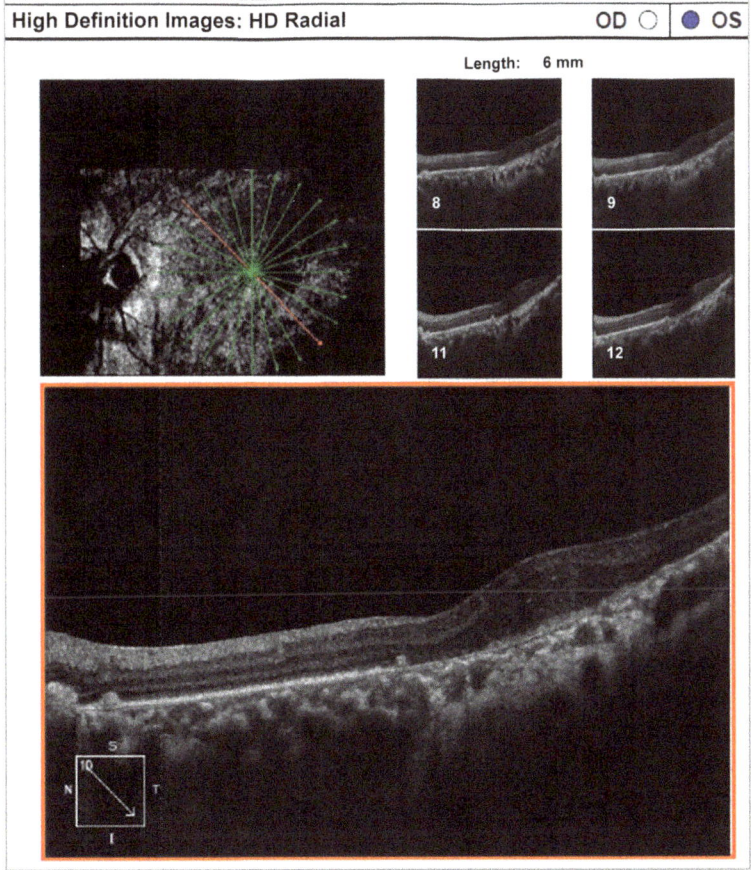

**Fig. 2:** Radial scan with axis focussed on the fovea; images at the top right-hand corner show radial scans (8–12 lines).

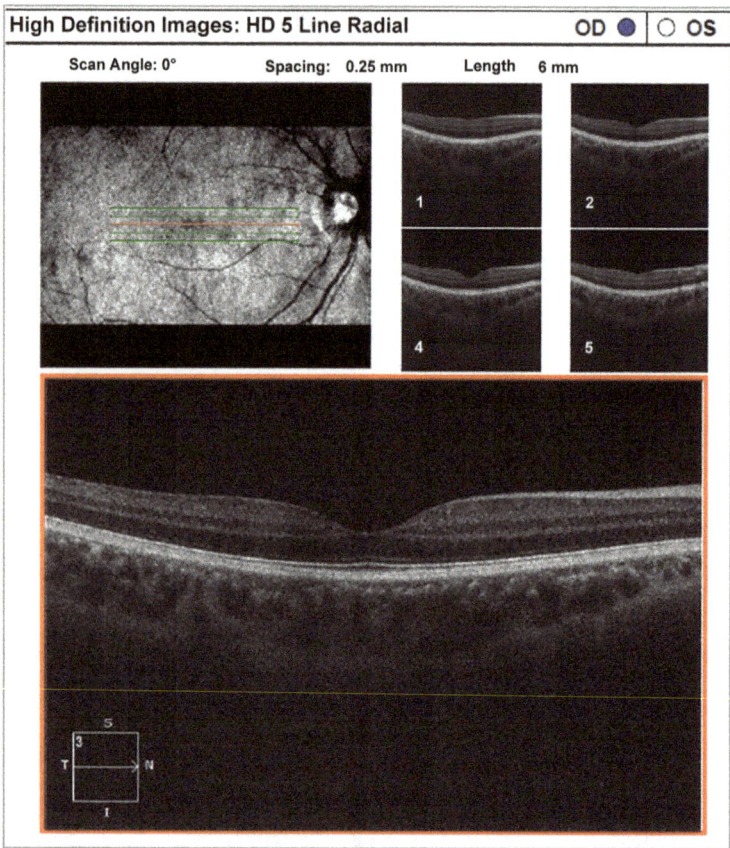

**Fig. 3:** Raster scan from temporal to nasal direction; image at top left corner shows orientation of parallel lines in the scan.

## Raster Scan

Raster scan consists of a series of parallel lines that can be oriented at a desired angle **(Fig. 3)**. This scan has a higher resolution. It can pick up even small lesions that may be missed on radial scan.[1]

## En Face Scan

En face scan combines confocal ophthalmoscopy and OCT. *"En face"* images are produced, which are comparable to an orientation similar to confocal microscopy **(Fig. 4)**.

The *en face* image is examined to ensure the absence of any media opacity, such as a posterior vitreous detachment (PVD), within the circumpapillary scan area. In areas overshadowed by opacity, some data will be missing and, therefore, it appears as a black patch. The overlying PVD can lead to a falsely thin retinal nerve fiber layer (RNFL) value in the underlying area.

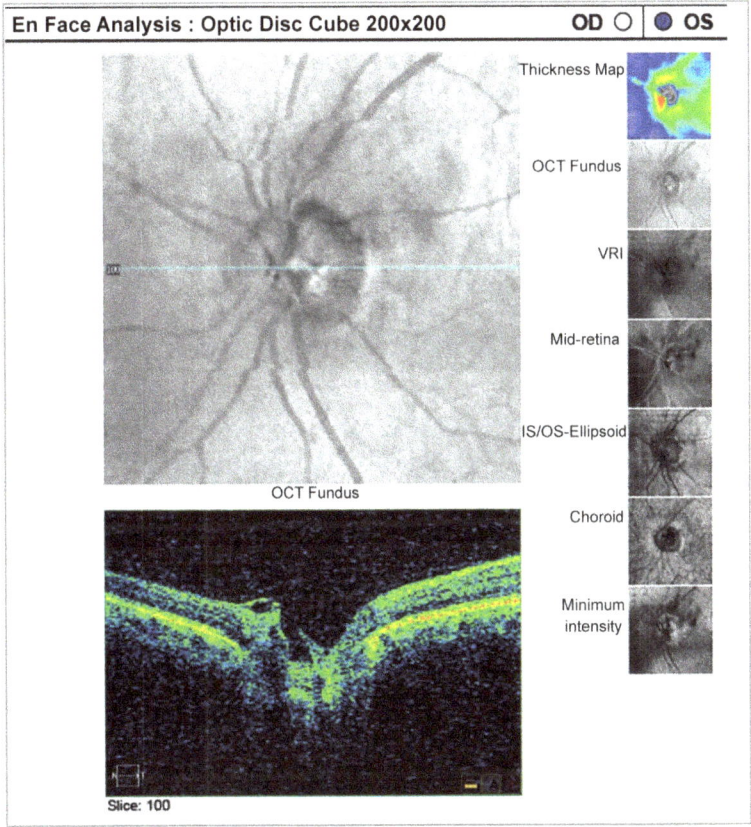

**Fig. 4:** En face image using optic disk cube showing a motion artifact in the top image. (OCT: optical coherence tomography; VRI: vitreoretinal interface)

## Enhanced Depth Imaging

Conventional OCT fails to image choroid accurately due to absorption by the retinal pigment epithelium (RPE) and also light scattering due to dense vascular structures.[2] Enhanced depth imaging (EDI)-OCT images deeper structures such as choroid by slightly modifying the conventional OCT system **(Fig. 5)**. It has been used to assess the position of LC in glaucoma patients. Researchers have observed that in patients who have mild glaucoma, LC is displaced posteriorly, while those who are affected by more advanced disease have an anteriorly displaced LC.[3]

Cirrus uses a disk cube 200 × 200 protocol that scans a 6 × 6 mm area and allows for RNFL thickness and ONH parameters **(Fig. 6)**. Cirrus OCT uses a reference plane of 200 mm above the RPE to calculate optic disk parameters, and it uses macular cube 200 × 200 protocol and 512 × 128 protocol for ganglion cell analysis (GCA). The GCA algorithm can also calculate the ganglion cell complex (GCC) or a summation that includes the combined thickness of the

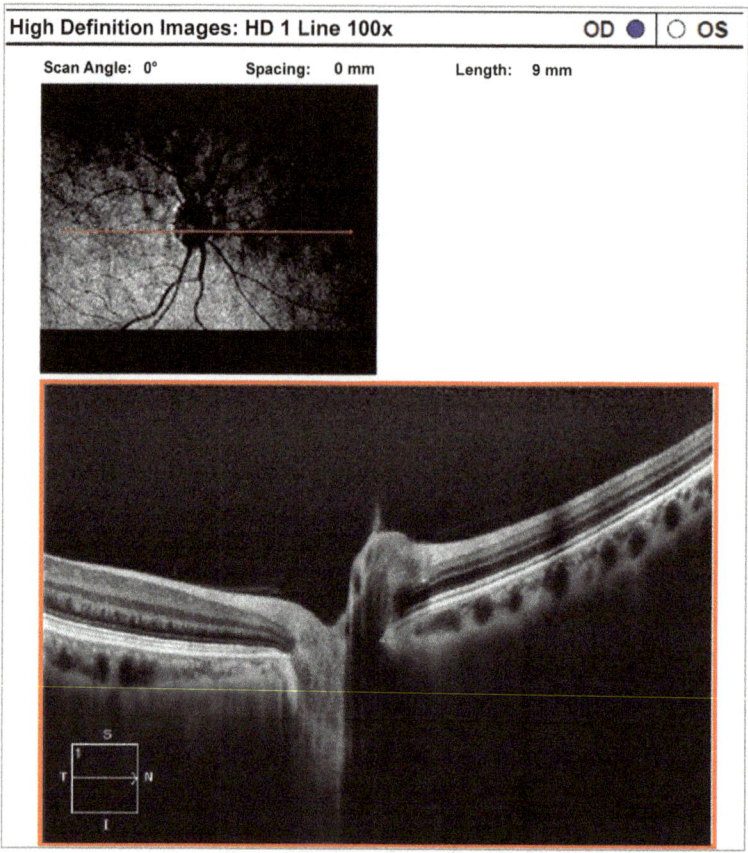

**Fig. 5:** Enhanced depth imaging (EDI) of the optic disk; structure of the choroid is visible in the image.

RNFL, ganglion cell layer (GCL), and inner plexiform layer (IPL). The best evidence-based parameters include RNFL thickness, ganglion cell-inner plexiform layer (GCIPL) thickness, rim area, and vertical CDR, with evidence of damage primarily manifesting in the inferior, superior, inferotemporal, and superotemporal regions.

RTVue ONH scan protocol is a combination of 12 radial scans (3.4 mm in length, 452 A-scans each) and 6 concentric circle scans ranging from 2.5 to 4 mm in diameter or 13 concentric circle scans ranging from 1.3 to 4.9 mm in diameter. From the ONH scan protocol, RNFL thickness values are generated along a 3.45-mm diameter circle. Disk parameters are generated using a reference plane 150 mm above the RPE.

SPECTRALIS OCT uses the RNFL circle scan protocol wherein RNFL thickness measurements are obtained along a peripapillary scan circle spanning 12° of arc. These RNFL measurements are obtained directly from manual centration of a circular RNFL scan.

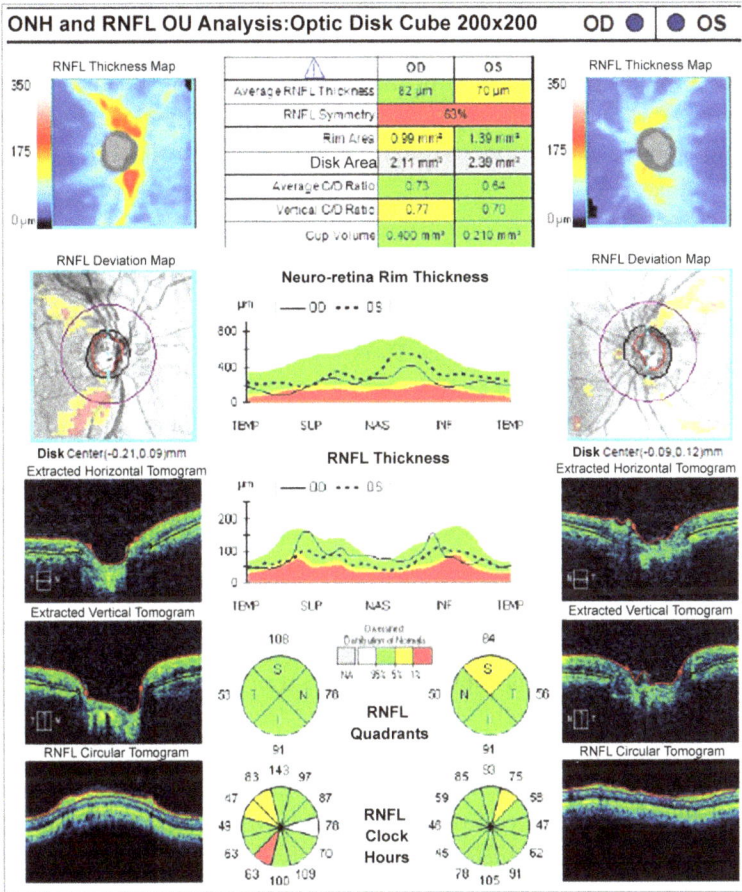

**Fig. 6:** Optical coherence tomography (OCT) image showing retinal nerve fiber layer (RNFL) thickness analysis scan using optic disk cube. (C/D: cup-to-disk; ONH: optic nerve head; RNFL: retinal nerve fiber layer; SUP: superior; TEMP: temporal)

Data of the neuroretinal rim (NRR) and RNFL thickness is presented in a "*temporal-superior-nasal-inferior-temporal (TSNIT)*" pattern, starting with the temporal thickness, followed by superior, nasal, inferior, and then temporal for both NRR and RNFL thickness. A newer presentation for profile map is the "*NSTIN*" curve, which splits the RNFL in the nasal hemifield rather than temporal. The tomogram is arranged with the most vulnerable region placed centrally.

The new SPECTRALIS Glaucoma Module Premium Edition (GMPE) software uses the GMPE scan protocol wherein three circumpapillary scans are obtained with diameters of 3.5, 4.1, and 4.6–4.7 mm, with scan circles centered over Bruch's membrane opening (BMO).

With this protocol, an NRR parameter, BMO-minimum rim width (MRW), can be calculated. BMO-MRW is a 360° region bordered internally by the cup surface and externally by the BMO, and BMO-MRW represents the minimum distance between these two boundaries. In the SPECTRALIS, a grid showing the thickness of macula is superimposed on a confocal scanning laser ophthalmoscopy image of the macula. The OCT compares the thickness between the superior and inferior halves of the macula.

## ◾ ALGORITHMS

### Optical Coherence Tomography Image Preprocessing

Intrinsic speckle noise in the OCT system compromises the quality of image and affects image analysis. Thus, a preprocessing step is done before the main processing of an OCT image. A good denoising algorithm should not compromise the image resolution. Nonlinear anisotropic filters and wavelet diffusion are the two most popular preprocessing algorithms as they preserve the edge information.[4] In recent times, graph-based algorithms have been used that do not suffer from noise and do not require a denoising algorithm.

### Optical Coherence Tomography Image Segmentation

Segmentation algorithms allow measurement of the thickness of the RNFL, which appears as the highly backscattering "red" layer at the vitreoretinal interface. Segmentation and measurement of RNFL are important because they are more sensitive and specific discriminator of glaucomatous damage than measurement of the entire retinal thickness. Macular segmentation is more complicated than pRNFL as numerous layers need to be segmented besides the RPE.

Intrinsic noise interference and intensity fluctuation have been known to hinder a good-quality image. Intensity fluctuation can arise due to intrinsic noise or light scattering. Intensity reduces as we go deeper into the layers of the retina. Blood vessels also generate discontinuity in the retinal layers, and motion artifacts compromise image quality. To counter all these difficulties, certain algorithms have been established for segmentation of OCT images. Segmentation approaches that have been developed use algorithm methods for A scan or B scan, active contour approaches, artificial intelligence-based methods, or 3D graph-based methods. Details of these methods are outside the scope of this chapter.

### Glaucoma Progression Analysis Algorithms

Studies have noted that SD-OCT progression is significantly more common than visual field progression in glaucomatous eyes.[5]
- *Cirrus:* Both event and trend-based analyses are done. RNFL thickness of each pixel is compared from baseline to follow-up images. Coding

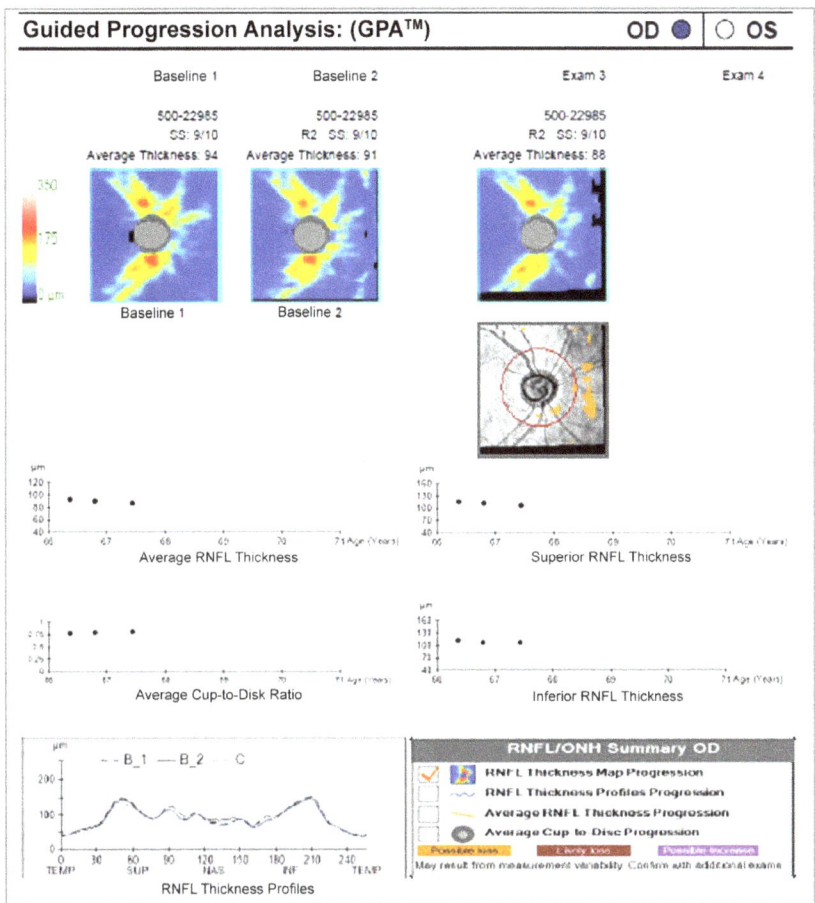

**Fig. 7:** Glaucoma progression analysis (GPA) of a glaucoma clinic patient on Cirrus optical coherence tomography (OCT) using scans of three consecutive visits, showing comparison of average retinal nerve fiber layer (RNFL) thickness, average cup-to-disk ratio (CDR), and superior and inferior RNFL thicknesses at each visit. (ONH: optic nerve head; SUP: superior; TEMP: temporal)

in yellow is done when there occurs a test–retest variability between a follow-up and baseline image, while red color indicates that identical change is apparent on three consecutive scans. The changes in the thickness of RNFL and trend reports are plotted over time in order to compare the rate of change **(Fig. 7)**.

- *SPECTRALIS:* Both event and trend-based analyses are performed.
- *RTVue:* RTVue software also performs a trend-based analysis that incorporates consecutive global RNFL thicknesses, analysis of thickness of six sectors, and a regression line for determination of the slope and standard error.

## Algorithms Used in Glaucoma Prediction

### Linear Discriminant Analysis

Linear discriminant analysis (LDA) uses a predictive analysis mechanism in order to point out the occurrence or absence of a characteristic based on preset values of variables. Its ability to distinguish eyes with visual field defects due to glaucoma from healthy eyes has been studied. It has been noted that all ONH parameters evaluated with OCT, with the exception of disk area, carried a good ability to distinguish healthy individuals from those with glaucoma using this method.[6]

### Artificial Neural Networks

Artificial neural network (ANN) refers to a system of information processing containing certain performance characteristics that are similar to biological neural networks. It contains several processing units analogous to neurons in the brain. These networks can be trained to perform a particular function.

### Classification and Regression Tree

Classification and regression tree (CART) refers to a predictive algorithm used in machine learning. It predicts the value of a target variable based on other values. It contains a decision tree having forks that split a predictor variable and, at the end, has a prediction for the target variable.

Researchers have used Cirrus HD-OCT for evaluating classification algorithms against distinct ONH and RNFL parameters for detection of glaucoma. ONH parameters such as disk area, rim area, CDR, and RNFL thickness in each quadrant were analyzed in normal subjects as well as in diagnosed cases of glaucoma. Classification algorithms utilized both ONH and RNFL parameters for diagnosing glaucoma, with the help of OCT, keeping in view improvisation in diagnostic accuracy. They concluded that CART and LDA showed a better performance than individual ONH and RNFL parameters, while CART had the highest performance among all parameters while detecting mild or early glaucoma.[7]

## ■ NEWER PARAMETERS

The usual two-dimensional parameters are susceptible to artifacts that can adversely compromise their diagnostic ability. This becomes more relevant in cases with variations in ONH tilt, peripapillary atrophy, myopia, and optic disk size. These may lead to inaccurate assessments because of erroneous RNFL measurements. The introduction of 3D volume scans has enabled high-density sampling of nerve tissue and 3D reconstruction of the NRR anatomy.

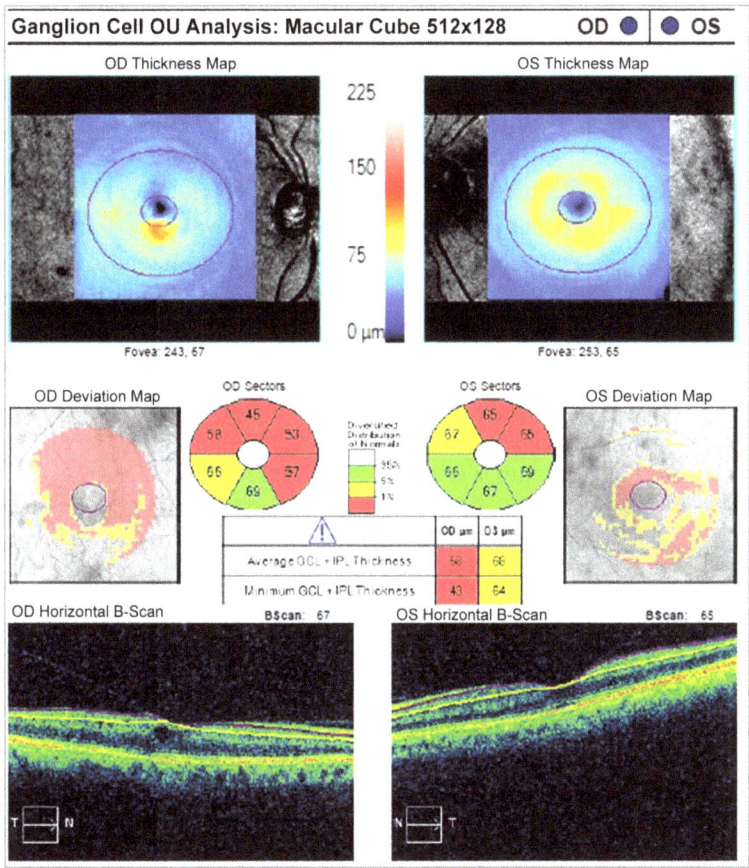

**Fig. 8:** Macular ganglion cell complex analysis showing reduced thickness in the right eye [average as well as minimum ganglion cell layer (GCL) + inner plexiform layer (IPL) thickness].

## Macular Ganglion Cell Complex Analysis

It is known that glaucoma damages the retinal ganglion cells (RGCs). Macular SD-OCT measurements may reflect RGC loss as the macular region contains approximately 50% of the RGCs, and here the GCL is more thick than a single cell layer.

Ganglion cell complex comprises a combination of GCIPLs. Analysis of this parameter helps to quantify the innermost layers of retina, which get potentially damaged with the progression of glaucoma **(Fig. 8)**. Few researchers have claimed that macular changes may be seen earlier and more consistently in glaucoma than RNFL changes, hence suggesting that macular OCT can prove to be a more sensitive tool for glaucoma screening. It can help in more accurate judgment of glaucomatous damage in eyes with myopia when compared to the traditional RNFL thickness as it does not get affected by increase in the axial length of the eye.[8] In myopes, asymmetry between superior and inferior GCIPL thickness may be seen in early glaucoma, and a difference of 5 μm is considered suspicious for glaucoma.

The average GCIPL thickness in normal individuals has been reported to be 82.1 ± 6.2 μm. The superonasal sector has been found to be the thickest and the inferior sector the thinnest. Macular GCIPL undergoes age-related attrition at a rate of about –0.31 μm/year.[9]

Macular GCC analysis has also been utilized to detect preperimetric glaucoma and may show progression earlier than pRNFL in preperimetric glaucoma.[10] A recent study has evaluated macular vessel density along with GCC in primary open-angle glaucoma (POAG) patients and concluded that both of these factors show significant decrement in preperimetric and early POAG patients.[11] Most accurate GCC parameters for detecting early glaucomatous changes are average and inferior GCC thicknesses.

In recent years, OCT manufacturers are incorporating macular scans as part of their glaucoma imaging protocols and analyses such as Carl Zeiss Meditec's PanoMap, the Hood report from both Heidelberg and Topcon, and Optovue's ONH/GCC report.[8]

## DETECTING PROGRESSION

Retinal nerve fiber layer progression patterns include widening of an existing RNFL defect, deepening without widening of an existing RNFL defect, or development of a new RNFL defect.

A comment on glaucoma progression using the RNFL thickness provided by the OCT can be made after accounting for thinning due to normal aging and the *"floor effect"* of RNFL in advanced cases, both globally and sectorally, and then correlation of this RNFL loss with corresponding visual field loss.

In healthy eyes, age-associated attrition of RNFL occurs at a mean rate of –0.48 μm/year for Cirrus SD-OCT and –0.60 μm/year for SPECTRALIS SD-OCT images. Glaucoma progression has a faster rate of RNFL thinning, ranging from –0.98 μm/year for the Cirrus SD-OCT to –2.12 μm/year for the SPECTRALIS SD-OCT. As glaucoma progresses, RNFL continues to thin out, but it never becomes zero, which is known as the *"floor effect,"* as the architectural support by astroglia, microglia, Müller cells, and blood vessels does not degenerate entirely.[12]

Average RNFL floor values range from 64.7 μm for the RTVue, 57 μm for the Cirrus, and 49.2 μm for the SPECTRALIS. For advanced glaucoma, once the floor thickness is reached, RNFL will no longer serve as an ideal parameter to monitor progression, but macular OCT can still be helpful, in addition to Humphrey 10-2 visual field test.

Two strategies for detecting change are event-based analysis and trend-based analysis.

1. *Event-based analysis:* In event-based analysis, one OCT test is compared to another. Since measurement error occurs in every test, therefore, in order to decide whether a change has actually occurred between the two tests, it needs to be decided what amount of change in the measurement is likely to be greater than the instrument's potential error. Some current studies indicate that SD-OCT has about a 4-µm intervisit reproducibility.[13] So, to be sure that a change is real, it should be twice 4 µm (8 µm).
2. *Trend-based analysis:* It identifies progression by monitoring the slope of RNFL thickness over time, which has already been mentioned in glaucoma progression analysis algorithms.

## BEYOND SPECTRAL DOMAIN OPTICAL COHERENCE TOMOGRAPHY

### Swept Source Optical Coherence Tomography

Swept source optical coherence tomography utilizes a longer wavelength than the conventional SD-OCT machine and has a deeper penetration. It helps in enhanced visualization of structures such as angle of the eye, LC, choroid, and sclera. SS-OCT can detect microarchitectural alterations between eyes with glaucomatous changes and healthy eyes by means of automated segmentation of the LC.[14]

Glaucoma leads to degenerative changes in ONH, for instance, retrograde bowing of LC and disorganization of its structure, along with axonal loss. Variances in the shape of LC pores in glaucomatous eyes have been noted to occur in association with increase in the severity of the disease.[15] LC pores can be categorized as striate, oval, or circular based on their shape. Studies have noted that the size of individual pores falls in glaucomatous eyes while the total area of pores rises.[15] Another study utilizing SS-OCT noted beam remodeling along with decrement in LC pore size and higher variability in pore size in glaucomatous eyes.[14]

Swept source optical coherence tomography is also valuable for the clinical evaluation of the anterior segment of the eye as it can precisely spot and compute peripheral anterior synechiae.[14] Studies have proved that SS-OCT has a similar diagnostic ability to that of SD-OCT in picking up preperimetric glaucoma and early glaucoma.[16] Commercially available models of SS-OCT are DRI Triton (Topcon, Tokyo, Japan) and ZEISS PLEX Elite 9000 SS-OCT angiography (Carl Zeiss Meditec, Inc., 5160 Hacienda Dr, Dublin, CA, United States).

### Adaptive Optics Optical Coherence Tomography

By reducing the effect of wavefront distortions, adaptive optics (AO) has improved the performance of optical systems. This technique uses a deformable mirror in order to compensate for distortions of wavefronts in the optical system. Incorporating AO in fundus cameras can help in better resolution of structures at the cellular level. A combined AO-OCT system allows comprehensive assessment of discrete structures such as retinal vessel, RNFL bundles, and LC; thus, it is a valuable instrument in understanding the glaucomatous process. Assessment of damage to retinal structures at a microscopic level might have an upper hand than measurement of retinal thickness while detecting glaucoma.[17]

## Polarization-sensitive Optical Coherence Tomography

In addition to detection of scattered/reflected light by standard OCT machines, this prototype technique also detects polarization state of tissues. It creates images based on the polarization state altering properties of the structure being evaluated. It carries the ability to distinguish individual retinal layers and has been utilized in experimental studies by incorporation of this technology in OCT machines. Studies have noted statistically significant enhancement in images obtained from polarization-sensitive (PS)-OCT when compared with conventional OCT images. This technology also improves the evaluation of the anterior chamber angle.[18] PS-OCT can also be utilized for subjective documentation of bleb status and for objective evaluation of its functionality. Therefore, it may be used as an effective tool for optimization of the postoperative course of trabeculectomy.[19]

## Doppler Optical Coherence Tomography

Doppler optical coherence tomography (DOCT) enables continuous measurement of the retinal blood flow (RBF) in the retinal arterioles and venules during one cardiac cycle. The loss of RGCs may result in a decrease in the RBF via autoregulatory mechanisms by responding to a decreased regional demand for oxygen; thus, by estimating alterations in tissue perfusion, we might be able to detect glaucoma earlier. Studies have observed correlation of reduced blood flow in retina with visual field changes, pRNFL thinning, and macular GCC thinning.[20] Decrease in RBF associated with RNFL thinning and GCC thinning has also been observed in glaucomatous eyes with apparently normal visual hemifield, thus implying that DOCT might pick up even subtle changes in early glaucoma.[14] In a recent Japanese study, DOCT showed that the RBF was significantly reduced in the damaged hemisphere compared with the normal one in normal tension glaucoma (NTG) eyes with single-hemifield damage.[21] Additionally, the RBF was found to be reduced in both the normal and the damaged hemispheres of NTG eyes when compared with the healthy hemisphere independent of the RNFL thickness.

## LIMITATIONS OF SPECTRAL DOMAIN OPTICAL COHERENCE TOMOGRAPHY

It is important that every clinician be aware of the limitations of every technology that influences clinical decision-making. SD-OCT image output can be affected by artifacts, such as those produced by eye movements (saccades, blink), or by media opacities (cataract). Additionally, artifacts may result from failure in the SD-OCT algorithm that delineates the retinal layers resulting in spurious thickness measurements of different layers.[22] Ocular pathologies such as myopia, age-related macular degeneration, or the presence of PVD or drusen may also introduce artifacts and confound the interpretation of results. OCT image truncation may commonly occur in myopic eyes with steep retinal curvature or peripapillary staphylomas.

## CONCLUSION

Optical coherence tomography has proven to be a quantitative and reliable tool for diagnosing as well as monitoring progression of glaucoma. However, it should always be used in conjunction with clinical evaluation and visual field testing. Understanding the limitations of imaging technologies coupled with structure–function correlation is important.

## REFERENCES

1. Bhende M, Shetty S, Parthasarathy MK, Ramya S. Optical coherence tomography: a guide to interpretation of common macular diseases. Indian J Ophthalmol. 2018;66:20-35.
2. Wang RK. Signal degradation by multiple scattering in optical coherence tomography of dense tissue: a Monte Carlo study towards optical clearing of biotissues. Phys Med Biol. 2002;47:2281-99.
3. Lopes FS, Matsubara I, Almeida I, Dorairaj SK, Vessani RM, Paranhos Jr A, et al. Structure-function relationships in glaucoma using enhanced depth imaging optical coherence tomography-derived parameters: a cross-sectional observational study. BMC Ophthalmol. 2019;19:52.
4. Kafieh R, Rabbani H, Kermani S. A review of algorithms for segmentation of optical coherence tomography from retina. J Med Signals Sens. 2013;3:45-60.
5. Nguyen AT, Greenfield DS, Bhakta AS, Lee J, Feuer WJ. Detecting glaucoma progression using guided progression analysis with OCT and visual field assessment in eyes classified by International Classification of Disease Severity Codes. Ophthalmol Glaucoma. 2019;2:36-46.
6. Pablo LE, Ferreras A, Pajarín AB, Fogagnolo P. Diagnostic ability of a linear discriminant function for optic nerve head parameters measured with optical coherence tomography for perimetric glaucoma. Eye. 2010;24:1051-7.
7. Baskaran M, Ong EL, Li JL, Cheung CY, Chen D, Perera SA, et al. Classification algorithms enhance the discrimination of glaucoma from normal eyes using high-definition optical coherence tomography. Invest Ophthalmol Vis Sci. 2012;53:2314.

8. Scuderi G, Fragiotta S, Scuderi L, Iodice CM, Perdicchi A. Ganglion cell complex analysis in glaucoma patients: what can it tell us? Eye Brain. 2020;12:33-44.
9. Lee WJ, Baek SU, Kim YK, Park KH, Jeoung JW. Rates of ganglion cell-inner plexiform layer thinning in normal, open-angle glaucoma and pseudoexfoliation glaucoma eyes: a trend-based analysis. Invest Ophthalmol Vis Sci. 2019;60(2):599-604.
10. Bhagat PR, Deshpande KV, Natu B. Utility of ganglion cell complex analysis in early diagnosis and monitoring of glaucoma using a different spectral domain optical coherence tomography. J Curr Glaucoma Pract. 2014;8:101-6.
11. Wang Y, Xin C, Li M, Swain DL, Cao K, Wang H, et al. Macular vessel density versus ganglion cell complex thickness for detection of early primary open-angle glaucoma. BMC Ophthalmol. 2020;20(1):17.
12. Leung CK, Yu M, Weinreb RN, Ye C, Liu S, Lai G, et al. Retinal nerve fiber layer imaging with spectral-domain optical coherence tomography: a prospective analysis of age-related loss. Ophthalmology. 2012;119:731-7.
13. Ghasia FF, El-Dairi M, Freedman SF, Rajani A, Asrani S. Reproducibility of spectral-domain optical coherence tomography measurements in adult and pediatric glaucoma. J Glaucoma. 2013;24:55-63.
14. Kostanyan T, Wollstein G, Schuman JS. Evaluating glaucoma damage: emerging imaging technologies. Expert Rev Ophthalmol. 2015;10:183-95.
15. Tezel G, Trinkaus K, Wax MB. Alterations in the morphology of lamina cribrosa pores in glaucomatous eyes. Br J Ophthalmol. 2004;88:251-6.
16. Lee WJ, Oh S, Kim YK, Jeoung JW, Park KH. Comparison of glaucoma-diagnostic ability between wide-field swept-source OCT retinal nerve fiber layer maps and spectral-domain OCT. Eye. 2018;32:1483-92.
17. Dong ZM, Wollstein G, Wang B, Schuman JS. Adaptive optics optical coherence tomography in glaucoma. Prog Retin Eye Res. 2017;57:76-88.
18. Mohana KP, Das D, Bhende M. Optical coherence tomography: newer techniques, newer machines. Sci J Med Vis Res Foun. 2015;33:75-9.
19. Kasaragod D, Fukuda S, Ueno Y, Hoshi S, Oshika T, Yasuno Y. Objective evaluation of functionality of filtering bleb based on polarization-sensitive optical coherence tomography. Invest Ophthalmol Vis Sci. 2016;57(4):2305-10.
20. Sehi M, Goharian I, Konduru R, Tan O, Srinivas S, Sadda SR, et al. Retinal blood flow in glaucomatous eyes with single-hemifield damage. Ophthalmology. 2014;121:750-8.
21. Yoshioka T, Song Y, Kawai M, Tani T, Takahashi K, Ishiko S, et al. Retinal blood flow reduction in normal-tension glaucoma with single-hemifield damage by Doppler optical coherence tomography. Br J Ophthalmol. 2021;105(1):124-30.
22. Somfai GM, Salinas HM, Puliafito CA, Fernández DC. Evaluation of potential image acquisition pitfalls during optical coherence tomography and their influence on retinal image segmentation. J Biomed Opt. 2007;12(4):041209.

CHAPTER 6

# Pitfalls in the Diagnosis of Glaucoma by Artificial Intelligence

*Mohana Sinnasamy, Murali Ariga, Nishanth Murali*

## ABSTRACT

Glaucoma leads to irreversible blindness that presents with symptoms in advanced stage of the disease. Early identification and prompt intervention are crucial in preventing visual impairment. Artificial intelligence (AI) holds promise to aid in diagnosing glaucoma in its early stages through its ability to learn from the images on par with human brain. But it is not without its limitations. This chapter aims to discuss the pitfalls in using AI to diagnose glaucoma, the extent to which these limitations can influence the results from these systems, and future of it in the diagnosis and management of glaucoma.

***Keywords:*** Artificial intelligence; glaucoma; machine learning; deep learning; diagnosis of glaucoma; black box.

## ■ INTRODUCTION

Glaucoma is one of the leading causes of irreversible blindness worldwide.[1] It may lead to visual impairment in around six million population and blindness in three million population worldwide.[2] This condition remains asymptomatic during the major portion of its time course presenting in advanced stage with irreversible visual impairment.[3] This implies that a significant proportion of patients with glaucoma remains undiagnosed till the advanced stage.[4] Hence, early diagnosis and intervention are crucial in preventing irreversible loss of vision. In this context, it is also worthwhile to mention that increasing life expectancy due to advances in healthcare has led to increase in population aged over 60 years. The health needs of this growing population will create an additional demand for glaucoma care, which may exceed the capacity of the ophthalmologists.[5] This has created a need for a solution to bridge the gap between the health-care needs and its delivery.

Artificial intelligence (AI) is increasingly being explored to bridge this gap between demand and supply. It can aid in screening and expedite the diagnosis by the health-care professionals. This has been possible largely due to the advancements in the processing ability of the machines and the availability of imaging studies that can be used to train the algorithms in diagnosis and predictive analysis. In ophthalmology, the retinal images have been the perfect study ground for the machine learning (ML) algorithms and retinal conditions such as diabetic retinopathy (DR), retinopathy of prematurity (ROP), and age-related macular degeneration (AMD), among others, are being extensively studied by ML algorithms.[6] This has also led to studies on other ophthalmic conditions such as cataract, glaucoma, keratoconus, and ocular oncology.

## ARTIFICIAL INTELLIGENCE IN THE DIAGNOSIS OF GLAUCOMA

Glaucoma is a diagnosis derived from combining multiple parameters such as intraocular pressure (IOP), visual fields (VFs), and optic nerve head (ONH) changes from the fundus examination, gonioscopy, and optical coherent tomography (OCT).[7] Hence, it is optimally suited to be studied with AI algorithms.[8] AI can aid the glaucoma specialists with its ability to combine data from multiple imaging modalities and deriving meaningful results to predict the progression of the glaucoma in a particular patient.

Artificial intelligence algorithms have begun to step in the clinical practices. IDx-DR, an AI device, is the first of its kind to be approved for the screening of DR in a primary care setting. In DR, this algorithm will classify the fundus images as one of the two classes: "More than mild DR detected: Refer to an eye care professional" or "negative for more than mild DR: Rescreen in 12 months."[9] Fundus photography may be used to screen glaucoma in a large volume of patients and is simple and relatively inexpensive which shows some promise when used with AI. A similar algorithm can be designed that can classify the fundus images as "glaucoma" and "not glaucoma" based on multiple characteristics of the fundus images and relationships between them.

Diagnosis and assessment of glaucoma using AI are primarily through interpreting the multiple modalities used in the diagnosis of glaucoma such as:
- Identifying glaucomatous optic nerve damage from fundus images[10]
- Analyzing the VF images for progression of glaucoma[11]
- Quantifying the retinal nerve fiber layer (RNFL) thickness from OCT images[12]
- Interpreting the angle structures in anterior segment OCT (AS-OCT)[13]

In addition to these modalities, incorporating data such as genomic data, lifestyle, and medical history among others in these systems may allow better estimation of the disease course and the need for surgical interventions in the future.[14] The basics of AI and the details of studies using AI in glaucoma diagnosis and predicting progression have been discussed in the chapter Artificial Intelligence in Glaucoma (in the volume 15 of Recent Advances in Ophthalmology). The readers are referred to this chapter on the various

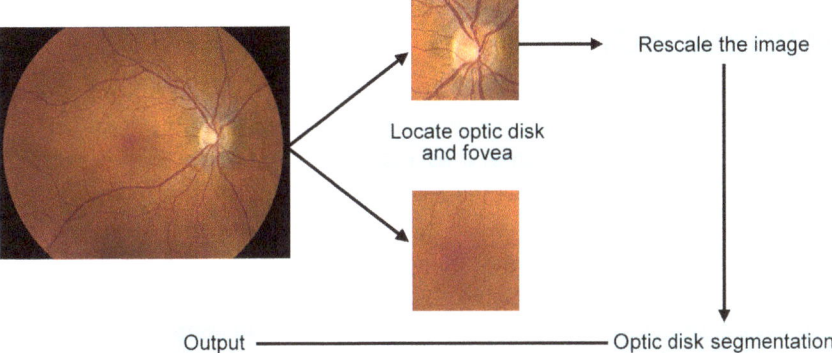

**Fig. 1:** Schematic representation of artificial intelligence (AI) model in glaucoma diagnosis.

**TABLE 1:** Challenges in implementing artificial intelligence in the diagnosis of glaucoma from bench to bed.

| Steps in implementing AI | Possible challenges |
| --- | --- |
| Identification of datasets | • Obtaining consent and maintaining confidentiality<br>• Difficulties in acquiring data for rare types of glaucoma |
| Validation of datasets | Difficulties in generalizability |
| Deciphering output | Understanding the black box outputs |
| Implementation in clinical practice | • Identifying areas of implementation<br>• Ethical challenges<br>• Legal implications |

(AI: artificial intelligence)

studies on AI in the diagnosis of glaucoma.[15] **Figure 1** shows a workflow in the diagnosis of glaucoma with AI.

# CHALLENGES IN GLAUCOMA DIAGNOSIS WITH ARTIFICIAL INTELLIGENCE

Multiple studies have been conducted on the diagnosis of glaucoma with AI. The ability of AI algorithms in differentiating two diagnostic groups is best described by the sensitivity, specificity, and area under the receiver-operating characteristic curve (AUC). It is considered that closer the AUC result to 1.0, the better is the diagnostic performance compared to the correct diagnosis. Majority of the important studies were able to demonstrate values at or above 0.80 suggesting that AI shows promises as a diagnostic aid in the screening, diagnosis, and predicting the progression of glaucoma.[16,17] Nevertheless, clinical and technical challenges **(Table 1)** exist in its translation to clinical practice.[14]

## Effects of Physiological Variations and Comorbidities in Using Artificial Intelligence

The AI algorithms are trained with labeled data that contains images with the characteristic features of the glaucomatous optic neuropathy (GON). In real-world settings, fundus images may have normal variations in the peripapillary region and optic disk that may lead to inaccuracy in its interpretation.

Another factor that may lead to inaccuracy in diagnosing glaucoma from fundus images is high myopia.[10] Being a risk factor for glaucoma by itself, a myopic disk frequently looks like glaucomatous and the true glaucomatous changes may be attributed to comorbid myopia. Other confounding features such as anomalous disks or high axial length may be misdiagnosed as glaucoma due to its similarity to the GON.

In addition, training of AI programs with datasets of a specific disease may lead to specific yes or no output; instead, they need to be trained to understand the influence of other factors such as age, hypertension, and diabetes on progression of glaucoma and their implication in medical and surgical management.[6]

## Inaccuracies in Labeling

When comparing computer programming and ML algorithms, programming is like explaining what a cat is and then help it identify the cats in the database but in ML we supply images of cats labeled as cat and the machine learns itself to identify cat from the images supplied. This process depends on the accuracy of human grader. Supervised learning involves feeding the ML algorithm images which are labeled by human graders. This labeling is referred to as "ground truth," i.e., the gold standard in ML.[18]

To label the training dataset, the human graders need defined criteria of the condition. In case of glaucoma, it does not have an approved criterion for diagnosis unlike DR. This is reflected in the consistency of labeling data in glaucoma training sets. Different experts may label differently for a same fundus image leading to discrepancies in labeling. This results in inaccurate learning by the AI systems and, therefore, may lead to errors in the output.[19]

## Reliance on Image Details

Studies using AI in the diagnosis and prognosis of glaucoma have claimed similar or better results than human graders in terms of sensitivity and specificity.[20] But in an experimental study conducted by Abramoff, a minor change in the pixels of fundus images was made, which are referred to as *adversarial images*. These images were presented to the human graders, image-based AI systems, and hybrid systems. Image-based systems rely on the images while hybrid systems train on features of focal lesions. It was seen that both image-based and hybrid systems were equally accurate in validated datasets, but the image-based system was inaccurate in the interpretation of adversarial images compared to the hybrid systems. Image-based systems identified the small changes in the pixels of the image and failed to interpret the pathology in the image which led to false negatives.[21]

## Influences of Image Quality on Artificial Intelligence Models

The ML algorithms rely on the images fed as input to learn the features of normal and diseased conditions. Hence, the quality of the images determines the accuracy of diagnostic ability learned by the algorithms. ML is entirely dependent on the dataset that is being input. Hence, understanding the *garbage in, garbage out* (*GIGO*) rule is vital when training the systems. The images in the training dataset need to be of high quality and validated to ensure that ML algorithms learn accurately. However, images acquired clinically are subject to variations in the width of the field, field of view, magnification of image, quality of the image, and range of variation in ethnicity of the patients.[14] Images which are blurry or those that do not completely show the entire retina may not be ideal images for these algorithms. In such cases, these algorithms need to identify that the error is of the quality and not the pathology in the retina. In the absence of this recognition, it can lead to equivocal results or errors in its processing.[18]

## Translation to Real-life Scenarios

Most of the AI studies use homogenous datasets to train their algorithms. As a result, the validation of these algorithms with real-world population is crucial as they may be less accurate when employed in clinical practice that may encounter a variety of patients with multiple comorbidities whose data may be significantly deviated from those of the training set data.[22,23]

To explain this with an example, the AI model DeepMind by Google exhibited high levels of accuracy in both sensitivity and specificity in the studies under controlled conditions. To apply the algorithms in real time, a study was conducted in selected primary care centers of Thailand with DeepMind. AI algorithms were unable to produce results similar to those obtained in the controlled settings with validated datasets during the training.[24] This lack of generalizability is one of the important hurdles in translating the results obtained with AI under controlled conditions with trained dataset to the real-world clinical practice with variations in patient data, testing conditions, and operator methods among others.

## Need for Large Volumes of Dataset

To ensure accurate learning, large datasets up to 100,000 images containing all stages of glaucoma are needed not only to train the algorithms but also for validation of the algorithms. This involves significant time to collect and validate before this can be translated into clinical practice. In this context, it is to be mentioned that the increasing volumes alone may not necessarily increase the accuracy. It is to be taken into account that increasing the volume may also result in the incorrect connections deduced by the algorithms and identifying nonretinal-related features as a part of learning.[22,25] This highlights the need for deducing the optimal volume of dataset needed for training that can produce accurate results.[26]

## ■ BLACK BOX—THE ENIGMA OF ARTIFICIAL INTELLIGENCE

Artificial intelligence is unique in its ability to learn from the data fed as training dataset. This process of learning can be supervised or unsupervised. In supervised learning, the algorithm is fed with datasets that are "labeled" or referred to as "ground truth," and in the unsupervised learning, the system learns details which are not labeled by the experts **(Flowcharts 1 and 2)**.[27,28]

During training with certain AI models, it was observed that systems produced results that could not be explained by the experts. This may be due to self-generated rules by the algorithms in learning the characteristics of the images. This was termed *"black box."* These rules remain unknown and cannot be validated by the specialists. Hence, its use in clinical practice is contended due to reliability of such systems that may learn from features that are not part of the actual disease process **(Flowchart 3)**.[14] This may pose difficulty in the acceptance of AI by treating clinician as the ultimate responsibility of care rests on the clinician.[29]

## Pitfalls Inherent in Using Software

In any method using software, some issues are inherent which include the possibility of the data being subjected to adversarial attacks such as hacking and data leakage that may threaten the privacy of the patient. Another factor that needs to be considered is the initial cost and investment needed to set up the system. In addition, the images in AI are uploaded in the cloud

**Flowchart 1:** Workflow of supervised learning.

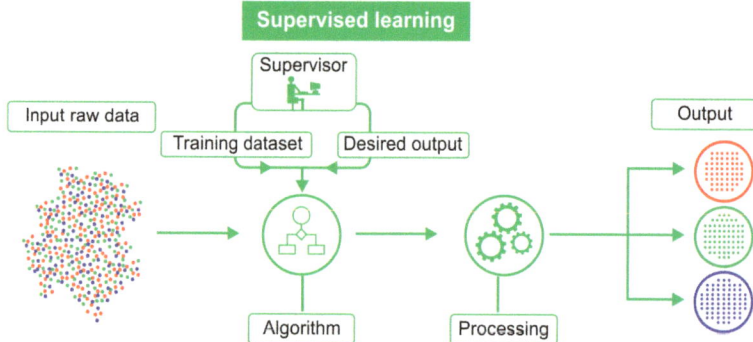

**Flowchart 2:** Workflow of unsupervised learning.

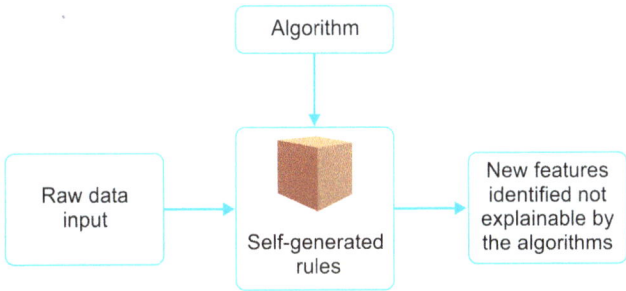

**Flowchart 3:** Illustration of black box—the unexplainable artificial intelligence (AI).

and, therefore, the use of internet to access images and to produce results becomes mandatory. In cases in which access to internet is inconsistent, systems should be developed that can work in an offline mode.

# Ethics and Medicolegal Implications in Using Artificial Intelligence

Introduction of AI-based methods in clinical practice must be gradual to be acceptable. In a field that involves years of human learning, to trust AI-based decisions may not be acceptable initially. In this context, any inaccurate conclusions by AI-based techniques can result in resistance in its acceptance. Also, patients' concerns regarding their data privacy need to be considered. Hence, regulations are made to ensure the privacy of the patient including devising laws to protect the privacy, ensuring that informed consents are obtained and accountability from all stakeholders who have access to the data.

As we start to consider AI in clinical practice, ophthalmologists may want to know how the legal system may embrace AI. Regulations about the liability for any injuries occurring because of the interaction between the treating physician and AI system need to be developed.[30]

## CONCLUSION

The capacity to learn like a human brain by AI systems has intrigued both the experts and public likewise. The volume of studies that attempt to validate the output from AI is unprecedented. AI holds promise to be the major gamechanger in screening, diagnosis, and predicting progression of glaucoma. It can help us identify new biomarkers, discover more about the pathophysiology of glaucoma, optimize health resources, train health-care teams, and reduce human errors.

Glaucoma is a silent thief of vision and needs early identification and intervention to prevent visual impairment. AI can be an effective diagnostic aid in the management of glaucoma. But there are limitations in using AI that need to be addressed such as validation with real-world patients' data, explaining the concept of black box, ensuring data privacy, and improving patients' acceptability. Further research is needed to overcome these limitations and study the cost-effectiveness of different AI systems in real-world settings. Nevertheless, AI promises to revolutionize the management of glaucoma in future.

## REFERENCES

1. Tham YC, Li X, Wong TY, Quigley HA, Aung T, Cheng CY. Global prevalence of glaucoma and projections of glaucoma burden through 2040: a systematic review and meta-analysis. Ophthalmology. 2014;121(11):2081-90.
2. Pascolini D, Mariotti SP. Global estimates of visual impairment: 2010. Br J Ophthalmol. 2012;96:614-8.
3. Bourne RR, Stevens GA, White RA, Smith JL, Flaxman SR, Price H, et al. Causes of vision loss worldwide, 1990-2010: a systematic analysis. Lancet Glob Health. 2013;1(6):e339-49.
4. De Voogd S, Ikram MK, Wolfs RC, Jansonius NM, Hofman A, de Jong PT. Incidence of open-angle glaucoma in a general elderly population: the Rotterdam Study. Ophthalmology. 2005;112(9):1487-93.
5. Resnikoff S, Felch W, Gauthier TM, Spivey B. The number of ophthalmologists in practice and training worldwide: a growing gap despite more than 200,000 practitioners. Br J Ophthalmol. 2012;96:783-7.
6. Kapoor R, Walters SP, Al-Aswad LA. The current state of artificial intelligence in ophthalmology. Surv Ophthalmol. 2019;64:233-40.
7. Weinreb RN, Garway-Heath DF, Leung C, Medeiros FA, Liebmann J. Diagnosis of Primary Open Angle Glaucoma: WGA Consensus Series 10. Amsterdam, The Netherlands: Kugler Publications; 2017.
8. Kapoor R, Whigham BT, Al-Aswad LA. The role of artificial intelligence in the diagnosis and management of glaucoma. Curr Ophthalmol Rep. 2019;7(2):136-42.
9. Roach L. Artificial Intelligence. AI is poised to revolutionize medicine. An overview of the field, with selected applications in ophthalmology. EyeNet Magazine. 2017, [online] Available from: https://www.aao.org/eyenet/article/artificial-intelligence. [Last accessed November, 2022].

10. Li Z, He Y, Keel S, Meng W, Chang RT, He M. Efficacy of a deep learning system for detecting glaucomatous optic neuropathy based on coloured fundus photographs. Ophthalmology. 2018;125(8):1199-206.
11. Li F, Wang Z, Qu G, Song D, Yuan Y, Xu Y, et al. Automatic differentiation of glaucoma visual field from non-glaucoma visual field using deep convolutional neural network. BMC Med Imaging. 2018;18(1):35. [Erratum in: BMC Med Imaging. 2019;19(1):40].
12. Asaoka R, Murata H, Hirasawa K, Fujino Y, Matsuura M, Miki A, et al. Using deep learning and transfer learning to accurately diagnose early-onset glaucoma from macular optical coherence tomography images. Am J Ophthalmol. 2019;198:136-45.
13. Niwas SI, Lin W, Bai X, Kwoh CK, Kuo C-CJ, Sng CC, et al. Automated anterior segment OCT image analysis for angle closure glaucoma mechanisms classification. Comput Methods Programs Biomed. 2016;130:65-75.
14. Ting DSW, Pasquale LR, Peng L, Campbell JP, Lee AY, Raman R, et al. Artificial intelligence and deep learning in ophthalmology. Br J Ophthalmol. 2019;103(2):167-75.
15. Ariga M, Sinnasamy M, Nivean PD, Henderson H. Artificial intelligence in the diagnosis of glaucoma. In: Nema HV, Nema N (Eds). Recent Advances in Ophthalmology, 15th edition. India: Jaypee Brothers Medical Publishers Pvt. Limited; 2019.
16. Shibata N, Tanito M, Mitsuhashi K, Fujino Y, Matsuura M, Murata H, et al. Development of a deep residual learning algorithm to screen for glaucoma from fundus photography. Sci Rep. 2018;8:14665.
17. Goldbaum MH, Sample PA, White H, Côlt B, Raphaelian P, Fechtner RD, et al. Interpretation of automated perimetry for glaucoma by neural network. Invest Ophthalmol Vis Sci. 1994;35:3362-73.
18. Schena LB. (2020). AI in the clinic: eye care's pioneering use of Big Data. [online] Available from: https://www.aao.org/eyenet/article/ai-in-the-clinic. [Last accessed February, 2023].
19. Azuara-Blanco A, Katz LJ, Spaeth GL, Vernon SA, Spencer F, Lanzl IM. Clinical agreement among glaucoma experts in the detection of glaucomatous changes of the optic disk using simultaneous stereoscopic photographs. Am J Ophthalmol. 2003;136:949-50.
20. Jammal AA, Thompson AC, Mariottoni EB, Berchuck SI, Urata CN, Estrela T, et al. Human versus machine: comparing a deep learning algorithm to human gradings for detecting glaucoma on fundus photographs. Am J Ophthalmol. 2020;211:123-31.
21. Lynch SK, Shah A, Folk JC, Wu X, Abramoff MD. Catastrophic failure in image-based convolutional neural network algorithms for detecting diabetic retinopathy. Invest Ophthalmol Vis Sci. 2017;58(8):3776.
22. Date RC, Jesudasen SJ, Weng CY. Applications of deep learning and artificial intelligence in retina. Int Ophthalmol Clin. 2019;59:39-57.
23. Ting DSW, Cheung CY-L, Lim G, Tan GSW, Quang ND, Gan A, et al. Development and validation of a deep learning system for diabetic retinopathy and related eye diseases using retinal images from multiethnic populations with diabetes. JAMA. 2017;318:2211-23.

24. Beede E, Baylor E, Hersch F, Iurchenko A, Wilcox L, Ruamviboonsuk P, et al. A human-centered evaluation of a deep learning system deployed in clinics for the detection of diabetic retinopathy. In: CHI '20: Proceedings of the 2020 CHI Conference on Human Factors in Computing Systems, April 25–30, 2020. pp. 1-12.
25. Ting DSW, Peng L, Varadarajan AV, Keane PA, Burlina PM, Chiang MF, et al. Deep learning in ophthalmology: the technical and clinical considerations. Prog Retin Eye Res. 2019;72:100759.
26. Campbell CG, Ting DSW, Keane PA, Foster PJ. The potential application of artificial intelligence for diagnosis and management of glaucoma in adults. Br Med Bull. 2020;134(1):21-33.
27. Morris J. What is the difference between supervised and unsupervised machine learning? [online] Available from: https://www.vproexpert.com/what-is-the-difference-between-supervised-and-unsupervised-machine-learning/. [Last accessed February, 2023].
28. Kolonin A. How SingularityNET is advancing unsupervised language learning. 2018 [online] Available from: https://blog.singularitynet.io/how-singularitynet-is-advancing-unsupervised-language-learning-2679dbfca645. [Last accessed November, 2022].
29. Mursch-Edlmayr AS, Ng WS, Diniz-Filho A, Sousa DC, Arnold L, Schlenker MB, et al. Artificial intelligence algorithms to diagnose glaucoma and detect glaucoma progression: translation to clinical practice. Transl Vis Sci Technol. 2020;9(2):55.
30. Price 2nd WN, Gerke S, Cohen IG. Potential liability for physicians using artificial intelligence. JAMA. 2019;322:1765-6.

# CHAPTER 7

# Optimizing Intraocular Lens Power Calculation in Eyes with Posterior Segment Diseases and Following Posterior Segment Surgery

*Meena Chakrabarti, Arup Chakrabarti*

## ABSTRACT

This chapter deals with factors that should be considered to facilitate a precise estimation of intraocular lens (IOL) power in postvitrectomy eyes as well as eyes undergoing phacovitrectomies with and without silicone oil or gas tamponade.

***Keywords:*** Silicone oil; postvitrectomy cataract; ultrasound biometry; optical biometry.

## ■ INTRODUCTION

With the advent of a better understanding of the underlying pathophysiology of retinal diseases, availability of better instrumentation, and refinement of available technologies and techniques, the visual outcome following surgical management of patients with vitreoretinal pathologies has improved by leaps and bounds. The indications for vitreoretinal surgeries have expanded tremendously, resulting in a greater number of patients requiring cataract surgery either in combination with the vitreoretinal procedure or later on as a second-stage procedure. Coupled with these developments is the welcome trend of novice surgeons choosing to specialize in vitreoretinal surgery, resulting in an exponential increase in the number of vitreoretinal procedures performed annually.

One of the most common complications of vitrectomy is the earlier onset and more rapid progression of lenticular opacity, especially nuclear sclerotic cataract and posterior subcapsular opacification.[1] Studies have suggested that light toxicity, oxidation of lens proteins, use of intraocular gas or silicone oil, length of surgery, mechanical trauma, and increased postoperative oxygen tension within the eye may be the causative factors of cataract following vitrectomy. Postvitrectomy cataract, such as nuclear sclerotic cataract, is clinically challenging due to the lack of vitreous support in the posterior segment and the relatively harder nucleus than in age-related cataract, which increase the risk of surgical complications.[2-8] With appropriate surgical techniques, cataract surgery in vitrectomized eyes can be safe and effective with refractive outcomes similar to nonvitrectomized eyes, although the underlying retinal pathology may limit the functional outcome and increase the risks for intraoperative and postoperative complications. Presence of dense nuclear sclerosis, hard cataract, preexisting zonular dialysis or posterior capsular rent as well as higher incidence of postoperative cystoid macular edema and earlier onset of posterior capsular opacification and capsular bag contracture can complicate the intraoperative and postoperative course.[9] Another major challenge is obtaining an accurate biometry and axial length measurement as well as precise calculation of intraocular lens (IOL) power in these eyes.[10,11]

This chapter will deal with all factors that should be considered to facilitate a precise estimation of IOL power for achieving the desired refraction after cataract surgery. IOL consideration in eyes with posterior segment pathology or following posterior segment surgeries is associated with challenges for axial length determination and inaccuracies regarding the choice of an appropriate IOL power.

## CHALLENGES INVOLVED IN AXIAL LENGTH MEASUREMENT

Errors in axial length measurement contribute maximally to inaccurate IOL power estimation in eyes with postvitrectomy cataracts. Olsen and McEwan et al. have conclusively reported that >54% of errors are attributable to inaccurate axial length measurement.[12,13]

Errors in axial length measurement can arise due to:
- Overestimation of axial length in silicone oil-filled eyes.[14,15]
- Underestimation of axial length in eyes with macular edema when ultrasound biometry is used.[14]
- Underestimation of axial length in eyes with bullous rhegmatogenous retinal detachment when optical biometry is performed.[16]

### Axial Length Measurement in Silicone Oil-filled Eyes

Biometry in silicone oil-filled eyes is difficult to perform, and an axial length measurement may not be obtainable when an ultrasound biometry is used for this purpose.[17]

### Axial Length Measurement in Silicone-filled Eyes Using Ultrasound A-scan Biometry

- Using ultrasound biometry for axial length measurement in silicone oil-filled eyes has several disadvantages. Silicone oil slows down the speed of sound and produces an apparent lengthening of the globe, resulting in longer axial length measurements.[3,4] The speed of sound in silicone

oil (for 1,000 cSt silicone oil, it is 980 m/s and for 5,000 cSt silicone oil, it is 1,040 m/s) is much slower when compared to that in normal vitreous, which is 1,532 m/s.[18]
- The absorption of sound waves in silicone oil results in poor penetration, thereby further impairing accurate measurements with low reflective retinal echoes.[19]
- Incomplete silicone oil fill may result in the presence of pooled posteriorly circulating aqueous when the axial length is measured in supine position. In this situation, the ultrasound waves will first traverse the silicone oil-filled vitreous cavity, the silicone oil–aqueous interface, followed by the pooled posteriorly circulating aqueous to reach the retinal surface. Hence, it is advisable to perform axial length measurements with the patient sitting up so that most part of posterior pole is covered with the silicone oil bubble.[14,20]
- Axial length that is obtained using an ultrasound biometer is the apparent axial length, and it has to be converted into the true axial length by making adjustment for the slow speed of ultrasound waves in silicone oil.[21]

## Axial Length Measurement in Silicone-filled Eyes Using Optical Biometry[22,23]

- Axial length measurement in silicone oil-filled eyes is best accomplished using optical coherence interferometry. The axial length obtained is a true and accurate measurement as the distance from cornea to the retinal pigment epithelium (RPE) is measured.
- Measurement in eyes with advanced/total cataract or thick posterior subcapsular lenticular opacity or poor fixation is most challenging.
- Axial length measurement in silicone oil-filled eyes was found to be more accurate using swept-source optical coherence tomography (OCT) in a few single-center studies with small sample sizes. The OA-2000 optical biometer when compared to IOL Master 700 was found to be ideal for axial length measurement in silicone oil-filled eyes.[23]

The presence of silicone oil in the vitreous cavity appears to increase the axial length and alter the eye's optics. Before the surgeon can calculate the correct IOL power, he or she must convert the apparent axial length to the true measurement.
- *Step 1: Measuring the apparent axial length in silicone oil-filled eye:*[24] To measure the vitreous cavity depth in an eye filled with silicone oil using the ultrasound biometer, the velocity gate should be readjusted based on the viscosity of silicone oil (1,040 m/s for 5,000 cSt silicone oil and 980 m/s for 1,000 cSt silicone oil).
- *Step 2: Converting apparent axial length to true axial length (when A scan is used)*

**TABLE 1:** Conversion factors available for silicone oil of different viscosities.

| Type of silicone oil (SO) | Conversion factor |
|---|---|
| • SO 1000 | • 0.63 |
| • SO 1300 | • 0.71 |
| • SO 5000 | • 0.36 |
| • Densiron 68 | • 0.597 |

The conversion can be done by the following two methods:
1. *Using a conversion factor:* The viscosities of silicone oil vary from 1,000 to 5,000 cSt, and in general, the higher the viscosity, the greater the change in refraction and axial length. If 1,300 cSt silicone oil is used for semipermanent tamponade, the apparent axial length obtained using ultrasonic biometry can be converted to true axial length by multiplying with a conversion factor of 0.71 **(Table 1)**.[25]
2. *Formula-based calculation:* The formula to calculate axial length in eyes with silicone oil tamponade is as follows. The corrected vitreous chamber depth (VCD) is first determined by the following formula:[26]

$$\text{VCD corrected} = \frac{\text{Velocity of sound in silicone oil}}{\text{Velocity of sound in normal vitreous}} \times \text{calculated vitreous chamber length}$$

Total axial length (TAL) = ACD + LT + VCD corrected

where ACD is the anterior chamber depth and LT is the lens thickness.

In situations where axial length measurement is not possible, by the method described above, any one of the following options may be resorted to:
- Axial length measurement may be carried out prior to the vitreoretinal surgery and archived in the hospital records.
- By using axial length of the fellow eye (which is not a very desirable option)
- Intraoperative biometry for IOL power calculation following silicone oil removal. The biometry is performed using a sterile probe after silicone oil removal and prior to cataract surgery. This technique provides good predictability and reasonable accuracy, and in various studies on this technique, the mean postoperative refractive error was only 0.77 diopters with no significant difference in long eyes and eyes with average normal axial length.[27]
- Intraoperative retinoscopy was used to calculate the IOL power in cases of combined phacoemulsification and silicone oil removal, using theoretical formulas based on aphakic refractive error.[28]

   The various formulas that are available in the literature are:
   - *Ianchulev et al.:*[29] Aphakic refraction × 2.01
   - *Mackool:*[30] Aphakic refraction × 0.75

- *Leccisotti et al.:*[31] 0.07 × (2) + 1.27X + 1.22, where X is the aphakic refraction
- In cases with partial silicone oil fill, the axial length may be obtained from a computed tomography (CT) scan.[20]
- The least desirable option is to implant a standard power IOL.

Accurate prediction of refractive outcomes in vitrectomized eyes is difficult due to multiple factors. First, the absence of vitreous in the posterior segment can result in an unusually deep and fluctuating anterior chamber, which increases the mobility of the posterior capsule and IOL movement after surgery. Furthermore, the high risk of zonular weakness and injury in vitrectomized eyes may lead to the instability of the lens capsular bag and the misalignment of IOL. In addition, the replacement of the vitreous with aqueous humor or silicone oil tamponade changes the refractive index of the posterior segment, which could influence the accuracy of axial length measurement. A relatively higher percentage of highly myopic or staphylomatous eyes in this population also aggravates the inaccuracy of IOL power calculation. And in all, these factors make it difficult to predict the accurate effective lens position (ELP) and refractive outcomes for patients with previous vitrectomy.[32-35] Furthermore, there can be errors in axial length measurement due to the presence of macular thickening which may also be a reason for concern.

## Axial Length Measurement Errors Associated with Vitrectomy for Macular Diseases

With a better understanding of the pathogenesis and clinical course of vitreoretinal interface disorders (such as diabetic macular edema, macular holes, vitreomacular traction, and epiretinal membrane), more number of macular surgeries are performed, and whenever required, these surgeries are usually combined with cataract extraction. This ensures early visual rehabilitation of patients with coexisting visually significant cataract and macular pathologies.

When these patients are being worked up preoperatively, it is best to perform axial length measurement using an optical biometer as it takes into account the distance from the cornea to the RPE. Most of these eyes will have thickened and edematous macula, and if ultrasound biometry is performed, the measured axial length will be erroneously short. In this situation, the corrected axial length is obtained by the following formula:[36]

Corrected axial length = Measured axial length (using ultrasound biometer A-scan) + Central foveal thickness (obtained from OCT scan)

Unless this correction is factored in, a postoperative myopic refractive surprise should be expected due to the underestimation of the cornea-photoreceptor layer (or RPE) distance in eyes with thickened macula.

Several studies have shown that the actual value of this predicted myopic shift is 0.50 diopter; hence, if the corrected axial length is not used for IOL power calculations, it is prudent to use a slightly hyperopic IOL in combined phacovitrectomy procedures. Thus, the myopic refractive shift after a combined single-stage phacovitrectomy performed for a vitreoretinal interface pathology can be compensated by either of these two strategies:
1. Adding the central foveal thickness measurement on OCT to the ultrasound axial length
2. Implanting an IOL that has a power that is 0.50 diopter less than the IOL power targeted for postoperative emmetropia.

The need to utilize these strategies does not arise if one resorts to measuring the axial length using the optical biometer.

### Errors in Axial Length Measurement in Eyes with Previous Scleral Buckling Procedure

In eyes that have undergone scleral buckling procedures, there is a definite increase in the axial length by nearly 1 mm due to elongation of the back of the globe. This elongation of the globe is not associated with any change in the anterior chamber depth. Hence, postoperatively buckled eyes show a myopic refractive shift. The elongation in axial length stabilizes by 3 months after scleral buckling surgery. 360° scleral buckling in conjunction with use of adjunctive cryoretinopexy is associated with a greater increase in axial length. In a buckled eye, cataract surgery is, therefore, usually delayed until at least 3 months after the primary buckle surgery. Taking into account the axial elongation of the globe following the scleral buckle procedure, the IOL power is adjusted down (for IOL power >14 diopters) by 0.50 diopter. This rule is incorporated into the Holladay constant, where the IOL power one gets on clicking the "scleral buckled button" is the one that has been adjusted down by 0.50 diopter.[37,38]

## EFFECT OF GAS TAMPONADE ON INTRAOCULAR LENS POSITION AND ITS EFFECT ON REFRACTIVE ERROR AFTER PHACOVITRECTOMY AND GAS TAMPONADE

Shiraki et al. used swept-source anterior segment OCT to calculate the anterior chamber depth, lens thickness, and the relative IOL position in eyes with gas tamponade.[40] They reported that even in eyes without gas tamponade, a forward displacement of the IOL occurred at the conclusion of the first postoperative month, relative to its position in the immediate postoperative period. This forward movement was more common in eyes with gas tamponade and persisted to a lesser degree even after the gas filling the vitreous cavity got reabsorbed. The forward movement of IOL pushes

the lens–iris diaphragm forward, leading to a shallower anterior chamber. Thus, the myopic postoperative refractive shift can be attributed to two factors:[39-41]
1. Anterior shift of IOL
2. Change in refractive index of intraocular medium as the vitreous cavity gets filled by posteriorly circulating aqueous after the intraocular gas has disappeared.

## ADJUSTING INTRAOCULAR LENS POWER IN SILICONE OIL-FILLED EYES

The refractive index of silicone oil (1.405) is higher than that of normal vitreous (1.336) and almost similar to that of the IOL (1.401). Because the index of refraction of silicone oil is higher than that of the vitreous gel, this optical medium behaves like an intraocular minus lens. When the IOL power is not adjusted to account for this difference, standard theoretical and regression lens power formulas predict a lens power that is less than needed to achieve emmetropia. The result is a significant postoperative hyperopic refractive error. As a rule of thumb, if more power is incorporated into the posterior surface of the chosen IOL, the greater the postoperative error. When a patient with silicone oil semipermanent tamponade has either a primary or a secondary IOL implant, there is an increase in the refractive power of the posterior surface of the IOL, which is in contact with the silicone oil. The quantum of increase in the refractive power of the implanted IOL is greatly influenced by the type of IOL used. It is greatest with biconvex lenses, least with meniscus lenses, and in between for plano-convex lenses with the plane surface facing posteriorly. Therefore, if silicone oil tamponade is necessary for an indefinitely long period of time (as determined by the stability of the retina), 3–8 diopters should be added to the calculated IOL power (for emmetropic refraction) to compensate for the alteration in the refractive power of the implanted IOL in silicone oil-filled eye, with the exact amount depending on the specific lens shape. With a convex-plano IOL, add 3 diopters to the calculated IOL power, and with a biconvex lens, add 6 diopters. Patients who will have the silicone oil removed at a later date should be warned about the possibility of a myopic shift of 2–5 diopters. The shift will be greater for an eye with a biconvex lens than for an eye with a plano-convex lens with a posteriorly facing planar surface; with the smallest change occurs in eyes with posterior-meniscus IOLs.[42]

The additional power that should be added to the calculated IOL power can also be determined using the following formula:[43]

$$\text{Additional power} = \frac{N_s - N_v}{AL - ACD} \times 1{,}000$$

where $N_s$ is the refractive index of silicone oil (1.405), $N_v$ is the refractive index of vitreous (1.336), and AL is the axial length (in millimeters).

Thus, if silicone oil removal is performed in these eyes at a later date, a myopic shift is to be expected. Hence, proper patient counseling is a very important aspect before planning surgery in these cases.

## ACCURACY OF INTRAOCULAR LENS FORMULA IN COMBINED PHACOVITRECTOMY

The correctness of IOL formula in phacovitrectomy surgery was analyzed and reported in several studies by comparing preoperative optical biometry and postoperative outcomes. The authors compared the prediction accuracy of new IOL calculation formulas, such as Barrett Universal 11 (BU11), emmetropia verifying optical (EVO), Kane and Ladas Super, and traditional formulas (Haigis, Hoffer Q, Holladay 1, and SRK/T) with Wang-Koch (WK) axial length adjustment in vitrectomized eyes. The BU11, EVO, Kane, and Haigis exhibited comparable performance in vitrectomized eyes with optimized constants. In vitrectomized highly myopic eyes, the new formulas as well as the traditional formulas with WK adjustment exhibited satisfactory prediction accuracy. Silicone oil or intraocular gas tamponade did not affect the prediction accuracy of formulas using optical biometry.[41]

It is observed that in different categories of patients (vitrectomized eyes, eyes undergoing combined phacoemulsification with IOL implantation and silicone oil removal, or when phacovitrectomy is performed as a single-stage procedure for vitreomacular interface pathologies), newer IOL formulas exhibited comparative or even better prediction accuracy compared to traditional formulas. For highly myopic eyes with axial length >26 mm, applying the WK axial length adjustment could correct the hyperopic bias of traditional formulas.

## CHOICE OF INTRAOCULAR LENS

In postvitrectomy eyes, hydrophobic and hydrophilic acrylic IOLs can have successful outcomes. Rigid polymethyl methacrylate (PMMA) IOLs may also be considered; however, silicone IOLs should never be implanted in vitrectomized eyes with silicone oil tamponade. This is also true for IOLs with a one-piece plate haptic design and those with small and ovoid optics. Lenses with a 360° square-edge design and an optic diameter of 6-6.5 mm provide greater area for fundus visualization and, therefore, are preferable in patients with retinal pathology.[42,43]

## CONCLUSION

Optimizing visual recovery in eyes with vitreoretinal pathologies is of paramount importance, and majority of these patients will require cataract surgery along with the primary vitreoretinal surgery in the same sitting or on a later date. Precise estimation of IOL power can be achieved by accurate measurement of axial length. The protocol to be adopted in silicone oil-filled eyes has been described in-depth taking into account the hyperopic refractive shift under oil and the myopic shift following silicone oil removal.

## ■ REFERENCES

1. Cherfan GM, Michels RG, de Bustros S, Enger C, Glaser BM. Nuclear sclerotic cataract after vitrectomy for idiopathic epiretinal membranes causing macular pucker. Am J Ophthalmol. 1991;111:434-8.
2. Jackson TL, Nicod E, Angelis A, Grimaccia F, Prevost AT, Simpson ARH, et al. Pars plana vitrectomy for vitreomacular traction syndrome: a systematic review and meta-analysis of safety and efficacy. Retina. 2013;33:2012-7.
3. Chang MA, Parides MK, Chang S, Braunstein RE. Outcome of phacoemulsification after pars plana vitrectomy. Ophthalmology. 2002;109:948-54.
4. Thompson JT. The role of patient age and intraocular gas use in cataract progression after vitrectomy for macular holes and epiretinal membranes. Am J Ophthalmol. 2004;137:250-7.
5. Biro Z, Kovacs B. Results of cataract surgery in previously vitrectomized eyes. J Cataract Refract Surg. 2002;28:1003-6.
6. Titiyal JS, Agarwal E, Angmo D, Sharma M, Kumar A. Comparative evaluation of outcomes of phacoemulsification in vitrectomized eyes: silicone oil versus air/gas group. Int Ophthalmol. 2017;37:565-74.
7. Truscott RJW. Age-related nuclear cataract-oxidation is the key. Exp Eye Res. 2005;80:709-25.
8. Holekamp NM, Shui YB, Beebe DC. Vitrectomy surgery increases oxygen exposure to the lens: a possible mechanism for nuclear cataract formation. Am J Ophthalmol. 2005;139:302-10.
9. Elhousseini Z, Lee E, Williamson TH. Incidence of lens touch during pars plana vitrectomy and outcomes from subsequent cataract surgery. Retina. 2016;36:825-9.
10. Lamson TL, Song J, Abazari A, Weissbart SB. Refractive outcomes of phacoemulsification after pars plana vitrectomy using traditional and new intraocular lens calculation formulas. J Cataract Refract Surg. 2019;45(3):293-7.
11. Faraldi F, Lavia CA, Nassisi M, Kilian RA, Bacherini D, Rizzo S. Swept-source OCT reduces the risk of axial length measurement errors in eyes with cataract and epiretinal membranes. PLoS One. 2021;16(9):e0257654.
12. Olsen T. Sources of error in intraocular lens power calculation. J Cataract Refract Surg. 1992;18(2):125-9.
13. McEwan JR, Massengill RK, Friedel SD. Effect of keratometer and axial length measurement errors on primary implant power calculations. J Cataract Refract Surg. 1990;16(1):61-70.
14. Murray DC, Potamitis T, Good P, Kirkby GR, Benson MT. Biometry of the silicone oil-filled eye. Eye (Lond). 1999;13(Pt 3a):319-24.
15. Kanclerz P, Grzybowski A. Accuracy of intraocular lens power calculation in eyes filled with silicone oil. Semin Ophthalmol. 2019;34(5):392-7.

16. Pongsachareonnont P, Tangjanyatam S. Accuracy of axial length measurements obtained by optical biometry and acoustic biometry in rhegmatogenous retinal detachment: a prospective study. Clin Ophthalmol. 2018;12:973-80.
17. Hoffer KJ. Special circumstances silicone oil power. In: Hoffer KJ (Ed). IOL Power. Thorofare, NJ: SLACK; 2011. pp. 221-2.
18. Hoffer KJ. Ultrasound velocities for axial eye length measurement. J Cataract Refract Surg. 1994;20:554-62.
19. Siddiqui MAR, Awan MA, Fairhead A, Atta H. Ultrasound velocity in heavy ocular tamponade agents and implications for biometry. Br J Ophthalmol. 2011;95:142-4.
20. Takei K, Sekine Y, Okamoto F, Hommura S. Measurement of axial length of eyes with incomplete filling of silicone oil in the vitreous cavity using X-ray computed tomography. Br J Ophthalmol. 2002;86(1):47-50.
21. Ghoraba HH, El-Dorghamy AA, Atia AF, Ismail Yassin AEA. The problems of biometry in combined silicone oil removal and cataract extraction: a clinical trial. Retina. 2002;22(5):589-96.
22. El-Baha SM, Hemeida TS. Comparison of refractive outcome using intraoperative biometry and partial coherence interferometry in silicone oil-filled eyes. Retina. 2009;29(1):64-8.
23. Zhang J, Han X, Zhang M, Liu Z, Lin H, Qiu X, et al. Comparison of axial length measurements in silicone oil-filled eyes using SS-OCT and partial coherence interferometry. J Cataract Refract Surg. 2022;48:1375-80.
24. Habibabadi HF, Hashemi H, Jalali KH, Amini A, Esfahani MR. Refractive outcome of silicone oil removal and intraocular lens implantation using laser interferometry. Retina. 2005;25(2):162-6.
25. Murray DC, Durrani OM, Good P, Benson MT, Kirkby GR. Biometry of the silicone oil-filled eye: II. Eye (Lond). 2002;16(6):727-30.
26. Kasturi N, Chakrabarti A. Demystifying intraocular lens power calculation. DJO. 2022;32:69-76.
27. Kunavisarut P, Poopattanakul P, Intarated C, Pathanapitoon K. Accuracy and reliability of IOL master and A-scan immersion biometry in silicone oil-filled eyes. Eye (Lond). 2012;26(10):1344-8.
28. Elbendary AM, Elwan MM. Predicted versus actual intraocular lens power in silicon-oil-filled eyes undergoing cataract extraction using automated intraoperative retinoscopy. Curr Eye Res. 2012;37(8):694-7.
29. Ianchulev T, Salz J, Hoffer K, Albini T, Hsu H, Labree L. Intraoperative optical refractive biometry for intraocular lens power estimation without axial length and keratometry measurements. J Cataract Refract Surg. 2005;31(8):1530-6.
30. Mackool RJ. Intraoperative retinoscopy. J Cataract Refract Surg. 2006;32(4):548-9.
31. Leccisotti A. Intraocular lens calculation by intraoperative autorefraction in myopic eyes. Graefes Arch. Clin. Exp. Ophthalmol. 2008;246:729-33.
32. Kanclerz P, Grzybowski A, Schwartz SG, Lipowski P. Complications of cataract surgery in eyes filled with silicone oil. Eur J Ophthalmol. 2018;28(4):465-8.
33. Hoffer KJ. The Hoffer Q formula: a comparison of theoretic and regression formulas. J Cataract Refract Surg. 1993;19(6):700-12.
34. Suk KK, Smiddy WE, Shi W. Refractive outcomes after silicone oil removal and intraocular lens implantation. Retina. 2013;33(3):634-41.

35. Hou Y, Liu L, Wang G, Xie J, Wang Y. Different lens power calculation formulas for the prediction of refractive outcome after phacoemulsification with silicone oil removal. BMC Ophthalmol. 2022;22:74.
36. Frings A, Dulz S, Skevas C, Stemplewitz B, Linke SJ, Richard G, et al. Postoperative refractive error after phacovitrectomy for epiretinal membrane with and without macular oedema. Graefes Arch Clin Exp Ophthalmol. 2015;253(7):1097-104.
37. Ophir SS, Friehmann A, Rubowitz A. Circumferential silicone sponge scleral buckling induced axial length changes: case series and comparison to literature. Int J Retina Vitreous. 2017;3:10.
38. Lee DH, Han JW, Kim SS, Byeon SH, Koh HJ, Lee SC, et al. Long-term effect of scleral encircling on axial elongation. Am J Ophthalmol. 2018;189:139-45.
39. Gülkilik G, Erdur SK, Özbek M, Özsütcü M, Adabasi M, Demirci G, et al. Changes in anterior chamber depth after combined phacovitrectomy. Turk J Ophthalmol. 2016;46:161-4.
40. Shiraki N, Wakabayashi T, Sakaguchi H, Nishida K. Effect of gas tamponade on the intraocular lens position and refractive error after phacovitrectomy: a swept-source anterior segment OCT analysis. Ophthalmology. 2020;127(4):511-5.
41. Schweitzer KD, García R. Myopic shift after combined phacoemulsification and vitrectomy with gas tamponade. Can J Ophthalmol. 2008;43(5):581-3.
42. Tan X, Zhang J, Zhu Y, Xu J, Qiu X, Yang G, et al. Accuracy of new generation intraocular lens calculation formulas in vitrectomized eyes. Am J Ophthalmol. 2020;217:81-90.
43. Patel AS. IOL power selection for eyes with silicone oil used as vitreous replacement. Abstract #163. Symposium on Cataract and Refractive Surgery, April 1-5, San Diego, California. 1995. p. 41.

CHAPTER

# 8

# Management of Uveitic Cataract

*Mohan Rajan, Arthi Mohankumar, Rakesh K*

## ABSTRACT

Cataract causes significant visual impairment in patients with uveitis. It may also hamper the evaluation of posterior segment by significantly affecting the media clarity. Cataract may occur as the result of prolonged or recurrent episodes of inflammation or due to long-term steroid therapy. Uveitic cataract is frequently complicated by the presence of corneal haze, band-shaped keratopathy, posterior synechiae, iris bombe, fibrin membrane, ocular hypertension, hypotony, and cystoid macular edema (CME). Intraocular lens (IOL) placement is still debated, especially in pediatric uveitis such as juvenile idiopathic arthritis (JIA), and may have to be decided by an individualized approach. Aggressive perioperative inflammation control in these cases using corticosteroids, immunosuppressants and nonsteroidal anti-inflammatory agents, cautious intraoperative maneuvers to reduce the risk of posterior capsular rent and other intraoperative complications, and concurrent management of associated ocular pathologies may help achieve visual gains almost similar to senile cataracts.

***Keywords:*** Uveitic cataract; complicated cataract; posterior subcapsular cataract; posterior synechiae; pediatric uveitic cataract; corticosteroids; immunosuppressants.

## ■ INTRODUCTION

Cataract is the most common cause of decreased vision in uveitis patients accounting up to 40% and contributing to 1.2% of all cataract surgeries.[1] Opacification of the lens is caused either by repeated or sustained intraocular inflammation or by prolonged corticosteroid usage. Cataract surgery in the setting of uveitis may pose a daunting challenge to the surgeon due to a high incidence of intra- and postoperative complications. Nearly one-third of all uveitis patients have small pupil, which necessitates additional intraoperative techniques.[2] Therefore, identifying the cause of uveitis, extent of preexisting damage to ocular structures, control of inflammation before surgery, surgical planning, and solving intra- and postoperative complications are necessary

Management of Uveitic Cataract

**TABLE 1:** Incidence of cataract in various uveitic entities.

| Uveitis | Incidence of cataract |
| --- | --- |
| Fuchs heterochromic iridocyclitis | 15–75% |
| Juvenile idiopathic arthritis | 40–60% |
| Intermediate uveitis | 40–50% |
| Behçet's disease | 21–36% |
| Herpetic uveitis | 20–75% |
| Sarcoidosis | 21% |

to ensure optimal visual recovery post surgery. Various myths revolving around uveitis cataract surgery include absolute contraindication of intraocular lens (IOL) implantation and chronic postoperative inflammation resulting in phthisis bulbi. In recent times, due to better surgical techniques, biocompatible IOLs, perioperative inflammation control, and prompt management of postoperative complications have led to better visual gains comparable to senile cataracts.[3]

## ■ EPIDEMIOLOGY

Uveitic cataracts generally occur in younger individuals. Complicated cataract is common in 50% of patients with anterior and intermediate uveitis and may be seen in up to 80% of patients with Fuchs heterochromic iridocyclitis (FHI). Thirty to thirty-five percent of children with chronic uveitis are found to be having complicated cataract. In juvenile idiopathic arthritis (JIA), the prevalence of cataract is around 40–60%.[4] The incidence of cataract in various uveitic entities is shown in **Table 1**.

## ■ PATHOPHYSIOLOGY

The critical factors in the formation and progression of uveitic cataract include duration, severity, and location of intraocular inflammation, and duration and route of corticosteroid therapy.[5] The cataractous changes usually originate in the posterior cortex and spread axially. This is because the posterior lens capsule is thinner and the epithelial barrier is absent through which the inflammatory cytokines gain access to lens material. Anterior capsular opacification associated with posterior synechiae and fibrin membrane is also not uncommon. Uveitic cataracts may begin as posterior subcapsular cataract and may develop bread crumb appearance or polychromatic luster. The clinical spectrum of uveitic cataracts is shown in **Figures 1A to F**.

# Management of Uveitic Cataract

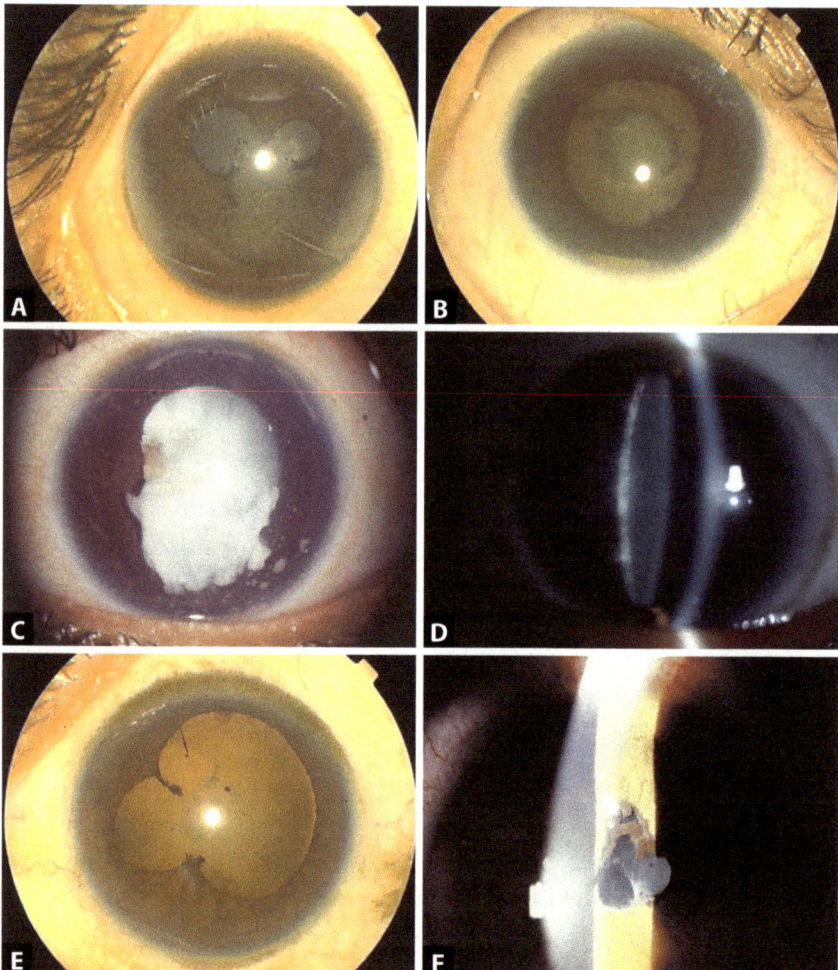

**Figs. 1A to F:** (A) Complicated cataract with posterior synechiae and band-shaped keratopathy; (B) Posterior subcapsular cataract with hypopyon; (C) Total cataract with posterior synechiae and Busacca nodules; (D) Bread crumb appearance of posterior subcapsular cataract; (E) Complicated cataract with posterior synechiae; (F) Seclusio pupillae.

## ■ INDICATIONS FOR CATARACT SURGERY

Common indications for cataract surgery in uveitis are mentioned below.[6] They include:
- Active inflammation secondary to leakage of lens proteins, i.e., phacoantigenic uveitis
- Visually significant cataract with good inflammation control
- Cataract impairing the assessment of posterior segment and treatment of fundus pathologies

- Cataract impairing posterior segment visualization in patients requiring posterior segment surgery when cataract surgery is combined with pars plana vitrectomy.

## ■ PREOPERATIVE EVALUATION

Meticulous ophthalmic and systemic evaluation preoperatively aids in planning surgery, minimizing postoperative complications, and prognosticating the patient. A patient with active inflammation is not suitable for cataract surgery because of a higher incidence of postoperative complications. A quiet eye for the past 3 months is a basic requirement for surgery for uveitic cataract and this period may be longer up to 12 months, especially in patients suffering from Behçet's disease.[7] On examination, chronic vitreous cells, choroidal detachment, lower intraocular pressure (IOP), band-shaped keratopathy, macular changes, and optic nerve atrophy may indicate a guarded postoperative visual prognosis. Management of IOP fluctuations, glaucoma, and hypotony, associated with inflammation should be treated appropriately.[8] B-scan ultrasonography (USG) is a very useful tool in the assessment of posterior segment in the presence of vitreous haze, retinal detachment, and choroidal detachments. Potential acuity meter and laser interferometer can be useful to assess the visual potential in uveitic cataract.

*Prerequisites for uveitic cataract surgery*
- Quiet eye for the past 3 months
- Preoperative steroids for inflammation control
- *Systemic investigations:* Blood sugar, blood pressure, liver function test (for patients on immunosuppressants)
- *Ocular investigations:* Potential acuity meter, optical coherence tomography, B-scan USG, electroretinogram

## ■ PREOPERATIVE CONTROL OF INFLAMMATION

The key to surgical success in patients with uveitic cataract is the absolute control of inflammation. Active uveitis during the time of cataract surgery has been associated with poor visual outcomes due to increased incidence of inflammatory episodes and postoperative complications.[2] In FHI, minimal but persistent anterior chamber cells and flare are frequently seen despite intensive treatment. Lesser than 10 cells per slit lamp field for >8 weeks is desirable for intraocular surgery. A steroid regimen for preoperative inflammation control depends specifically on the type and etiology of uveitis. For uncomplicated anterior uveitis such as Fuchs uveitis, prednisolone acetate 1% six times a day initiated a week before surgery is sufficient to avoid an outburst of postoperative inflammation. Oral steroids may be required in cases such as JIA, anterior granulomatous iridocyclitis, intermediate uveitis, posterior and panuveitis. Oral prednisolone (1 mg/kg/day) is usually started 1-2 weeks prior to surgery, continued for a week after surgery, and then tapered slowly. Subtenon injection of triamcinolone acetate and intravitreal dexamethasone implants have also shown to be effective alternatives in patients in whom systemic steroid therapy cannot be tolerated.[9,10] Patients who are on immunosuppressive therapy and biologics should continue the current dosage. The use of topical nonsteroidal anti-inflammatory drugs (NSAIDs) such as ketorolac 0.4% and nepafenac 0.15% have become standard of practice for perioperative management of inflammation, pain, surgically induced miosis, and cystoid macular edema (CME). In cases such as herpetic uveitis, prophylactic antiviral therapy with acyclovir or valacyclovir should be considered at least 1 week before surgery in order to avoid remission of viral infection. Reactivation of toxoplasmosis is also common postoperatively and needs administration of antibiotics perioperatively.[11] Cataract and glaucoma coexist as uveitis complication and a combined surgical procedure may be associated with an increased risk of failure. Posterior vitrectomy and cataract extraction may be an alternative for patients with posterior segment pathology such as vitreous opacities, vitreous hemorrhage, tractional retinal detachment, epiretinal membranes, and macular hole.

*Challenges in uveitic cataract surgery*
- Decompensated cornea, band-shaped keratopathy
- Pupil—posterior synechiae, fibrin membrane, occlusio pupillae, iris bombe
- Fragile iris vessels
- Cyclitic membrane
- Anterior capsule calcification
- Posterior capsule plaque
- Intraocular pressure fluctuations—raised IOP or hypotony

## ■ SURGICAL TECHNIQUES

Various challenges are faced while operating uveitic cataracts. The visualization of cataract and its access are challenging due to band-shaped keratopathy, miotic pupil, posterior synechiae, pupillary membrane, and calcified anterior capsule. Phacoemulsification with IOL is preferred over extracapsular cataract extraction (ECCE).[12] Conventional procedures of cataract extraction such as ECCE may require a larger incision and, hence, are associated with intense inflammation; however, this procedure is inevitable in patients with dense brown cataracts. Studies have shown decreased incidence of clinically significant inflammation requiring treatment in phacoemulsification as compared to ECCE as well as a decreased rate of postoperative CME, epiretinal membrane formation, and posterior synechiae formation. Intraoperative complications such as corneal stromal edema, hyphema, pigment dispersion, and posterior capsule rupture with vitreous loss occur in increased frequency and have to be anticipated and managed accordingly.[13]

## PUPIL MANAGEMENT

### Posterior Synechiolysis and Peripupillary Membranectomy

Posterior synechiae can severely limit pupillary dilation and often require lysis intraoperatively if they do not respond to pharmacological mydriasis. Synechiolysis is best performed by placing a viscoelastic cannula or iris spatula underneath the openings in the pupillary margin and sweeping laterally to free adhesions. Viscodissection can also be done using a high molecular weight cohesive expansive viscoelastic. In patients with previous uveitis, a thick fibrotic peripupillary membrane can get formed alongside synechiae and cause adhesions between the iris and the lens. This membrane may often be peeled away using intraocular or capsulorhexis forceps.[14]

### Small Pupil

Bimanual pupil stretching (stretch pupilloplasty) using hooks or choppers to pull the pupillary border in opposite directions is a relatively quick means of mechanically enhancing dilation. However, this technique creates microtears in sphincter pupillae muscle but tends to preserve more sphincter tissue and is, therefore, more cosmetically appealing than sphincterotomies. Self-retaining iris hooks are another effective way of maintaining a dilated pupil intraoperatively. Pupil expansion rings are devices placed on the pupillary margin and intended to maintain pupil throughout the surgical procedure.[15] Various pupil-enlarging devices are shown in **Figures 2A to C**.

## CHOICE OF INTRAOCULAR LENS

Intraocular lens implantation can be done during primary cataract extraction or it may be deferred and planned as a separate procedure in patients in whom excessive postoperative inflammation is anticipated. In-the-bag IOL, implantation is ideal in uveitic patients. In case of posterior capsular rupture (PCR) or zonular dehiscence, scleral fixated IOLs may be the best approach. Sulcus-placed IOLs are relatively contraindicated in uveitic cataract as haptics may erode the iris and cause persistent inflammation and can even result in optic capture. Iris-fixated and anterior chamber IOLs are contraindicated due to the increased risk of inflammation conferred by them. Acrylic lenses have a lower rate of inflammation and relapse rate when compared to other lens materials. Heparin surface modified (HSM) poly(methyl methacrylate) (PMMA) IOLs are preferred as they are associated with lesser anterior chamber flare and IOL surface deposits. Acrylic and HSM PMMA IOLs are associated with reduced chances of posterior synechiae

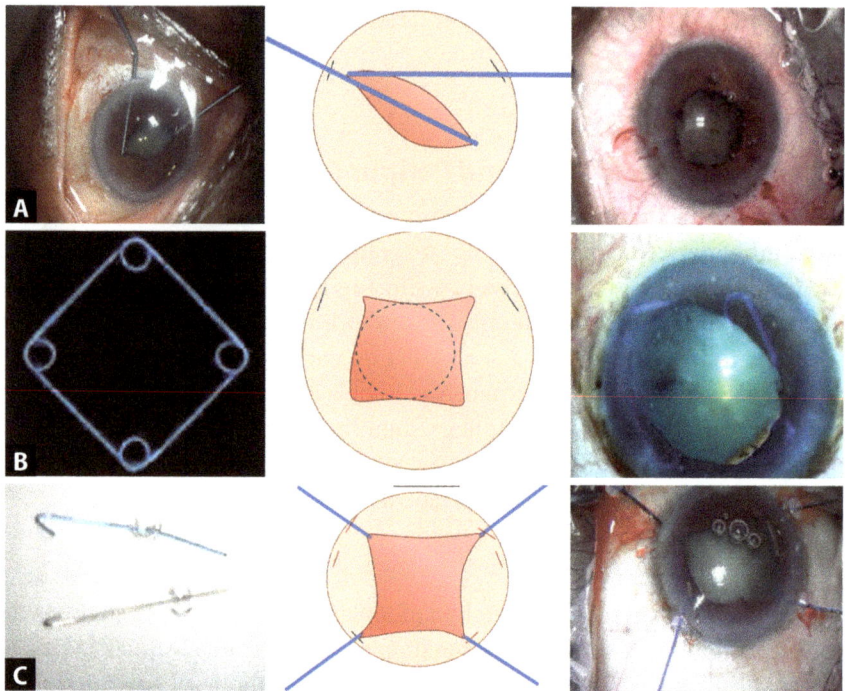

**Figs. 2A to C:** (A) Stretch pupilloplasty—illustration demonstrates the technique and figure on the right indicates pupil size post procedure; (B) Malyugin ring—figure on the left shows intraoperative appearance of Malyugin ring; (C) Self-retaining iris hooks—figure on the right shows intraoperative positioning of iris hooks.

formation and recurrent inflammation.[16,17] IOLs with sharp edges may reduce the incidence of posterior capsular opacification. Silicone IOLs are relatively contraindicated as they are associated with a slightly higher incidence of inflammation and considering the possibility that some uveitic patients may need a vitreoretinal surgical procedure in future with silicone oil injection.

*Tips and tricks for uveitic cataract surgery*
- Use of pupil-expanding devices—iris hooks and pupil-expanding rings
- Good capsulorhexis
- Adequate hydrodissection
- Thorough cortical cleanup
- Avoid posterior capsular rupture
- Use of heparin surface-modified PMMA IOLs/foldable hydrophobic acrylic IOLs

## ■ POSTOPERATIVE OUTCOME

Cataracts associated with FHI have good visual prognosis when compared to other causes of anterior uveitis. Behçet's disease-associated cataract has a poor prognosis. The common causes of decreased vision in these patients are postoperative macular edema, occurring due to severe inflammation,

**TABLE 2:** Surgical expectations in different uveitic entities.

| Type of uveitis | Projected outcome |
| --- | --- |
| Fuchs iridocyclitis, HLA-B27 uveitis | Fairly good without much postoperative inflammation |
| Pars planitis | Guarded visual prognosis; postoperative inflammation; possible CME or rise in IOP |
| Sarcoidosis | Guarded visual prognosis; postoperative inflammation, posterior uveitis, possible CME or rise in IOP |
| Juvenile rheumatoid arthritis | Guarded visual prognosis; postoperative inflammation, possible CME, rise in IOP or cyclitic membrane formation, challenges in IOL implantation may result in phthisis |

(CME: cystoid macular edema; HLA: human leukocyte antigen; IOL: intraocular lens; IOP: intraocular pressure)

and preexisting conditions such as optic atrophy and epiretinal membrane **(Table 2)**. Aggressive topical steroid therapy along with systemic steroids or immunosuppressants may help tackle postoperative flare-up of inflammation and associated complications **(Figs. 3A to F)**. These patients need a slow tapering of steroids over 2–4 weeks. Frequent postoperative follow-ups may help in early identification of postoperative complications.[17]

## ■ POSTOPERATIVE COMPLICATIONS

A number of postoperative complications are reported in the literature after uveitic cataract extraction.[18-21] The commonly encountered complications that may affect the visual outcome after cataract surgery are described below.

### Postoperative Inflammation

Postoperative flare-up of inflammation is of utmost concern in patients undergoing uveitic cataract extraction. Patients may have to be maintained on a higher dose of systemic and topical steroids compared to their preoperative doses with slow tapering over 12 weeks. This may be augmented by supplementing with subtenon triamcinolone acetonide injection and intravitreal dexamethasone implant wherever indicated, but increase in IOP is a concern with these alternatives. Rapid tapering and inadequate dosing of steroids may cause increased inflammation and its associated complications. Systemic immunosuppressive drugs are continued in the preoperative doses and usually not altered. Topical and oral NSAIDs may also help to some extent to control the inflammation **(Figs. 4A to D)**.

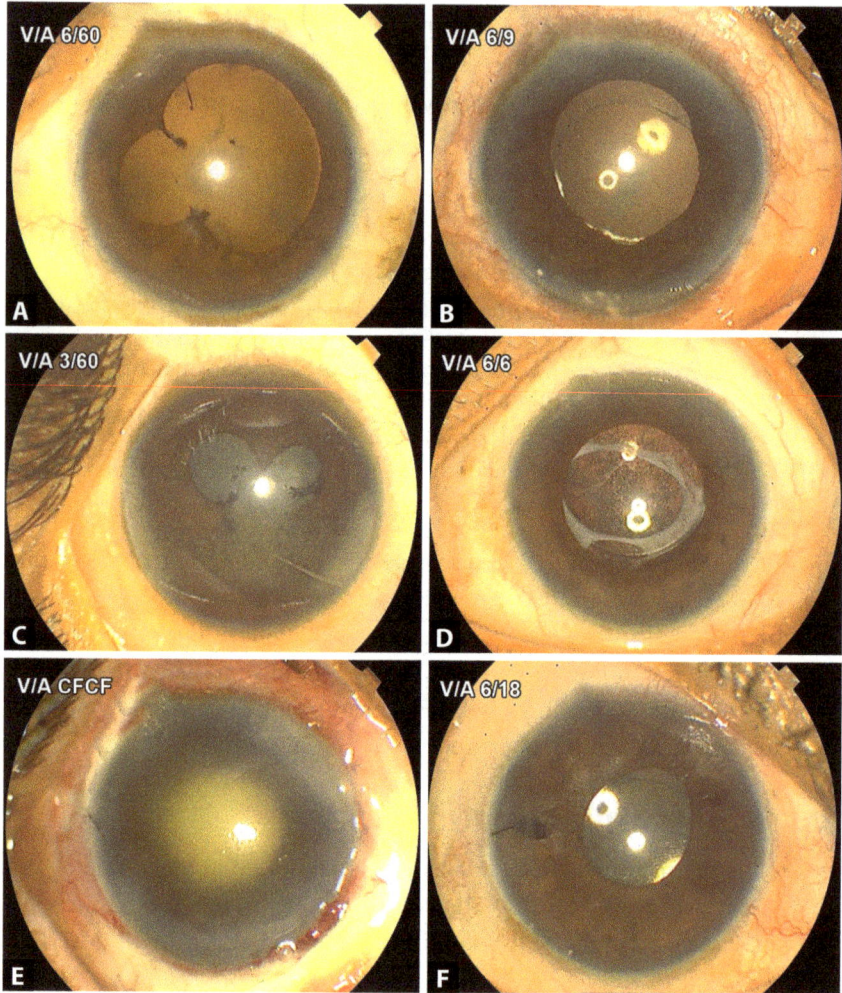

**Figs. 3A to F:** Preoperative appearance and postoperative outcome with visual acuity in uveitis. (CFCF: counting of fingers close to face; V/A: visual acuity)

## Elevated Intraocular Pressure

Raised IOP post-uveitic cataract extraction could be due to both open-angle and angle-closure mechanisms. Inflammatory glaucoma occurs because of blockage of a trabecular meshwork by inflammatory cells, fibrin, debris, and red blood cells (RBCs). Pupillary block may result from 360° synechiae and fibrin membrane formation. IOP control is achieved by inflammation control and topical antiglaucoma medications. Surgical interventions such as trabeculectomy and glaucoma drainage devices are indicated in cases of refractory and neovascular glaucoma.

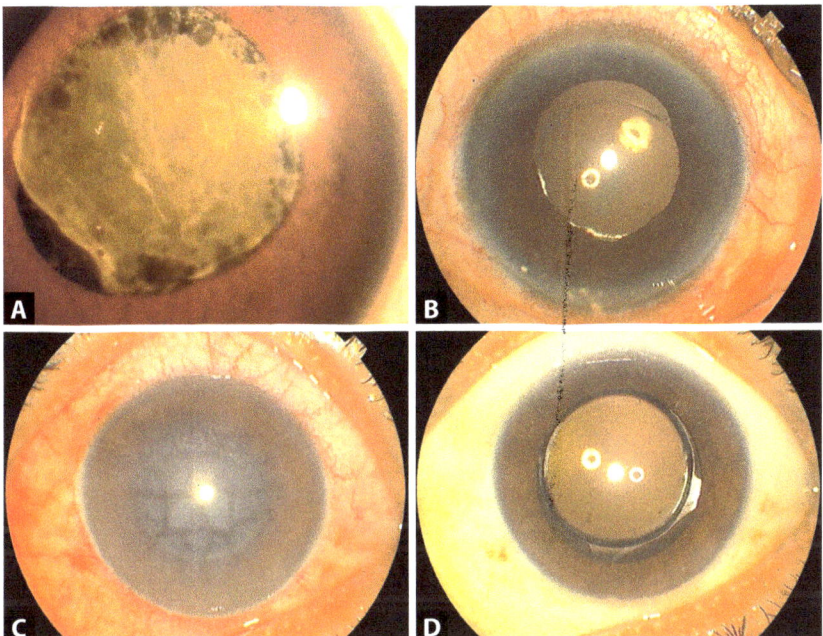

**Figs. 4A to D:** (A) Patient with fibrin membrane post-uveitic cataract extraction; (B) Complete resolution of fibrin membrane following aggressive steroid treatment; (C) Striate keratopathy post-cataract extraction in a uveitic patient; (D) Clear cornea post treatment.

## Hypotony

Ocular hypotony may occur due to either wound leak or intraocular inflammation, causing cyclitic membrane formation or ciliary dysfunction. Intraoperative suturing of all surgical wounds is recommended to avoid wound leak. Adequate inflammation control may help combat hypotony. Persistent hypotony mostly culminates in phthisis bulbi and silicone oil injection may be required for reattachment of ciliary body and countering phthisis.

## Posterior Capsule Opacification

Posterior capsule opacification (PCO) formation is one of the common postoperative complications in uveitic cataracts. Its incidence ranges from 23 to 96% as mentioned in different studies. PCO, if visually disturbing, can be treated by neodymium-doped yttrium aluminum garnet (Nd:YAG) laser capsulotomy with adequate inflammation control.

## Cystoid Macular Edema

Cystoid macular edema is another sight-threatening complication of uveitic cataract surgery. Its incidence ranges between 21 and 50%. Treatment

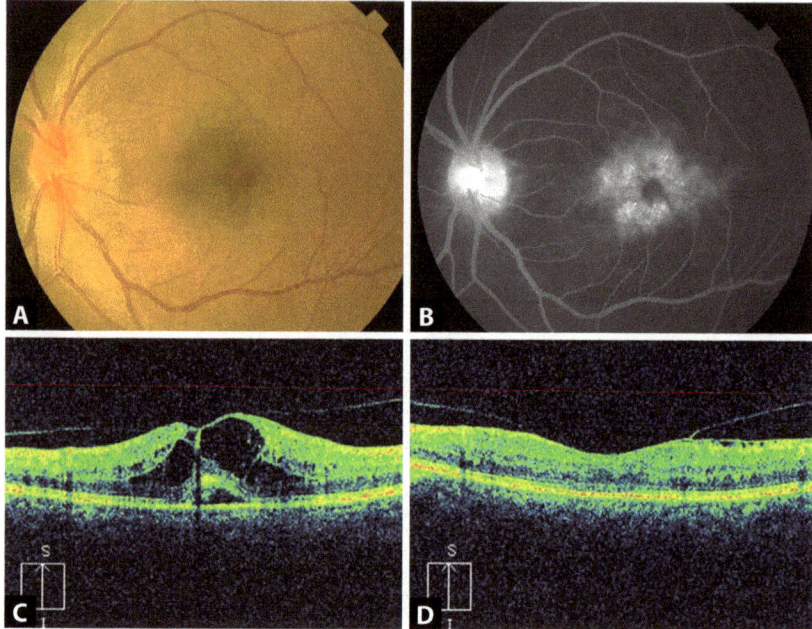

**Figs. 5A to D:** (A) Cystoid macular edema (CME) post-cataract surgery in uveitis; (B) Petaloid leakage in fundus fluorescein angiography (FFA); (C) Optical coherence tomography (OCT) macula shows CME with predominantly cysts in outer nuclear layer; (D) Resolution of CME post-treatment with intravitreal injection Ozurdex.

of postoperative CME includes topical NSAIDs and steroids. Intravitreal and orbital floor triamcinolone acetonide can also be given. A sustained drug delivery implant could provide long-term benefits with control of inflammation **(Figs. 5A to D)**.

*Spectrum of postoperative complications expected in uveitic cataract surgery*
- Flare-up of the uveitis
- IOP increase—steroid responders, neovascular glaucoma, refractory glaucoma
- Corneal edema—endothelial decompensation
- Pupillary capture of implant
- Posterior capsular opacification
- Cystoid macular edema
- Exudative retinal detachment
- Choroidal detachment
- Cyclitic membrane, chronic hypotony, and phthisis bulbi

## ■ PEDIATRIC UVEITIC CATARACT SURGERY

Management of pediatric uveitic cataracts is challenging with IOL implantation being still more controversial. The timing of surgery is of utmost importance in children with uveitic cataract due to concerns of amblyopia. The most common cause of pediatric uveitic cataract is JIA where the children are antinuclear antibody positive.[22] Other causes include sarcoidosis, tuberculosis, pars planitis, toxoplasmosis, and toxocariasis along with prolonged steroid treatment for the control of inflammation. Though various studies have shown good visual outcomes following IOL implantation in a subgroup of pediatric uveitis, children with JIA may have suboptimal visual outcomes due to unrelenting postoperative inflammation and associated complications.[23] Factors such as age of the child at the time of surgical intervention, preexisting amblyopia, nature of underlying uveitis, baseline visual acuity, and current therapeutic regimen must be considered before planning cataract surgery in pediatric uveitis. Postoperative course may be complicated by pathologies such as band-shaped keratopathy, glaucoma, rubeosis, cyclitic membranes, hypotony, and phthisis. CME and epiretinal membrane formation may lead to reduced visual gains even in children with low-grade inflammation. Hence, IOL implantation cannot be generalized in pediatric uveitis cataracts and may have to be decided based on an individualized approach.[24]

## ■ CONCLUSION

Visual outcome post-uveitic cataract surgery does not only depend on excellent preoperative care, surgery, and postoperative control of inflammation but also depends on the type of uveitis the patient has. Cataract surgery in uveitis patients requires extensive diagnostic evaluation to determine the cause of uveitis, proper patient selection, zero tolerance to preoperative inflammation, vigilant use of immunomodulatory drugs wherever necessary to control the preoperative inflammation, meticulous surgery, thoughtful decision for implantation of IOL, and early detection and aggressive management of complications.

*Pearls in the management of uveitic cataract*
- Thorough evaluation of basic uveitic pathology
- Operate on a quiet eye
- Corticosteroids—mainstay in the management of preoperative and postoperative inflammation and related complications
- Phacoemulsification with in-the-bag hydrophobic acrylic foldable IOL for the best possible outcome
- Minimal surgical manipulation
- Aggressive management of postoperative inflammation
- Anticipate the worst and be equipped to avoid/manage complications
- Children with uveitic cataracts may need a staged procedure

## ■ REFERENCES

1. Chan NSW, Ti SE, Chee SP. Decision-making and management of uveitic cataract. Indian J Ophthalmol. 2017;65:1329-39.

2. Chen JL, Bhat P, Lobo-Chan AM. Perioperative management of uveitic cataracts. Adv Ophthalmol Optom. 2019;4:325-39.
3. Agrawal R, Murthy S, Ganesh SK, Phaik CS, Sangwan V, Biswas J. Cataract surgery in uveitis. Int J Inflam. 2012;2012:548453.
4. Nicholson BP, Zhou M, Rostamizadeh M, Mehta P, Agrón E, Wong W, et al. Epidemiology of epiretinal membrane in a large cohort of patients with uveitis. Ophthalmology. 2014;121:2393-8.
5. Jancevski M, Foster CS. Cataracts and uveitis. Curr Opin Ophthalmol. 2010;21(1):10-4.
6. Pålsson S, Andersson Grönlund M, Skiljic D, Zetterberg M. Phacoemulsification with primary implantation of an intraocular lens in patients with uveitis. Clin Ophthalmol. 2017;11:1549-55.
7. Bhargava R, Kumar P, Bashir H, Sharma SK, Mishra A. Manual suture less small incision cataract surgery in patients with uveitic cataract. Middle East Afr J Ophthalmol. 2014;2:77-82.
8. Chu CJ, Dick AD, Johnston RL, Yang YC, Denniston AK, UK Pseudophakic Macular Edema Study Group. Cataract surgery in uveitis: a multicentre database study. Br J Ophthalmol. 2017;101:1132-7.
9. Ren Y, Du S, Zheng D, Shi Y, Pan L, Yan H. Intraoperative intravitreal triamcinolone acetonide injection for prevention of postoperative inflammation and complications after phacoemulsification in patients with uveitic cataract. BMC Ophthalmol. 2021;21:245.
10. Sudhalkar A, Vasavada A, Bhojwani D, Vasavada V, Vasavada S, Vasavada V, et al. Intravitreal dexamethasone implant as an alternative to systemic steroids as prophylaxis for uveitic cataract surgery: a randomized trial. Eye (Lond). 2020;34:491-8.
11. Mora P, Gonzales S, Ghirardini S, Rubino P, Orsoni JG, Gandolfi SA, et al. Perioperative prophylaxis to prevent recurrence following cataract surgery in uveitic patients: a two-centre, prospective, randomized trial. Acta Ophthalmol. 2016;94:e390-4.
12. Bhargava R, Kumar P, Sharma SK, Kumar M, Kaur A. Phacoemulsification versus small incision cataract surgery in patients with uveitis. Int J Ophthalmol. 2015;8:965-70.
13. Jinagal J, Gupta G, Agarwal A, Aggarwal K, Akella M, Gupta V, et al. Safety and efficacy of dexamethasone implant along with phacoemulsification and intraocular lens implantation in children with juvenile idiopathic arthritis associated uveitis. Indian J Ophthalmol. 2019;67:69-74.
14. Chakraborty D, Mohanta A, Bhaumik A. B-HEX pupil expander in vitreoretinal surgery—a case series. Indian J Ophthalmol. 2020;68:1188-91.
15. Uy HS, Cruz FM, Kenyon KR. Efficacy of a hinged pupil expansion device in small pupil cataract surgery. Indian J Ophthalmol. 2021;69:2688-93.
16. Leung TG, Lindsley K, Kuo IC. Types of intraocular lenses for cataract surgery in eyes with uveitis. Cochrane Database Syst Rev. 2014;3:CD007284.
17. Süllü Y, Oge I, Erkan D. The results of cataract extraction and intraocular lens implantation in patients with Behçet's disease. Acta Ophthalmol Scand. 2000;78:680-3.
18. Shaw E, Patel BC. Complicated cataract. StatPearls [Internet]. Treasure Island, FL: StatPearls Publishing; 2022.

19. Macarie SS, Macarie DM. Phacoemulsification in adult patients with post-uveitis complicated cataract. Rom J Ophthalmol. 2018;62:135-7.
20. Zhang Y, Zhu X, He W, Jiang Y, Lu Y. Efficacy of cataract surgery in patients with uveitis: a STROBE-compliant article. Medicine (Baltimore). 2017;96:e7353.
21. Hazari A, Sangwan VS. Cataract surgery in uveitis. Indian J Ophthalmol. 2002;50:103-7.
22. Schmidt DC, Al-Bakri M, Rasul A, Bangsgaard R, Subhi Y, Bach-Holm D, et al. Cataract surgery with or without intraocular lens implantation in pediatric uveitis: a systematic review with meta-analyses. J Ophthalmol. 2021;2021: 5481609.
23. Clarke SL, Sen ES, Ramanan AV. Juvenile idiopathic arthritis-associated uveitis. Pediatr Rheumatol Online J. 2016;14:27.
24. Jancevski M, Foster CS. Cataracts and uveitis. Discov Med. 2010;9(44):51-4.

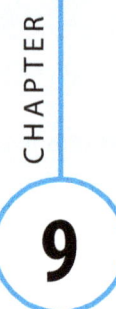

# Artificial Intelligence in Diabetic Retinopathy

*Payal Naresh Shah, Divyansh Kailashchandra Mishra, Mahesh Shanmugam Palanivelu*

## ABSTRACT

With increasing burden of diabetes, the burden of screening for diabetic retinopathy (DR) has also become very high. Since early detection and routine screening can prevent progression to sight-threatening blindness from DR, a lot of emphasis on automated screening is being laid. While technology to capture fundus color photographs (CP) has evolved from bulky fundus cameras to portable handheld and smartphone-based cameras, automated detection methods of DR based on various machine learning (ML) and artificial intelligence (AI) based systems are developing.

This chapter explains the basic terminology which helps to understand AI and how AI helps to screen, diagnose, and predict treatment outcomes in DR along with a brief review on existing literature.

***Keywords:*** Artificial intelligence; diabetic retinopathy; machine learning in diabetic retinopathy; deep learning in diabetic retinopathy.

## ■ INTRODUCTION

With increasing burden of diabetes, diabetic retinopathy (DR) is also on the rise. The global prevalence of DR among diabetics is 22.7% and of vision-threatening diabetic retinopathy (VTDR) is 6.7%.[1] China and India have the highest number of diabetic population; hence, the burden of screening also remains very high.[2]

## ■ DIABETIC RETINOPATHY SCREENING

The major causes of vision loss in DR include diabetic macular edema (DME), preretinal hemorrhage involving the macula, vitreous hemorrhage (VH), and retinal detachment (RD). Based on the Early Treatment Diabetic Retinopathy Study (ETDRS) study, the progression of eyes from severe nonproliferative diabetic retinopathy (NPDR) to proliferative diabetic retinopathy (PDR) and high-risk PDR (HR-PDR) is 50 and 17%, respectively, within 1 year and 71 and 44% within 3 years.[3] Also, unless a patient develops DME or PDR, the patient may remain asymptomatic despite the disease being silently progressive.

Hence, a periodic retina screening is necessary to identify the disease at an early stage and manage appropriately.

## Challenges Faced in Diabetic Retinopathy Screening

These challenges can be broadly classified into patient related and system related. *Patient-related challenges* include lack of awareness and economic constraints for periodic follow-up.

*System-related challenges* are screening burden on the healthcare professionals, lack of trained retina specialists, lack of trained paramedical staff to capture fundus color photographs (CP), poor image quality for telescreening, lack of access to fundus cameras, and limited motivation among treating physicians/diabetologists to refer patients for routine fundoscopy. As a result, the majority of patients end up presenting in the late stages.

## Evolution of Diabetic Retinopathy Screening

Apart from routine ophthalmoscopy performed by ophthalmologists, optometrists and paramedical staff are being trained to diagnose DR. With the increasing burden of diabetes and screening, a paradigm shift has been noted from a seven-field stereoscopic FP-based classification system to single-field nonmydriatic fundus camera and smartphone-based photographs.[4-7] Today, there are various adapters available to fix to the smartphone to convert them into fundus cameras.[8]

While technology to capture FP has evolved from bulky fundus cameras to portable handheld and smartphone-based cameras, ways of detection of DR have also evolved tremendously from manual grading systems to automated detection systems and further into machine learning (ML) and artificial intelligence (AI) based identification systems. Thus, the integration between newer cameras and newer software technologies is now enabling us to screen DR in more efficient ways. AI-based solutions are built in with fundus cameras, for example, EyeArt™, Medios DR app on Remidio™ fundus on phone camera, and Aurora IQ™ handheld fundus camera by Optomed technologies.[9,10]

The main focus of this chapter is to understand the application of AI to identify DR.

## ■ UNDERSTANDING THE TERMINOLOGY

*Artificial intelligence:* It is the ability of a computer program or a machine to think like humans.

*Machine learning:* It is a subfield of AI enabling the computer/machine to learn from examples without being explicitly programmed. However, the algorithms require human supervision to improvise the predictions or feature extraction.

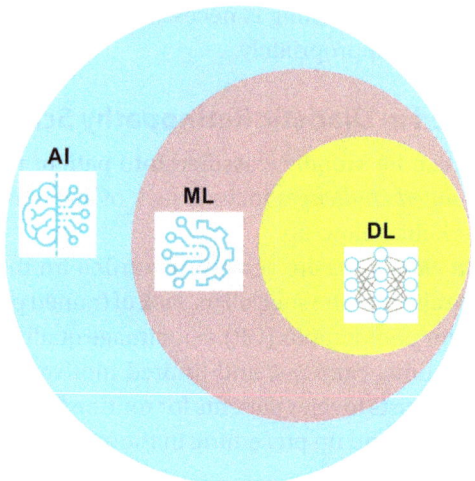

**Fig. 1:** Artificial intelligence (AI) and its subclasses.
(DL: deep learning; ML: machine learning)

*Deep learning (DL):* It is a specialized subfield of ML, enabling the computer/machine to learn by itself using neural networks. The algorithm can determine by itself whether the prediction is accurate or not and improvise by itself without any human interference **(Fig. 1)**.

*Ensemble ML:* Ensemble methods use multiple learning algorithms to obtain better predictive performance by combining various models.

*Computer vision:* It is a subfield of AI that enables computers to understand/extract meaningful data from digital images.

*Data training set:* It includes the set of images used as input to train the model.

*Validation sets:* They are classified into internal and external validation. *Internal validation* involves splitting the input data initially into a training set and a test set. The training set is used to train the model, while the test set is used to check the accuracy of the model once it has been trained.

*External validation* uses the entire input data for model training, and the validation is done using an independently derived dataset(s) **(Flowchart 1)**.

*Overfitting:* When a model performs very well for training data but has poor performance with test or new data, it is known as *overfitting*.

*Ground truth:* The annotation/labeling done by humans (ophthalmologists in this case) to train the input data is called *ground truth*.

*Layers:* A layer is a network that usually receives weighted input, transforms it with a set of mathematical functions, and then passes these values as output to the next layer. In general, the more the number of layers or the deeper that

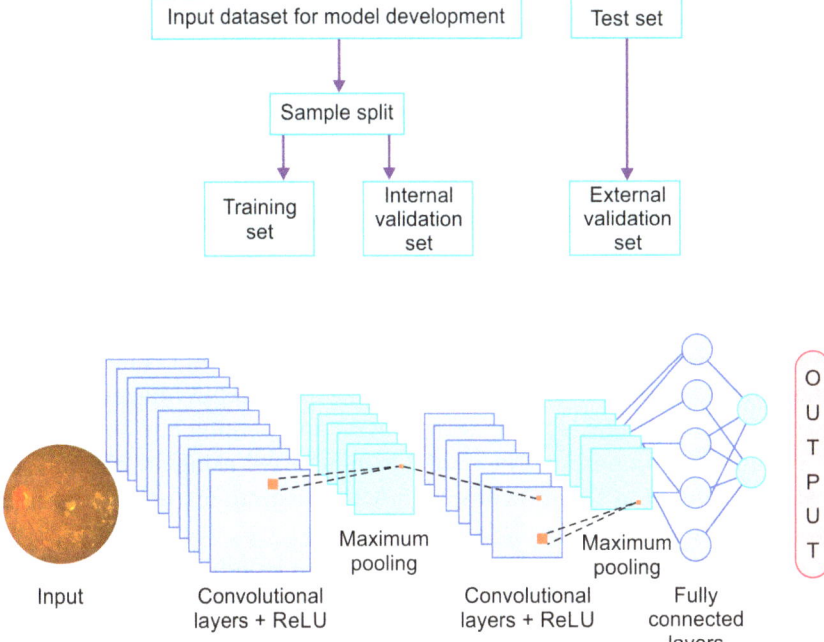

**Flowchart 1:** Various data models used in artificial intelligence (AI).

**Fig. 2:** Working of deep convolutional neural networks (CNN).
(ReLU: rectified linear unit)

you go, the more specific or specialized is the feature extraction. Layers are also known as *kernels*.

*Convolutional neural networks (CNN):* It is the mathematical specialized operation called *convolution* that operates between the various layers of a neural network, which gives the name CNN.

*Max pooling:* A pooling layer is a new layer added after the convolutional layer. It reduces the size of each feature map and thus reduces the computational overload. Also, with max pooling, the most activated pixels or predominant features are preserved while discarding the lower valued pixels or minor features, thus reducing overfitting **(Fig. 2)**.

*Black box phenomenon:* In deep neural networks, sometimes we do not know how all the individual neurons work together to arrive at the final output. This is called a *black box phenomenon*, which is one of the limitations of AI.

*Downsampling the majority class and upsampling the minority class:* These techniques are used when there is class imbalance in the training set; for example, a majority of data has normal features while a small minority has positive or disease features. Hence, for effective training, the majority class is downsampled and the minority class is upsampled to train for positive features.

Some of the examples of deep network architectures used are LeNet, AlexNet, VGGNet, Inception v3, Inception v4, ResNet, DenseNet, SENet, ReLAy Net, GoogLeNet, MobileNet, and U-Net.

Although ML approaches involve supervised and unsupervised training, most often, the application of these models in retinal imaging involves supervised training where the input data is annotated or labeled and supplied as a ground truth.[11]

## ■ HOW DOES ARTIFICIAL INTELLIGENCE WORK?

A training set of images is fed into the computer as input. Now a series of mathematical operations are performed over these input images to extract features from various layers by convolution and pooling and thus classify them and give an output. The model is then tested using an internal and external validation set and compared with the ground truth to assess its performance.

While some AI models have been trained to identify any DR, some are trained for referrable DR, and some others are trained to classify sight-threatening DR (STDR). The input datasets used in these models are also immensely varied. Several datasets such as EyePACS, MESSIDOR, MESSIDOR-2, DIARETDB0, DIARETDB1, Singapore Eye Research Institute (SERI), and Kermany et al.'s datasets[12] are already available online which can be used to train the AI models. Alternatively, one can also use institutional datasets to train the AI.[13]

## ■ FACTORS TO CONSIDER ABOUT AN ARTIFICIAL INTELLIGENCE MODEL FOR DIABETIC RETINOPATHY

Since AI helps as a screening tool to identify DR, a good balance between high sensitivity and specificity will help to make the screening programs cost-effective. The robustness of any AI model depends mainly on its training dataset.
- The training set should be large and widely variable, i.e., images collected from various fundus cameras. Images should also be trained to distinguish between gradable and nongradable images.
- Variable or different sources of external validation set, so as to know that the model actually generalizes to a varied population.
- The training dataset should be annotated by multiple graders in order to improve the robustness and performance of the system.
- The performance of the model is assessed based on the sensitivity, specificity, receiver operating characteristic (ROC) curve, and area under the ROC (AUROC) curve.

- Other parameters which are often used are accuracy, precision, recall, and F-measure/F1-score, which combines both precision and recall into a single measure.

Accuracy = [True positive (TP) + True negative (TN)]/[True positive + True negative + False positive (FP) + False negative (FN)] OR
Number of correct predictions/Total number of predictions
Precision = TP/(TP + FP)
Also called *positive predictive value*
Recall = TP/(TP + FN)
F-Measure = (2 × Precision × Recall)/(Precision + Recall)

## ARTIFICIAL INTELLIGENCE IN IDENTIFYING DIABETIC RETINOPATHY FROM FUNDUS COLOR PHOTOGRAPHS

There are so far several robust models developed to identify DR from FP. Abràmoff et al. implemented one of the earliest DL models called IDx-DR, which achieved an area under the curve (AUC) of 0.980, a sensitivity of 96.8%, and a specificity of 87.0%. This is the first Food and Drug Administration (FDA)-approved AI-based medical device which is commercially available for DR screening.[14,15]

The second FDA-approved AI-based DR detection system, i.e., the EyeArt system, developed by Eyenuk™, reported a sensitivity of 95.5%, specificity of 87.8%, and imageability rate of 97.7% for referrable DR and a sensitivity and specificity of 96 and 88%, respectively, for STDR.[16]

Gulshan et al. from Google AI Healthcare™ developed a model using multiple datasets, which had an AUROC curve of 0.991 for detecting referrable DR and a sensitivity of 97% with a specificity of 93%.[17]

Another large-scale study from Singapore by Ting et al. demonstrated an AUC, sensitivity, and specificity of 0.936, 90.5%, and 91.6%, respectively, achieving reliable diagnosis in multiple ethnic groups.[18] A further validation study of this model conducted in the African population showed a sensitivity of 99.42% for STDR and 97.19% for DME.[19] The Singapore Eye Lesion Analyser Plus (SELENA+) AI model is now not only used as a nationwide screening tool in Singapore but also has received approval for clinical use in the European Union and has the ability to screen for DR, age-related macular degeneration, and glaucoma.

We have also validated a DL model, Netra.AI, developed by Leben Care Technologies™ and reported an overall sensitivity and specificity of 99.7 and 98.5%, respectively, for any DR detection and 98.9 and 94.84%, respectively, for referrable DR with an AUC of 0.991 and 0.969 for any DR detection and referrable DR, respectively **(Fig. 3)**.[20]

Another DL model, Medios™, which is integrated with Remidio™ and Intuvision™ smartphone-based fundus cameras, has shown a sensitivity

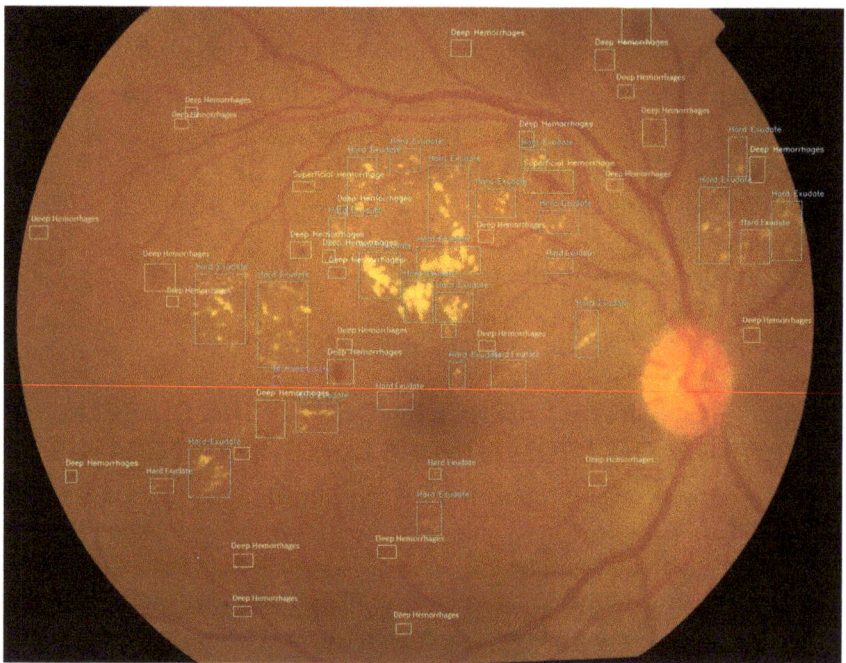

**Fig. 3:** Example of annotation of diabetic retinopathy (DR) lesions by a convolutional neural networks (CNN) model.

and specificity of 99 and 88%, respectively, with an AUC of 0.92 to detect referrable DR.[21,22]

Today, there are several companies across the world who have developed and validated various DL models to identify DR from color FP. Some of them are OphtAI, AEye, AirDoc, Cognizant, D-EYE, Diagnos, DreamUp Vision, Eyenuk, Google, IDx-DR, Intelligent Retinal Imaging Systems, Medios Technologies, Microsoft Corporation, Retina-AI Health, RetinAI Medical, RetinaLyze System, Retmarker, SERI, SigTuple Technologies, Spect, VisionQuest Biomedical, Leben Care Technologies, and Xtend.AI.

A brief summary of various DL models based on FP to identify DR is shown in **Table 1**. Although there is no head-to-head study to compare one DL model with the other, most models have shown overall good sensitivity to the use of AI as an efficient DR screening tool.[23] Yet, in real-world setting, a multicenter study comparing seven DL algorithms from five AI companies showed that AI showed low positive predictive value as compared with the human teleretinal grades.[24] Three out of seven algorithms showed comparable sensitivity and one out of seven comparable specificities to the teleretinal graders. This emphasizes the need for more external validation of the AI models to make them more robust.

**TABLE 1:** Comparison of various color fundus photograph-based artificial intelligence (AI) models.

| Authors and year of publication | Validation dataset | Sensitivity | Specificity | AUC |
|---|---|---|---|---|
| Gulshan et al.[17] (2016) (Google Inc.) | EyePACS-1 and MESSIDOR-2 | EyePACS-1: 97.5% MESSIDOR-2: 96.1% | EyePACS-1: 93.4% MESSIDOR-2: 93.9% | 0.99 |
| Abràmoff et al.[15] (2018) (IDx-DR) | MESSIDOR-2 | 96.8% | 87% | 0.98 |
| Van der Heijden et al.[25] (2018) (IDx-DR 2.0) | Hoorn Diabetes Eyecare | 91% | 84% | 0.94 |
| Bhaskaranand et al.[26] (2019) (EyeArt v2.0) | Multicentric | 91.3% | 91.1% | 0.96 |
| Ting et al.[18] (2017) (EyRIS SELENA+) | SiDRP and external validation sets (multicentric) | SiDRP: 90.5% External sets: 92–100% | SiDRP: 91.6% External sets: 76–92% | 0.93 0.89–0.98 |
| Gargeya et al.[27] (2017) | MESSIDOR-2 | 93% | 87% | 0.94 |
| Bawankar et al.[28] (2017) (BOSCH) | Multicentric (6 centers across India) | 91.2% | 96.9% | – |
| Li et al.[29] (2018) | NIEHS SiMES AusDiab | 92.5% | 98.5% | 0.95 |
| Keel et al.[30] (2018) (Eyegrader) | Labelme.org (Chinese online set) | 92% | 94% | – |
| Ramachandran et al. (2018)[31] (VISIONA) | ODEMS MESSIDOR-1 | 84.6% 96% | 79.7% 90% | 0.90 0.98 |
| Raumviboonsuk et al.[32] (2019) | Thailand national DR screening program | 96.9% | 95.3% | 0.99 |
| Shah et al.[20] (2019) (Netra.AI) | Sankara Eye Hospital, India and MESSIDOR-1 | 98.98% 94.68% | 94.84% 97.40% | 0.97 0.95-0.97 |
| Natarajan et al.[22] (2019) (Medios AI) | Multiple datasets from India: Dr Mohan's Diabetes Center Diacon Hospital Community based screening of patients (Aditya Jyot Hospital, India) | 95.9% 100% 100% | 81.3% 78.7% 88.4% | – |

*Contd...*

*Contd...*

| Authors and year of publication | Validation dataset | Sensitivity | Specificity | AUC |
|---|---|---|---|---|
| Zhang et al.[33] (2020) (VoxelCloud Retina) | Multicentric real-world study (across 155 centers in China) | 83.3% | 92.5% | – |

(AusDiab: Australian Diabetes, Obesity and Lifestyle Study; AUC: area under the curve; NIEHS: National Indigenous Eye Health Survey; ODEMS: Otago Diabetic Eye Monitoring Service; SELENA+: Singapore Eye Lesion Analyser Plus; SiDRP: Singapore Integrated Diabetic Retinopathy Screening Program; SiMES: Singapore Malay Eye Study)

## Artificial Intelligence in Identifying Vision-threatening Diabetic Retinopathy from Ultrawide Field Fundus Color Photographs

Artificial intelligence is also used to identify VTDR/PDR from widefield fundus images and has shown good results. A study by Nagasawa et al. has shown a sensitivity of 94.7% and specificity of 97.2%, with an AUC of 0.969 in identifying PDR from the ultrawide field (UWF)-FP using Optos™.[34] Another DL model on UWF-FP from a multicentric study showed AUROCs and accuracies for detecting both referrable DR and VTDR to be >0.9 and >80%, respectively, for the geographical external validation datasets.[35] Wang et al. have developed another DL model which showed a 91.7% sensitivity with a 50% specificity for detecting referrable DR using UWF-FP.[36]

## ARTIFICIAL INTELLIGENCE IN IDENTIFYING DIABETIC MACULAR EDEMA FROM OPTICAL COHERENCE TOMOGRAPHY

Identifying macular edema from a two-dimensional fundus image is a challenge. Most algorithms arbitrarily considered the presence of hard exudates around the fovea to be a predictor of macular edema. However, not only subsequent AI models on optical coherence tomography (OCT) images helped in diagnosis of DME but also models are being built on predicting treatment responses. DME has thus been diagnosed using AI from FP, OCT, and fluorescein angiograms (FA). A systematic review of AI in DME showed that 47% of studies have used FP images, 48% applied OCT images, and about 5% of studies used FA images for the classification and diagnosis of DME.[37]

As of today, two AI-enabled OCT systems are available for commercial use: Notal Vision™ and Altris AI™.

Notal Vison's home-based OCT is equipped with an ML algorithm that provides automated detection of pathological fluid in exudative retinal diseases **(Fig. 4)**.[38,39]

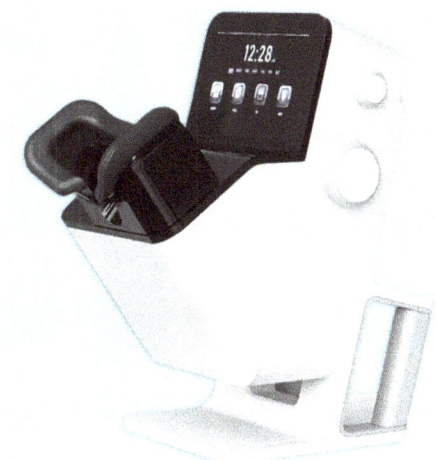

**Fig. 4:** Notal™ home-based optical coherence tomography (OCT) monitor with artificial intelligence (AI) integration.

Notal's novel OCT machine is meant to be used by high-risk patients at home. It allows monitoring of the disease activity in patients with DR and age-related macular degeneration. Once a patient completes the test, the Notal OCT Analyzer (NOA) performs an automated analysis. If retinal fluid is detected, a report is generated and conveyed to the physician, thereby reducing the time from fluid onset to the next treatment. A recent trial to evaluate the performance of NOA in sequential OCT examinations on an in-office Spectralis OCT and Notal Vision's home OCT system showed a strong correlation of retinal fluid quantification between NOA and human graders (correlation coefficient of 0.96).[40]

Another commercially available solution is Altris AI™.[41] Altris AI is trained using nearly 5 million OCT scans to identify over 50 retinal pathologies on OCT with an accuracy of 91%. In 2021, Altris partnered with Topcon Healthcare™ and Optopol™ to integrate AI with OCT scans. They also have an Altris Education OCT™ mobile application for segmentation and interpretation of OCT lesions for beginners **(Fig. 5)**.

## Brief Review of Algorithms Identifying Diabetic Macular Edema from Optical Coherence Tomography

To develop an AI model, the OCT images first undergo preprocessing (by grey-scale conversion, noise reduction, flattening of retinal contour, and cropping laterally and axially), followed by feature extraction and detection by various methods, and finally are classified.

Various AI-based algorithms are developed to identify DME on OCT[42-45] **(Table 2)**. These models use various automatic segmentation and edge

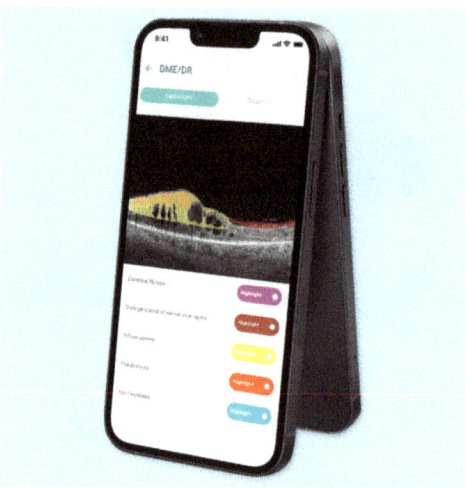

**Fig. 5:** Altris™ artificial intelligence (AI) education optical coherence tomography (OCT) mobile application.

**TABLE 2:** Sensitivity and specificity of various artificial intelligence (AI)-based algorithms to identify diabetic macular edema (DME) on optical coherence tomography (OCT).

| Authors and year of publication | Sensitivity | Specificity |
|---|---|---|
| Srinivasan et al.[42] (2014) | 68.8% | 93.8% |
| Lemaître et al.[52] (2015) | 87.5% | 75% |
| Sidibé et al.[53] (2017) | 81.3% | 62.5% |
| Alsaih et al.[43] (2017) | 87.5% | 87.5% |
| ElTanboly et al.[54] (2017) | 83% | 100% |
| Lu et al.[55] (2018) | 94.2% | 96.4% |
| Hwang et al.[46] (2020) | 96.4% | 86.7% |
| Luo et al.[56] (2021) | 94.2% | 97.9% |

detection methods to identify edema based on retinal thickness, intraretinal fluid (IRF)/cystoid spaces, subretinal fluid (SRF), layer boundary identification, and, also, layer disruption on OCT. Apart from DL CNN, other ML techniques, such as support vector machine (SVM) and random forest (RF) methods, are used for classification of OCT images.

Hwang et al. classified DME on OCT into mild DME, moderate DME, severe DME, DME with serous retinal detachment (SRD), DME with posterior hyaloid traction (PHT), and DME with traction retinal detachment (TRD) based on international classification of DR (ICDR) and OCT classification systems and built an AI model which showed a sensitivity of 96% and specificity of 87%.[46] Studies have also been published from India showing similar accuracy.[47,48]

A study by Wu et al. showed a mean accuracy of detection of various DME patterns (diffuse retinal thickening, cystoid macular edema, and SRD) on OCT to be 90.2-95.9%, with a mean AUC of 0.970-0.997.[49] Another study from Wang et al. showed the ability of AI to detect 15 various pathologies on OCT and identify cases requiring urgent referrals with an accuracy of 98%.[50]

Moreover, smartphone-based offline AI models (MobileNet architecture) and mobile applications have also been developed to identify DME from OCT images, with a comparable accuracy to that of Inception v3 and VGG16.[51]

## ARTIFICIAL INTELLIGENCE IN IDENTIFYING DIABETIC RETINOPATHY FROM OPTICAL COHERENCE TOMOGRAPHY ANGIOGRAPHY

Artificial intelligence is also used to identify microvascular biomarkers of DR using OCT angiography (OCTA) images. Various AI models have been developed to classify and identify early DR from OCTA images based on various parameters such as blood vessel tortuosity, caliber, density, vessel perimeter index, foveal avascular zone (FAZ) area, and FAZ contour irregularity from the superficial and deep capillary plexuses.

An SVM classification model was used to classify various DR stages using OCTA images and found that vessel density shows the best classification accuracies, 93.89 and 90.89% for control versus disease and control versus mild-NPDR, respectively.[57] Also, they suggested that the temporal perifoveal region was the most sensitive region for early detection of DR.

Another AI model used transfer learning model and found that the accuracy for differentiating among healthy, no DR, and DR eyes was 87.27%, with 83.76% sensitivity and 90.82% specificity.[58] Eladawi et al. showed an overall accuracy of 94.3%, a sensitivity of 97.9%, and a specificity of 87% in identifying early DR from OCTA images.[59]

Combined AI models using OCT and OCTA images have also been developed to classify healthy, no DR, and DR.[60] A study by Govindaswamy et al. showed that vascular changes precede tomographic changes in diabetic eyes without retinopathy.[61] Studies have also shown that the performance and accuracy of the AI models are better enhanced when OCTA models are combined with OCT to predict early DR changes, compared to OCT-based or OCTA-based AI models alone.[48,62]

## ARTIFICIAL INTELLIGENCE IN IDENTIFYING DIABETIC RETINOPATHY FROM FLUORESCEIN ANGIOGRAM

The role of FA in differentiating NPDR from DR is very well known. Ehlers et al. have proposed microaneurysm count, ischemic index, and leakage index to differentiate between NPDR and PDR.[63] Several AI models have been built based on ischemic index and leakage index, which differentiate NPDR and PDR.[64,65]

## ARTIFICIAL INTELLIGENCE TO PREDICT PROGNOSIS IN DIABETIC RETINOPATHY

Cao et al. have developed a model to predict the response of antivascular endothelial growth factor (VEGF) as good responders and poor responders based on various OCT baseline features such as layer disruption, area of IRF and SRF, optical density ratios of IRF and SRF, and number of hyperreflective dots, and found that the sum of hyperreflective dots in all layers was found to be the most relevant feature for prediction.[66]

Liu et al. have developed an ensemble model including both classic ML (CML) and DL to predict the posttreatment best-corrected visual acuity (BCVA) and central retinal thickness (CRT) on OCT based on various input clinical parameters and baseline OCT images.[67] Their study found that to predict posttreatment BCVA and CRT, the CML models outperformed the DL models and suggested that for tasks involving multifactorial conditions such as DME, CML algorithms should be used which consider multiple factors and are effective.

Chen et al. have developed a model using DRCR.net Protocol I patient database to predict visual outcomes in patients treated with ranibizumab for DME based on various input parameters such as baseline visual acuity, age, gender, lens status, and retinal thickness.[68]

Thus, AI has been proven to be a very effective tool for screening, diagnosis, and prediction of outcomes in DR based on FP, OCT, FA, UWF fundus images, smartphone-based FP, OCTA, and combined features **(Fig. 6)**. In future, AI

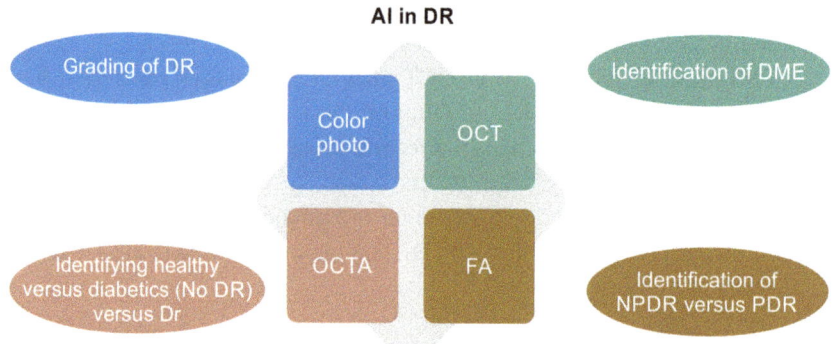

**Fig. 6:** Role of artificial intelligence (AI) in diabetic retinopathy (DR) based on various investigations. (DME: diabetic macular edema; FA: fluorescein angiograms; NPDR: nonproliferative diabetic retinopathy; OCT: optical coherence tomography; OCTA: optical coherence tomography angiography; PDR: proliferative diabetic retinopathy)

may be able to detect prognosis and outcomes and help the ophthalmologist to make better clinical decisions.[69] We conducted a study on acceptance of AI among patients for DR screening and found that 90% of patient population were willing for AI-based DR screening as it saves time and gives them better understanding of the disease.[70]

## PITFALLS OF ARTIFICIAL INTELLIGENCE-BASED DIABETIC RETINOPATHY DETECTION

- The results of an AI model largely depend on the size and quality of training datasets and balance of various categories/classes of images.
- Black box phenomenon, where we do not know why the AI algorithm has arrived at a particular decision, keeps the clinician in the dark. To address this concern, there is a push toward explainable AI (XAI) systems, where the systems are programmed, so as to describe their decision-making process. XAI is expected to provide accountability and transparency in ML.[71] Another way to overcome the black box phenomenon is generation of heatmaps.[72]
- Despite good performance of an AI model, human surveillance is still required.
- AI lacks human touch and affects patient-doctor relationships.[46]
- Legal accountability in cases of misdiagnosis with AI is an issue.[73]
- It can bring about a breach in data confidentiality, security, and privacy.
- AI algorithms trained to identify specific retinal lesions may not identify other coexisting retinal pathologies, which can compromise patient care.

## LOOKING INTO THE FUTURE

With the pandemic of COVID-19, telemedicine has gained a lot of popularity. Thus, AI can help as an effective first-line screening tool where there is no access to tertiary eyecare services. Home-based screening devices with integrated AI to identify referrable DR/DME may emerge and become more popular if provided at affordable costs. Further, smartphone-based fundus image capture with AI-integrated DR screening has a huge potential in a country like ours.

## CONCLUSION

Artificial intelligence is a great tool and can help to reduce the DR screening burden on our healthcare system. Although there are a few caveats, it can help in early identification of DR and in reducing blindness. This can revolutionize telescreening in ophthalmology, especially where people do not have access to specialized healthcare. In future, AI may not just be a screening tool but can even be able to detect prognosis and outcomes and help the ophthalmologist to make better clinical decisions.

## REFERENCES

1. Teo ZL, Tham YC, Yu M, Chee ML, Rim TH, Cheung N, et al. Global prevalence of diabetic retinopathy and projection of burden through 2045: systematic review and meta-analysis. Ophthalmology. 2021;128(11):1580-91.
2. Saeedi P, Petersohn I, Salpea P, Malanda B, Karuranga S, Unwin N, et al. Global and regional diabetes prevalence estimates for 2019 and projections for 2030 and 2045: results from the International Diabetes Federation Diabetes Atlas, 9th edition. Diabetes Res Clin Pract. 2019;157:107843.
3. Early Treatment Diabetic Retinopathy Study Research Group. Fundus photographic risk factors for progression of diabetic retinopathy. ETDRS report number 12. Ophthalmology. 1991;98(5 Suppl):823-33.
4. Davis MD, Norton EWD, Myers FL. The Airlie classification of diabetic retinopathy. In: Goldberg MF, Fine SL (Eds). Symposium on the Treatment of Diabetic Retinopathy: Public Health Service Publication No. 1890. Washington, DC: US Government Printing Office; 1969. pp. 7-22.
5. The Diabetic Retinopathy Study Research Group. A modification of the Airlie House classification of diabetic retinopathy. DRS report #7. Invest Ophthalmol Vis Sci. 1981;21:210-26.
6. Fenner BJ, Wong RLM, Lam WC, Tan GSW, Cheung GCM. Advances in retinal imaging and applications in diabetic retinopathy screening: a review. Ophthalmol Ther. 2018;7(2):333-46.
7. Early Treatment Diabetic Retinopathy Study Research Group. Grading diabetic retinopathy from stereoscopic color fundus color photographs—an extension of the modified Airlie House classification. ETDRS report number 10. Ophthalmology. 1991;98(5 Suppl):786-806.
8. Wintergerst MWM, Mishra D, Hartmann L, Shah P, Kumar V, Sagar P, et al. Smartphone-based fundus imaging in diabetic retinopathy screening in low- and middle-income countries: evaluation of four different devices. Invest Ophthalmol Vis Sci. 2019;60(9):1542.
9. Ruan S, Liu Y, Hu WT, Jia HX, Wang SS, Song ML, et al. A new handheld fundus camera combined with visual artificial intelligence facilitates diabetic retinopathy screening. Int J Ophthalmol. 2022;15(4):620-7.
10. Sosale B, Sosale AR, Murthy H, Sengupta S, Naveenam M. Medios—an offline, smartphone-based artificial intelligence algorithm for the diagnosis of diabetic retinopathy. Indian J Ophthalmol. 2020;68:391-5.
11. Schmidt-Erfurth U, Sadeghipour A, Gerendas BS, Waldstein SM, Bogunović H. Artificial intelligence in retina. Prog Retin Eye Res. 2018;67:1-29.
12. Kermany DS, Goldbaum M, Cai W, Valentim CCS, Liang H, Baxter SL, et al. Identifying medical diagnoses and treatable diseases by image-based deep learning. Cell. 2018;172(5):1122-31.e9.
13. Yang J, Fong S, Wang H, Hu Q, Lin C, Huang S, et al. Artificial intelligence in ophthalmopathy and ultra-wide field image: a survey. Expert Syst Appl. 2021;182:115068.
14. Abràmoff MD, Folk JC, Han DP, Walker JD, Williams DF, Russell SR, et al. Automated analysis of retinal images for detection of referable diabetic retinopathy. JAMA Ophthalmol. 2013;131(3):351-7.
15. Abràmoff MD, Lavin PT, Birch M, Shah N, Folk JC. Pivotal trial of an autonomous AI-based diagnostic system for detection of diabetic retinopathy in primary care offices. NPJ Digit Med. 2018;1:39.

16. Ipp E, Liljenquist D, Bode B, Shah VN, Silverstein S, Regillo CD, et al. Pivotal evaluation of an artificial intelligence system for autonomous detection of referrable and vision-threatening diabetic retinopathy. JAMA Netw Open. 2021;4(11):e2134254.
17. Gulshan V, Peng L, Coram M, Stumpe MC, Wu D, Narayanaswamy A, et al. Development and validation of a deep learning algorithm for detection of diabetic retinopathy in retinal fundus color photographs. JAMA. 2016;316:2402-10.
18. Ting DSW, Cheung CY, Lim G, Tan GSW, Quang ND, Gan A, et al. Development and validation of a deep learning system for diabetic retinopathy and related eye diseases using retinal images from multiethnic populations with diabetes. JAMA. 2017;318:2211-23.
19. Bellemo V, Lim ZW, Lim G, Nguyen QD, Xie Y, Yip MYT, et al. Artificial intelligence using deep learning to screen for referable and vision-threatening diabetic retinopathy in Africa: a clinical validation study. Lancet Digit Health. 2019;1(1):e35-44.
20. Shah P, Mishra DK, Shanmugam MP, Doshi B, Jayaraj H, Ramanjulu R. Validation of deep convolutional neural network-based algorithm for detection of diabetic retinopathy—artificial intelligence versus clinician for screening. Indian J Ophthalmol. 2020;68(2):398-405.
21. Bidwai P, Gite S, Pahuja K, Kotecha K. A systematic literature review on diabetic retinopathy using an artificial intelligence approach. Big Data Cogn Comput. 2022;6(4):152.
22. Natarajan S, Jain A, Krishnan R, Rogye A, Sivaprasad S. Diagnostic accuracy of community-based diabetic retinopathy screening with an offline artificial intelligence system on a smartphone. JAMA Ophthalmol. 2019;137(10):1182-8.
23. Grzybowski A, Brona P, Lim G, Ruamviboonsuk P, Tan GSW, Abràmoff M, et al. Artificial intelligence for diabetic retinopathy screening: a review. Eye (Lond). 2020;34(3):451-60.
24. Lee AY, Yanagihara RT, Lee CS, Blazes M, Jung HC, Chee YE, et al. Multicenter, head-to-head, real-world validation study of seven automated artificial intelligence diabetic retinopathy screening systems. Diabetes Care. 2021;44(5):1168-175.
25. Van der Heijden AA, Abràmoff MD, Verbraak F, van Hecke MV, Liem A, Nijpels G. Validation of automated screening for referable diabetic retinopathy with the IDx-DR device in the Hoorn Diabetes Care System. Acta Ophthalmol. 2018;96(1):63-8.
26. Bhaskaranand M, Ramachandra C, Bhat S, Cuadros J, Nittala MG, Sadda SR, et al. The value of automated diabetic retinopathy screening with the EyeArt system: a study of more than 100,000 consccutive cncounters from people with diabetes. Diabetes Technol Ther. 2019;21(11):635-43.
27. Gargeya R, Leng T. Automated identification of diabetic retinopathy using deep learning. Ophthalmology. 2017;124(7):962-9.
28. Bawankar P, Shanbhag N, Smitha KS, Dhawan B, Palsule A, Kumar D, et al. Sensitivity and specificity of automated analysis of single-field non-mydriatic fundus color photographs by Bosch DR Algorithm—comparison with mydriatic fundus photography (ETDRS) for screening in undiagnosed diabetic retinopathy. PLoS One. 2017;12(12):e0189854.
29. Li Z, Keel S, Liu C, He Y, Meng W, Scheetz J, et al. An automated grading system for detection of vision-threatening referable diabetic retinopathy on the basis of color fundus color photographs. Diabetes Care. 2018;41:2509-16.

30. Keel S, Lee PY, Scheetz J, Li Z, Kotowicz MA, MacIsaac RJ, et al. Feasibility and patient acceptability of a novel artificial intelligence-based screening model for diabetic retinopathy at endocrinology outpatient services: a pilot study. Sci Rep. 2018;8(1):4330.
31. Ramachandran N, Hong SC, Sime MJ, Wilson GA. Diabetic retinopathy screening using deep neural network. Clin Exp Ophthalmol. 2018;46(4):412-6.
32. Raumviboonsuk P, Krause J, Chotcomwongse P, Sayres R, Raman R, Widner K, et al. Deep learning versus human graders for classifying diabetic retinopathy severity in a nationwide screening program. NPJ Digit Med. 2019;2:25.
33. Zhang Y, Shi J, Peng Y, Zhao Z, Zheng Q, Wang Z, et al. Artificial intelligence-enabled screening for diabetic retinopathy: a real-world, multicenter and prospective study. BMJ Open Diabetes Res Care. 2020;8(1):e001596.
34. Nagasawa T, Tabuchi H, Masumoto H, Enno H, Niki M, Ohara Z, et al. Accuracy of ultrawide-field fundus ophthalmoscopy-assisted deep learning for detecting treatment-naïve proliferative diabetic retinopathy. Int Ophthalmol. 2019;39(10):2153-9.
35. Tang F, Luenam P, Ran AR, Quadeer AA, Raman R, Sen P, et al. Detection of diabetic retinopathy from ultra-widefield scanning laser ophthalmoscope images: a multicenter deep learning analysis. Ophthalmol Retina. 2021;5(11):1097-106.
36. Wang K, Jayadev C, Nittala MG, Velaga SB, Ramachandra CA, Bhaskaranand M, et al. Automated detection of diabetic retinopathy lesions on ultrawidefield pseudocolour images. Acta Ophthalmol. 2018;96(2):e168-73.
37. Shahriari MH, Sabbaghi H, Asadi F, Hosseini A, Khorrami Z. Artificial intelligence in screening, diagnosis, and classification of diabetic macular edema: a systematic review. Surv Ophthalmol. 2023;68:42-53.
38. Liu Y, Holekamp NM, Heier JS. Prospective, longitudinal study: daily self-imaging with home OCT for neovascular age-related macular degeneration. Ophthalmol Retina. 2022;6(7):575-85.
39. Keenan TDL, Goldstein M, Goldenberg D, Zur D, Shulman S, Loewenstein A. Prospective, longitudinal pilot study: daily self-imaging with patient-operated home OCT in neovascular age-related macular degeneration. Ophthalmol Sci. 2021;1(2):100034.
40. Chakravarthy U, Goldenberg D, Young G, Havilio M, Rafaeli O, Benyamini G, et al. Automated identification of lesion activity in neovascular age-related macular degeneration. Ophthalmology. 2016;123(8):1731-6.
41. Dahrouj M, Miller JB. Artificial intelligence (AI) and retinal optical coherence tomography (OCT). Semin Ophthalmol. 2021;36(4):341-5.
42. Srinivasan PP, Kim LA, Mettu PS, Cousins SW, Comer GM, Izatt JA, et al. Fully automated detection of diabetic macular edema and dry age-related macular degeneration from optical coherence tomography images. Biomed Opt Express. 2014;5:3568-77.
43. Alsaih K, Lemaitre G, Rastgoo M, Massich J, Sidibé D, Meriaudeau F. Machine learning techniques for diabetic macular edema (DME) classification on SD-OCT images. Biomed Eng Online. 2017;16:68.
44. Perdomo O, Otálora S, González FA, Meriaudeau F, Müller H. OCT-NET: a convolutional network for automatic classification of normal and diabetic macular edema using SD-OCT volumes. IEEE 15th International Symposium on Biomedical Imaging (ISBI 2018). 2018;1423-6.

45. Kamble RM, Chan GCY, Perdomo O, Kokare M, González FA, Müller H, et al. Automated diabetic macular edema (DME) analysis using fine tuning with Inception-ResNet-V2 on OCT images. IEEE-EMBS Conference on Biomedical Engineering and Sciences (IECBES). 2018;442-6.
46. Hwang DK, Chou YB, Lin TC, Yang HY, Kao ZK, Kao CL, et al. Optical coherence tomography-based diabetic macula edema screening with artificial intelligence. J Chin Med Assoc. 2020;83(11):1034-8.
47. Latha V, Ashok LR, Seerni KG. Automated macular disease detection using retinal optical coherence tomography images by fusion of deep learning networks. 2021 National Conference on Communications (NCC). 2021;1-6.
48. Dash P, Sigappi AN. Detection of DME in OCT images based on histogram descriptor. In: Chong PHJ, Kalam A, Pascoal A, Bera MK (Eds). Emerging Electronics and Automation: Lecture Notes in Electrical Engineering, Vol. 937. Singapore: Springer; 2022. pp. 357-71.
49. Wu Q, Zhang B, Hu Y, Liu B, Cao D, Yang D, et al. Detection of morphologic patterns of diabetic macular edema using a deep learning approach based on optical coherence tomography images. Retina. 2021;41:1110-7.
50. Wang L, Wang G, Zhang M, Fan D, Liu X, Guo Y, et al. An intelligent optical coherence tomography-based system for pathological retinal cases identification and urgent referrals. Transl Vis Sci Technol. 2020;9(2):46.
51. Hwang DK, Yu WK, Lin TC, Chou SJ, Yarmishyn A, Kao ZK, et al. Smartphone-based diabetic macula edema screening with an offline artificial intelligence. J Chin Med Assoc. 2020;83(12):1102-6.
52. Lemaître G, Rastgoo M, Massich J, Sankar S, Mériaudeau F, Sidibé D. Classification of SD-OCT volumes with LBP: application to DME detection. In: Chen X, Garvin MK, Liu JJ, Trusso E, Xu Y (Eds). Proceedings of the Ophthalmic Medical Image Analysis Second International Workshop, OMIA 2015, held in conjunction with MICCAI 2015. Munich, Germany; 2015. pp. 9-16.
53. Sidibé D, Sankar S, Lemaître G, Rastgoo M, Massich J, Cheung CY, et al. An anomaly detection approach for the identification of DME patients using spectral domain optical coherence tomography images. Comput Methods Programs Biomed. 2017;139:109-17.
54. ElTanboly A, Ismail M, Shalaby A, Switala A, El-Baz A, Schaal S, et al. A computer-aided diagnostic system for detecting diabetic retinopathy in optical coherence tomography images. Med Phys. 2017;44(3):914-23.
55. Lu W, Tong Y, Yu Y, Xing Y, Chen C, Shen Y. Deep learning-based automated classification of multi-categorical abnormalities from optical coherence tomography images. Transl Vis Sci Technol. 2018;7(6):41.
56. Luo Y, Xu Q, Jin R, Wu M, Liu L. Automatic detection of retinopathy with optical coherence tomography images via a semi-supervised deep learning method. Biomed Opt Express. 2021;12(5):2684-702.
57. Alam M, Zhang Y, Lim JI, Chan RVP, Yang M, Yao X. Quantitative optical coherence tomography angiography features for objective classification and staging of diabetic retinopathy. Retina. 2020;40(2):322-32.
58. Le D, Alam M, Yao CK, Lim JI, Hsieh YT, Chan RVP, et al. Transfer learning for automated OCTA detection of diabetic retinopathy. Transl Vis Sci Technol. 2020;9(2):35.
59. Eladawi N, Elmogy M, Khalifa F, Ghazal M, Ghazi N, Aboelfetouh A, et al. Early diabetic retinopathy diagnosis based on local retinal blood vessel analysis

in optical coherence tomography angiography (OCTA) images. Med Phys. 2018;45(10):4582-99.
60. Govindasamy N, Ratra D, Dalan D, Mochi TB, Roy AS. Artificial intelligence effectively combined OCT and OCTA indices to improve early detection of diabetic retinopathy (DR). Invest Ophthalmol Vis Sci. 2019;60(9):1434.
61. Govindaswamy N, Ratra D, Dalan D, Doralli S, Tirumalai AA, Nagarajan R, et al. Vascular changes precede tomographic changes in diabetic eyes without retinopathy and improve artificial intelligence diagnostics. J Biophotonics. 2020;13(9):e202000107.
62. Sandhu HS, Elmogy M, Taher Sharafeldeen A, Elsharkawy M, El-Adawy N, ElTanboly A, et al. Automated diagnosis of diabetic retinopathy using clinical biomarkers, optical coherence tomography, and optical coherence tomography angiography. Am J Ophthalmol. 2020;216:201-6.
63. Ehlers JP, Jiang AC, Boss JD, Hu M, Figueiredo N, Babiuch A, et al. Quantitative ultra-widefield angiography and diabetic retinopathy severity: an assessment of panretinal leakage index, ischemic index and microaneurysm count. Ophthalmology. 2019;126(11):1527-32.
64. Wang X, Ji Z, Ma X, Zhang Z, Yi Z, Zheng H, et al. Automated grading of diabetic retinopathy with ultra-widefield fluorescein angiography and deep learning. J Diabetes Res. 2021;2021:2611250.
65. Gao Z, Jin K, Yan Y, Liu X, Shi Y, Ge Y, et al. End-to-end diabetic retinopathy grading based on fundus fluorescein angiography images using deep learning. Graefes Arch Clin Exp Ophthalmol. 2022;260:1663-73.
66. Cao J, You K, Jin K, Lou L, Wang Y, Chen M, et al. Prediction of response to anti-vascular endothelial growth factor treatment in diabetic macular oedema using an optical coherence tomography-based machine learning method. Acta Ophthalmol. 2021;99(1):e19-27.
67. Liu B, Zhang B, Hu Y, Cao D, Yang D, Wu Q, et al. Automatic prediction of treatment outcomes in patients with diabetic macular edema using ensemble machine learning. Ann Transl Med. 2021;9(1):43. [Erratum in: Ann Transl Med. 2021;9(14):1215].
68. Chen SC, Chiu HW, Chen CC, Woung LC, Lo CM. A novel machine learning algorithm to automatically predict visual outcomes in intravitreal ranibizumab-treated patients with diabetic macular edema. J Clin Med. 2018;7(12):475.
69. Chakroborty S, Gupta M, Devishamani CS, Patel K, Ankit C, Ganesh Babu TC, et al. Narrative review of artificial intelligence in diabetic macular edema: diagnosis and predicting treatment response using optical coherence tomography. Indian J Ophthalmol. 2021;69(11):2999-3008.
70. Shah P, Mishra D, Shanmugam M, Vighnesh MJ, Jayaraj H. Acceptability of artificial intelligence-based retina screening in general population. Indian J Ophthalmol. 2022;70:1140-4.
71. Ahuja AS, Halperin LS. Understanding the advent of artificial intelligence in ophthalmology. J Curr Ophthalmol. 2019;31(2):115-7.
72. Lim G, Bellemo V, Xie Y, Lee XQ, Yip MYT, Ting DSW. Different fundus imaging modalities and technical factors in AI screening for diabetic retinopathy: a review. Eye Vis (Lond). 2020;7:21.
73. Padhy SK, Takkar B, Chawla R, Kumar A. Artificial intelligence in diabetic retinopathy: a natural step to the future. Indian J Ophthalmol. 2019;67(7):1004-9.

CHAPTER 10

# Artificial Intelligence in Retinopathy of Prematurity

*Lingam Gopal, Arjun Bamel, Anand Vinekar*

## ABSTRACT

Artificial intelligence (AI) has entered mainstream medical practice in a big way, thanks to some significant developments in technology. The major shift has been from computer programs that needed to be programmed at every step in the analysis of images to "deep learning"—a self-learning technology. Ophthalmology is a heavily image-dependent specialty and is elegantly suitable for this technology. AI has been explored in the diagnosis of diabetic retinopathy, age-related macular degeneration, glaucoma, and retinopathy of prematurity (ROP). The aim of use of this technology is not to replace a specialist but to aid in the overall care of patients. The technology has proved to be useful at the screening stage to detect patients that need to be referred versus normal subjects who need only follow-up. In ROP, deep learning programs have been explored to refine the diagnosis of plus disease, locating zone I and to some extent the stage of disease, and to evaluate the images and weed out those of poor quality. Studies on plus disease have proved that deep learning-based programs can outperform even experts. These studies have also led to the development of a continuous score for "vascular severity" from the three-class inputs for plus disease. Other applications that are being explored relate to improving image acquisition while handling handheld wide-angle cameras and to integrate data from other devices such as optical coherence tomography.

*Keywords:* Retinopathy of prematurity; artificial intelligence; machine learning; deep learning; computer-based image analysis.

### ■ INTRODUCTION

While intelligence refers to the ability to learn, understand, and think in a logical way, the term artificial intelligence (AI) refers in general to the development of computer programs that can mimic human behavior.[1]

Artificial intelligence as a concept was introduced in 1956.[1] Traditionally, computers had to be programmed to answer specific questions. Any improvement or variation had to be reprogrammed. However, the advent of "machine learning" permitted the program to learn from the previous data automatically.[2] Deep learning is a subfield of machine learning which is complex in terms of processing information in multiple layers using neural networks akin to human brain.[3] AI has already found significant use in the practice of medicine.[4]

Ophthalmology is a specialty that is heavily dependent on image analysis and, hence, is especially suited for application of AI. It has already been applied in the fields of glaucoma,[5] age-related macular degeneration (AMD),[6,7] diabetic retinopathy,[8] and retinopathy of prematurity (ROP). In this chapter, we will present the current status of use of AI in the area of ROP.

## ARTIFICIAL INTELLIGENCE

### History

In 1950, Alan Turing first discussed on the subject of building intelligent machines. But it was the Dartmouth Summer Research Project on Artificial Intelligence (DSPRAI) that kick-started the whole idea in 1955. John Hopfield and David Rumelhart introduced "deep learning."[9] Readers may remember the IBM deep blue computer that beat the World Chess Champion in 1997. From there, AI made its way into common man's home through Google Now, Amazon Alexa, Apple's Siri, etc.

Medicine did not lag in adopting this exciting new technology. One of the first applications was in the development of "the CASNET" model by Rutgers University—a consultation program for glaucoma.[10] Bakkar et al. used the IBM Watson program to identify altered ribonucleic acid (RNA) binding proteins in amyotrophic lateral sclerosis.[11] Deep learning is currently being applied in several medical specialties. "Arterys" is a company that offers deep learning-based analysis of images in various specialties—neuro, cardiac, chest, breast cancer, etc.[12]

Major developments in the field of AI took place since 2010, leading to diverse applications including those in medicine and specifically ophthalmology.[5-8] This chapter is targeted toward ophthalmologists and, hence, it is not important to dwell into the details of the technical aspects of AI. However, acquaintance with a few terms may be important.

### Machine Learning

Coined by Arthur Samuel, the term means "the computer should have ability to learn without being explicitly programmed."[2] Using machine learning algorithms, the program can learn and would be able to predict result based on data that have been previously fed into the system in either a supervised or an unsupervised manner. Such programs can be useful in prognosticating an event.

## Deep Learning

Deep learning is a category of machine learning in which features are not described by the programmer. The algorithm uses the datasets to create its own abstract features. This program is useful to classify diseases. One issue is that it may not be openly obvious as to how the deep learning program has come up with the conclusions from the images—a kind of black box in which the processing takes place.

## Artificial Neural Network

Artificial neural network (ANN) is a machine learning algorithm that is modeled after biological neural network taking advantage of Hebbian theory. Hebbian theory is a neuroscientific theory that claims that the efficacy of a synapse is increased when a presynaptic cell repeatedly and persistently stimulates the postsynaptic cell—a phenomenon aptly described as "neurons that fire together are wired together."[13] Artificial neural networks (ANNs) have many nodes analogous to axons and dendrites. The synapses are thus strengthened when their neurons have correlated output.

## Convolutional Neural Network

Convolutional neural network (CNN) is a variety of ANN where patches of specific nodes are fed the information instead of all the nodes. Hence, the spatial context is preserved in relation to where the feed was extracted. This process can lead to specific trained filters that pick up specific features from images and mark them on the feature map. Most computer-based image analysis (CBIA) systems utilize CNNs.

## Data Augmentation

Data augmentation describes the generation of new synthetic images from existing images by slightly altering them—such as rotating them and changing the width or height. This increases the number of images that can be used to train the program, although the original set of images was limited in number. Having more images for training reduces the risk of "overfitting."

## Pretrained Networks

There are several models available where the network is already trained with millions of images to help detect features, e.g., VGG-19, ResNet-101, DenseNet, GoogLeNet, Inception v3.

Using pretrained networks, one can:
- Directly classify images

- Adopt them as feature extractors, which can train another machine learning model such as support vector machine (SVM)
- Take layers from pretrained networks and fine-tune on new data (transfer learning)

### Transfer Learning

Transfer learning refers to transfer of previously acquired knowledge and applying it for the present problem. Large databases such as "ImageNet" are available that have been built with more than a million natural images of different categories. Models that have been already trained with these large databases (pretrained networks) can serve as the beginning for construction of deep learning neural networks being designed for a specific purpose such as ROP.

## ■ RETINOPATHY OF PREMATURITY

Retinopathy of prematurity is a major pediatric ophthalmic problem, almost reaching epidemic proportions in developing and underdeveloped countries.[14] The combination of some degree of improved neonatal care and inadequate facilities for timely screening for ROP has resulted in increase in the burden of unnecessary blindness. ROP is a vascular disease of the newborn that results from a combination of variable extent of the avascular retina at birth (due to prematurity) and a turbulent postnatal period. Various risk factors have been identified, including low gestational age, low birth weight, exposure to uncontrolled oxygen administration, respiratory distress syndrome, and number of days of ventilatory support.[15]

The International Classification of Retinopathy of Prematurity (ICROP) is a consensus statement that creates a standard nomenclature for the classification of ROP. First published in 1984, this has been revised several times with the last revision published in 2021.[16] ROP has been graded based on staging of the disease (stages 1–5), location of disease in the fundus (zone), and presence or absence of plus disease.

Stage 1 refers to the development of a sharp demarcation line separating the posterior vascularized retina from the anterior avascular retina. Stage 2 refers to the development of a ridge (conversion of the two-dimensional disease to a three-dimensional one). Stage 3 describes the advent of extraretinal proliferation of anomalous vasculature, and this can be subgraded as mild, moderate, and severe on a purely subjective basis. Stages 4 and 5 refer to the onset of retinal detachment. Partial retinal detachment not involving macula is termed 4a and that which involves macula is termed 4b, while total retinal detachment is termed stage 5.

Zone I is defined as a circle centered on the optic disc with its radius twice that of the distance between disc and macula. Zone II starts from zone I and extends to a circle concentric with zone I and abutting on the nasal ora serrata. Zone III refers to the residual temporal crescent. Zone II is broad and, hence, was further divided into posterior and anterior zone II. Posterior zone II refers to a region of two-disc diameters peripheral to the limit of zone I.

Plus disease defines the presence of dilated and tortuous retinal vessels in the posterior pole. It is usually compared with a standard reference photograph. Suspicious cases of plus disease that do not reach up to the severity noted in the standard reference photograph are termed "preplus."

Treatment-requiring ROP is defined based on the description of type 1 and type 2 ROP. Type 1 ROP refers to eyes with ROP in zone I of any stage with plus disease, ROP in zone I of stage 3 without plus disease, and ROP in zone II of stage 2 or 3 with plus disease. These eyes are considered an indication for immediate intervention rather than observation. By corollary, eyes with ROP in zone I of stages 1–2 without plus disease, eyes in zone II of stages 1–3 without plus disease, and eyes with ROP in zone III are usually observed rather than treated since they can regress spontaneously. They are followed up critically till the disease regresses along with normalization of retinal vascularization till periphery or treated if they convert to type 1 ROP.

## Evaluation of Infants for Retinopathy of Prematurity

The gold standard has been evaluation with a binocular indirect ophthalmoscope by a trained ophthalmologist. However, the advent of wide-field handheld cameras (RetCam, FORUS, etc.) gives additional methods for evaluation of the infants for ROP. Wide-field digital imaging has been modified and adopted for retinal imaging giving 120° imaging capability. In addition to documentation, the images can be transmitted immediately to a remote location where experts can view the images and advise accordingly - either observation or immediate direct evaluation by an ophthalmologist (teleophthalmology).

## Issues in the Management of Retinopathy of Prematurity and why Artificial Intelligence may be Useful

- *Burden of screening*: It is estimated that in the United Kingdom (UK), for every infant treated for ROP, at least 55 infants are screened.[17]
- *Feasibility of examining every infant at risk*: This is indeed a challenge and a strain on the health care system in most countries. The problem gets compounded when there is difficult access to health care for a significant section of the population (rural areas in developing and underdeveloped countries), even for routine illness. Obviously, access to good neonatal care would be even less in such circumstances, thus increasing the risk of ROP in these premature infants.[18]

- *Requirement of trained ophthalmologists*: ROP examination needs special skills and, hence, trained personnel are needed to ensure that the disease is not missed. In most countries, pediatric ophthalmologists or vitreoretinal surgeons tend to be involved in the detection and care of ROP patients. The number of such available trained personnel would again be a limiting factor to offer services to every infant at risk.[19]
- *Repeated ocular examination*: In most cases, more than one examination would be needed for every infant at risk. Even when there is no ROP, one would need to reexamine till the retina is normally vascularized up to the periphery. This again adds to the burden of screening.[20]
- *Subjectivity in clinical diagnosis*: Medicine is an imperfect science.[21] Hence, there is always room for difference of opinion for major as well as minor things. ROP is no exception. In a study by Campbell et al., of 1,553 eye examinations, comparing RetCam image evaluation (by two independent experts) with binocular indirect ophthalmoscope evaluation (by routine ophthalmologists caring for ROP babies in seven centers), there was 40% disagreement in staging classification, 18% disagreement in plus disease (including preplus) classification, 8% disagreement in zone classification, and 40% disagreement in overall staging.[22] Fleck et al. reported that treatment-requiring ROP was more often diagnosed by UK ophthalmologists versus ophthalmologists in Australia and New Zealand.[23]

## ARTIFICIAL INTELLIGENCE IN OPHTHALMOLOGY

As alluded to earlier, ophthalmology lends itself very well to the utilization of AI since a lot of subspecialties in ophthalmology depend on the analysis of images. Notably, AI has been used in the detection of diabetic retinopathy, glaucoma, AMD, and ROP. Use of AI is also inextricably linked to use of teleophthalmology for certain conditions. The combination provides a more complete package, especially for screening programs.

In the management of diabetic retinopathy, AI is mainly used for screening wherein coupled with teleophthalmology, larger populations can be reached effectively.[8,24] Currently, the approach is to identify "more than mild diabetic retinopathy" and "diabetic macular edema" so that potentially vision-threatening stages can be referred to an ophthalmologist at an appropriate time. In the field of AMD, algorithms based on color fundus images,[25] fundus autofluorescence (FAF), and optical coherence tomography (OCT) have been used to predict growth rates of areas of geographic atrophy and[26] identification of intraretinal and subretinal fluid, etc.[27] Deep learning models have also been used to diagnose pathological myopia.[28]

## UTILITY OF ARTIFICIAL INTELLIGENCE IN RETINOPATHY OF PREMATURITY

Retinopathy of prematurity is a disease with significant societal impact for the following reasons:
- It affects newborn infants and, hence, can affect the entire life of that individual.
- There is a narrow window of opportunity to detect and treat appropriately. If this opportunity is missed, it can lead to potential lifelong blindness.
- Considering that the disease is affecting a newborn infant, the emotional impact on the family is significant.
- A significant number of these children are born after a precious pregnancy—raising the emotional quotient even higher.
- Current approaches in management can only address fully formed disease but cannot prevent its occurrence in a majority of cases.
- Facilities for good neonatal care are not uniform across the world, and in developing countries, the facilities vary from excellent to nonexistent.
- The disease is not evident to the discerning parent on external examination till it has reached an advanced stage (stage 5 leading to leukocoria) and, hence, often lulls them into complacency and not keeping up to the schedule of timely eye examination.
- Similar complacency can creep into the routine of neonatal units, especially when overwhelmed by too many cases and too few trained personnel.

Under these circumstances, anything that can automate some steps in the detection, categorization, and prediction of ROP can be extremely useful in impacting the outcomes for these premature infants on a global scale.

Integral to the use of AI in ROP is the use of digital imaging to capture the retinal topography. As alluded to above, the gold standard for evaluating the retina for ROP is binocular indirect ophthalmoscopy with scleral indentation by a trained ophthalmologist. The advent of wide-angle digital imaging using handheld cameras has made it possible to image the retina in the neonatal intensive care unit by trained personnel.[29] This prompted the concept of teleophthalmology for ROP. Using trained nurses and store and forward system, teleophthalmology has been used successfully to screen infants for ROP.[30,31] Potentially, this reduces the number of visits an ophthalmologist has to make to see the infants. The images are still to be evaluated by a trained ophthalmologist although at a time of his/her convenience. Digital imaging enables documentation, provides ability to serially compare the images to identify progression or regression, and provides opportunity to take a second opinion. In the context of this chapter, digital imaging is crucial for application of any AI programs. Imaging and Informatics in ROP Research Consortium is a group formed in the United States to develop and validate computer-based methods for quantitative ROP diagnosis.[32] As part of this study, several landmark publications have come out. Wittenberg et al. in 2012 published a review of computer-based systems for ROP diagnosis available at that time.[33]

## The Plus Disease Conundrum

Defining plus disease happens to be the most important step toward identifying treatment requiring cases of ROP. Traditionally, it started with yes or no statements (plus disease present or absent). However, rapidly one realized that there are many cases between the two ends of the spectrum that defy uniform agreement among practitioners. Subsequent international classifications introduced the term "preplus disease," which gives an additional step to slot a given case into but does not remove the ambiguity entirely. It also does not tell us when one needs to treat if we use three steps instead of the two traditional steps to grade plus disease. It was realized that packaging a disease continuum into discrete steps may not be the right approach.[34]

Computer-based image analysis has been used for feature extraction as well as using deep learning programs to help identify several features of ROP. In the ensuing discussion, we will summarize important publications related to these areas.

- *Vessel finder (2002):*[35] In this computer program, the retinal vessels were segmented out from the retinal images, and the tortuosity and dilation were characterized. The computer analysis of the fundus pictures revealed that the mean vessel width of eyes that ultimately needed treatment was 96.8 versus 86.4 μm in those that did not need treatment. Similarly, the tortuosity was 1.125 in eyes needing treatment versus 1.097 for those that did not.
- *Retinal image multiscale analysis (RISA) (2005):* It was developed by Gelman et al.[36] This program measured the integrated curvature (IC) diameter and tortuosity of the vessels. The area under curve shows the best accuracy for curvature of the vessel (0.911 for arterioles and 0.824 for venules).
- *ROPtool:* Developed by Wallace, this tool permitted automated measurement of the retinal arteriolar width (dilation) and tortuosity.[37] There was good correlation ($r = 0.8$) with the clinician's judgment. The area under curve was 0.93 for diagnosing plus disease and 0.90 for preplus disease. The sensitivity was 89% and specificity was 83%.
- *Vessel map:* This program used the brightness indices perpendicular to the vessel lengths within two-disc diameter from the disc to measure the diameter of arterioles and venules.[38]

- *Computer-assisted image analysis of the retina (CAIAR):*[39] This computer-aided image analysis enabled semiautomatic detection of retinal vasculature and measurement of vessel width and tortuosity. The authors used computer-generated sinusoidal vessels for measurements with the program. There was moderate correlation with grading done by five expert ophthalmologists for tortuosity but not so good correlation for width of vasculature.

## Issues Arising out of the Experience with the Above-described Algorithms

The above-described algorithms generate quantitative measurements of individual retinal vessels. The issues with this approach can be summarized as follows:
- Which of the two—arteriole or venule—should be used for the evaluation?
- Is posterior pole evaluation enough or should the vasculature be evaluated even beyond? Evaluation of fundus images (nonwide-field) was mostly restricted to the posterior pole, while a clinician examining the fundus with a binocular indirect ophthalmoscope evaluates the vasculature much beyond the posterior pole.
- Can features other than just dilation and tortuosity be also used to label "plus" disease?
- Can information from serial examinations be combined for the diagnosis of plus disease instead of information from only one examination?
- Can combination of features be used instead of one?

## Use of Combination of Parameters

- Using the ROPtool, Johnston et al. showed that arteriolar tortuosity is better than venular tortuosity to diagnose plus disease although the combination is even better.[40] Tortuosity-weighted algorithms that increase the contribution of vessel width as the tortuosity increases yielded the highest diagnostic accuracy of plus disease.
- Chiang et al. have linearly combined different parameters.[41] In this study, they measured three parameters for each vessel, arteriole, and venule.
  - *IC:* This is a measure of the number of twists and turns a vessel takes in its path. Each bend is converted into an angle, and the sum of all the angles along the vessel normalized by its length gives the value of IC.
  - *Tortuosity index (TI):* This is obtained by dividing the length of the vessel by the line segment joining the two ends. The more the tortuosity, the greater the value of TI beyond 1. The minimum value is 1 (for a straight vessel).

- *Diameter:* This is the total area of the vessel divided by its length (effectively an average of all diameters taken across the length of the vessel).

Based on area under curve, specificity, and sensitivity, the authors found venular IC, venular diameter, and arteriolar IC to perform best individually. Various combinations of these parameters were also tried to improve diagnostic accuracy. The combination of arteriolar IC, venular IC, arteriolar TI, venular TI, and venular diameter gave the greatest area under curve of 0.967.

## ■ DEEP LEARNING IN RETINOPATHY OF PREMATURITY

The above discussion pertains to computer programs predominantly based on feature extraction and algorithms built around the extracted features. The success of these algorithms is dependent on the accuracy of vessel segmentation. This process, however, may involve time-consuming manual inputs. In recent years, there has been progress in the field of AI with the use of deep CNNs. The deep learning classifier has the capacity to learn without being told what to look for in terms of user-defined parameters. Worrall was the first to report the use of deep learning in ROP.[42] Since then, there has been tremendous progress in the application of deep learning in ROP. Investigators have focused on several key areas that can aid diagnosis and management.

### Identification of Stage of Disease

- *Automated ROP screening using deep neural networks:*[43]
  - Developed a deep neural network-based automated ROP detection system called "DeepROP." The system has two models—one for identification and one for grading, ID-Net and Gr-Net.
  - A sensitivity of 96.2% and specificity of 99.3% were achieved on the ID-Net for identifying the disease. The grading model had a sensitivity of 88.46% and specificity of 92.3%.
  - Subsequent investigations in 552 cases have shown that "DeepROP" performed better than some human graders.
  - The authors chose to classify the pictures as normal, minor ROP, and severe ROP. Minor ROP in this study was defined as zone II or zone III disease of stage 1 or 2. Severe ROP was defined by the authors as threshold disease, type I, type II, aggressive posterior retinopathy of prematurity (APROP), and stages 4 and 5 ROP.
  - It is not clear why the authors did not try to separate type I from type II ROP and also try to define plus disease.
  - Presumably, the purpose is to define ROP that needs a referral and not necessarily aid the ophthalmologist any further in defining plus disease.

- *Automated analysis of ROP by deep neural networks:*[44]
  - A two-step process was utilized—step 1 is designed to identify the presence or absence of ROP and step 2 to characterize the disease in terms of severity (stage).
  - When applied to test data from 406 examinations, the model correctly identified the presence or absence of ROP in 352 out of 356 images. While classifying ROP as mild and severe, the model misclassified only one image.
  - The authors felt that the reflection of light in the image may impact the recognition result of the model.
- *A deep learning framework for identifying zone I in RetCam images:*[45]
  - Concentrated on identifying zone I disease from RetCam pictures using deep CNNs
  - The algorithms automatically identify disc and macula. The results are compared with the gold standard of interpretation by six experts.
  - The model shows an accuracy of 91% in zone I identification when Intersection over Union (IOU) threshold is 0.8. IOU refers to an evaluation metric. Ground truth boundaries are the boundaries defined by the six experts and considered the gold standard. The predicted boundaries are defined by the software. IOU is the ratio of the numerator indicated by the area of overlap to the predicted and ground truth boundaries and denominator indicated by the total combined area occupied by both predicted and ground truth boundaries.
- *Deep learning models for automated diagnosis of ROP in preterm infants:*[46]
  - Used CNN to diagnose ROP versus no ROP and as the second stage identifying the severity of ROP (mild or severe ROP). Mild ROP was stage 1 or 2 and severe ROP was stage 3. No reference to plus disease.
  - Datasets from Japan and Taiwan used in the analysis
  - Data underwent preprocessing.
  - Transfer learning and data augmentation were used in this study.
  - The program identified ROP and no ROP with a sensitivity of 96.6% and specificity of 95.2%. The results were much worse when transfer technology was not used as well as when data augmentation was not done.
- *Automated identification of ROP by image-based deep learning:*[47]
  - The authors identified four grades of ROP—normal, mild (stage 1 or 2 with no plus disease), semiurgent (stage 1 or 2 with plus disease), and urgent (stages 3-5)
  - The system achieved an accuracy of 0.903, sensitivity of 0.778, and specificity of 0.932 for grading ROP cases in the four grades as described above.

- *Automated detection and classification of telemedical ROP images:*[48]
  - The authors reported an automated detection and classification approach to assess the severity of ROP using wide-field telemedical images using a Hessian analysis and SVM classifier.
  - They classified the normal, stage 2, and stage 3 images with an accuracy of 91.8%, sensitivity of 90.37%, specificity of 94.65%, false-positive rate of 5.35%, and false-negative rate of 9.63% using images from a telemedicine network.
- *Deep learning for the diagnosis of stage in ROP:*[49]
  - Two sets of images from two different populations (American and Nepali) were used.
  - Each dataset was acquired with different cameras.
  - Preprocessing of images was done to better define the stage using a contrast-limited adaptive histogram equalization to improve pigment differences between avascular and vascularized retina, green channel extraction to improve visibility of darker structures such as vessels and demarcation lines, and Wiener filter application to reduce noise and aberrations.
  - 90% images were used to train the system and 10% were used to test it.
  - Training and testing were done on each set of images (American and Nepali) separately and also as a combined set.
  - CNN could be trained to identify stages 1–3 of ROP with high accuracy.
  - CNNs trained on the American set did relatively poorly on Nepali images and vice versa, i.e., the system suffers when tested on external samples that differ from the training dataset.
  - However, if they are trained on a combined dataset (i.e., heterogeny introduced into the sets), the performance improves significantly.
  - The authors conclude that generalizability requires that the sets are trained on data belonging to different populations.

## Identification of Zones

Assistive framework for automatic detection of all the zones in ROP using deep learning:[50]
- The authors attempt to automatically detect the zones by a novel method using a combination of "U-Network" and "Circle Hough Transform."
- The purpose was to detect zones I–III from retinal images in which macula is not developed and they showed an accuracy of 98%.

## Identification of Plus Disease

- *Automated diagnosis of plus disease in ROP using deep CNNs:*[51]
  - This fully automated computer-based system, deep learning neural network (i-ROPDL algorithm) system, could diagnose plus disease.

- The i-ROPDL algorithm outperformed all previous CBIA systems for diagnosing ROP and was even better than most experts.
- The authors also state that although data was labeled as normal, preplus, or plus (categorical labels) without indicating the order of severity, the program learned the order of severity by itself.
- Hence, the system appears to have understood that the disease is a continuum.
- This is an important take-home message from this study—to try and create a continuous grading score for plus disease rather in to artificially created blocks.

▪ *A computer-aided diagnosis system for plus disease in ROP with structure adaptive segmentation and vessel-based features:* The authors developed and evaluated a computer-based analysis system for objective assessment of plus disease in ROP, which best mimics the clinical method of disease diagnosis by identifying unique vessel-based features:[52]
- The algorithm introduced the usage of additional retinal features, namely leaf node count and vessel density, to portray the abnormal growth and branching of the blood vessels and to complement the commonly used features, namely tortuosity and width.
- In this fully automated system, the test results show a better classification of plus disease in terms of sensitivity (95%) and specificity (93%), emphasizing the superiority of the proposed segmentation algorithm and vessel-based features.

▪ *A deep learning framework for the detection of plus disease in retinal fundus images of preterm infants:*[53]
- The authors used CNN to identify the tortuosity of retinal vasculature from fundus images with ROP. Image augmentation was used in this study.
- They compare the results obtained with the deep learning algorithm with those obtained using U-COSFIRE filters—an image processing algorithm.[54]
- The authors obtained a sensitivity of 0.99 and specificity of 0.98 with the CNN, which was better than what was obtained with the U-COSFIRE filter system.

## Vascular Severity Score

The deep learning program i-ROPDL was developed to diagnose plus disease as a three-class output, namely no plus, preplus, and plus. By comparing the output with that of experts and calculating the probabilities, the investigators could come up with a continuous score spread between 0 and 9. "0" indicates 100% probability of no plus disease and "9" indicates 100% probability of plus disease. This has been termed the *vascular severity score* and is expected to treat plus disease as a continuum rather than as discrete ordinals.

After the publication of the ICROP3 classification, a study to validate "vascular severity score" as an appropriate output for AI through comparison with ordinal disease severity labels for stage and plus disease was reported. All 34 members of the ICROP3 committee participated. The vascular severity score was found to be highly correlated with both the average plus disease classification and the ophthalmoscopic diagnosis of stage among all experts. This could portend that the generation of a consensus for a validated scoring system for ROP has the potential to facilitate global regulatory authorization of these technologies. The following publications have explored the validity of the "vascular severity score":

- *Validation of a vascular severity scale against international expert diagnosis:*[55]
  - Good correlation was seen between the vascular severity score generated by the algorithm and the average derived from experts' labels of the images.
  - Similar correlation was seen for staging also (1–3), excluding stages of retinal detachment.
  - Authors infer that although experts label plus disease as an ordinal (discrete labels), they probably agree that it is actually a continuum.
- *Variability in plus disease identified using a deep learning-based ROP severity scale:*[56]
  - The authors derived the vascularity severity score (a continuous score to evaluate the plus disease as a continuum) from the images procured as a part of routine management of ROP in real-life setting.
  - This vascularity severity score was compared with the clinician's diagnosis. Interclinician variability as well as intraclinician variability was assessed in comparison to the score from the algorithm.
  - Significant differences were seen between clinicians as well as between two examinations by the same clinician as evaluated by the vascular severity score. The same picture may trigger different labels from the same clinician at different times.
  - The authors feel that factors other than visible vascular dilation seem to influence the decision to label a case as plus disease. Possible factors include the following: (1) sense of overall disease severity based on clinical judgment, (2) the interpretation could be altered by additional information from zone and stage of disease, (3) clinicians who diagnosed stage 3 are more likely to diagnose plus disease compared to those who diagnosed stage 2 for the same picture, (4) internal cutoff point for plus disease, i.e., the inherent variability between examiners on when to call a case as plus disease. This is a systematically biased internal cutoff point.

- *Evaluation of a deep learning-derived ROP severity scale:*[57]
  - The authors tried to evaluate the relationship between a deep learning-derived vascular severity scale with zone, stage, and extent of stage 3 and plus disease.
  - Vascular severity scale was graded between 1 and 9 as in the previous publications.
  - Investigations have shown the following associations with vascular severity score:
    - Higher the stage of disease, greater the score, irrespective of the zones of involvement
    - Higher score seen in zone I (for stages 1–3) compared to similar stages in zone II
    - The more the circumferential extent of stage 3 disease, the higher the score. This applies to both zones I and II.
    - For the same amount of the circumferential extent of stage 3 disease (number of clock hours), the score was higher in zone I compared to zone II.
- *A quantitative severity scale of ROP using deep learning to monitor disease regression after treatment:*[58]
  - The authors applied the vascular severity score to images obtained before treatment, at the time of treatment, and after treatment.
  - Mean vascular severity score was 7.43 at the time of treatment. The mean increased significantly 2 weeks prior to treatment, peaked at treatment, and then reduced for at least 2 weeks after treatment. Bevacizumab-treated eyes had higher pretreatment vascular severity score compared to those treated with laser. A week after treatment, bevacizumab-treated eyes had greater reduction in vascular severity score.

## Assessing Image Quality Using Deep Learning

*Deep learning for image quality assessment of fundus images in ROP:*[59]
- CNNs were able to discriminate between gradable and nongradable images with area under receiver operating curve equal to 0.964.
- Potentially, CNN can be used to prescreen images for use in tele-ophthalmology for ROP.

So far, the evidence seems to suggest that deep learning-based algorithms have the potential to diagnose ROP reliably—comparable to or sometimes better than clinicians. However, there are obstacles for the implementation and integration of this technology into routine practice.

## Challenges in Incorporating Deep Learning-based Algorithms into Routine Practice

- *Applicability across different populations:* Studies across the world have shown significant differences between regions with regard to the occurrence of ROP, the profile of infants that develop ROP, the levels of neonatal care, ROP presentation, etc.[14] Hence, a program based on images from one community/geographical location may not necessarily work for another population.[49]

- *Quality of fundus camera:* The camera used may also influence the applicability. Different fundus cameras may have different levels of resolution, color rendition, etc. Programs developed using images from one camera perhaps work best with the same camera.
- *Quality of images captured:* In a study, one uses mostly the best images, thus discarding images of borderline value that may still yield useful information but are considered not good enough for the study purpose. However, in real life, one must contend with the use of these borderline images. The situation in the neonatal intensive care unit is not always congenial for the production of high-quality images. The small eye, the presence of various tubes around the head, the fragile systemic status of the infant (that may not permit prolonged examination), and a nondilating pupil may all interfere with the production of an ideal image for processing by AI-based software.
- *Need for shift in protocols:* Currently, most infants being screened and followed up for ROP have a physical examination by a trained ophthalmologist with a binocular indirect ophthalmoscope aided by scleral indentation. Photography is mostly resorted to as an addendum for documentation to aid teaching, seeking second opinion, or as a part of study protocols. Hence, the images are mostly not used to change one's clinical diagnosis or interpretation.

If CBIA is implemented, one would need to reverse this approach. The initial screening would then be through image acquisition by trained nursing personnel (not an ophthalmologist) and processed by the AI-based program. Further, follow-up and need for physical examination by an ophthalmologist would be decided based on the diagnosis arrived at by the CBIA. It obviously involves a degree of trust in the CBIA. This trust cannot be built overnight. Hence, it is more likely that one will see a slow evolution, perhaps on the following lines at each of the centers that are adopting CBIA:

- *Phase of testing the competence of the available CBIA:* The ophthalmologist in charge will physically examine each infant and also process the images through CBIA. Thus, the CBIA output will be tested against their own judgment. There is a possibility that this may be a learning process for the clinician as well if the CBIA really proves to be better at diagnosing plus disease.
- *Phase of initial acceptance of CBIA for preliminary screening:* Once the clinicians are more comfortable, they may use this system for the initial screening. However, it is more likely that there will be a

mix of teleophthalmology (clinician reading the images acquired) as well as giving weightage to the output from the CBIA. They may opt to confirm the findings in infants identified with ROP (any ROP) by ophthalmoscopy. Even in those with no ROP at initial examination by the CBIA-based evaluation, the second evaluation will probably be done by ophthalmologists directly.
- *Phase of full utilization of CBIA's competence:* It is only much later that the clinician may accept the CBIA output and resort to ophthalmoscopic verification only if ROP needing treatment is diagnosed or one is faced with the decision to discharge the patient from further follow-up.
- The role of CBIA, thus to begin with, is explorative, progresses to become additive and finally to being assistive and supportive.
- Fundamental to the success of CBIA is image acquisition, which is a manual process and heavily dependent on competence of the technician/nurse. Training of such a massive number of personnel who literally form the first defense against ROP is not a small task.

## APPLICATIONS OF ARTIFICIAL INTELLIGENCE IN RETINOPATHY OF PREMATURITY

Real-world testing of AI in ROP will define the utility of this new technology.

Some of the recent reports are mentioned below:
- *Applications of AI for ROP screening:*[60]
  - AI was used in an Indian ROP telemedicine program to determine whether differences in ROP severity between neonatal care units (NCUs) identified by using AI are related to differences in oxygen-titrating capability.
  - The area under the receiver operating characteristic curve for detection of treatment-requiring ROP was 0.98, with 100% sensitivity and 78% specificity.
  - They also found higher median (interquartile range) ROP severity in NCUs without oxygen blenders and pulse oxygenation monitors, most apparent in bigger infants.
- *Developing an ROP risk model:*[61]
  - In a telemedicine program in Nepal, Mongolia and India, the authors reported the development of an ROP risk model (using retinal images) to identify infants who are likely to develop treatment-requiring ROP.
  - The results suggested that the number of examinations for low-risk infants could be reduced without missing cases of those requiring treatment, and high-risk infants could be identified and closely monitored before the development of treatment-requiring ROP.

- *In training and improving interclinical variability:*[62]
  - The authors explored how experts' decision matches with other experts and with their respective trainees they are mentoring.
  - A completely automated algorithm quantifies the differences by using machine learning techniques and acts as a training and audit tool to address the differences, to measure the consistency objectively, and to help build more accurate automated diagnosis systems.

### ■ FUTURE OF DEEP LEARNING-BASED IMAGE ANALYSIS

One would envisage a better acceptance of the CBIA output and attempts at incorporating the same into overall strategy for the detection and management of ROP. The best utility would be in the communities that lack uniform access to prompt screening of at-risk babies. Mobile cameras manned by nonophthalmologists are already in vogue in some parts of the third-world countries, coupled with web-based teleophthalmology for the preliminary screening.[29] This process can be made more robust by coupling it with AI-based software that eliminates the immediate need for the images to be read by a remotely located ophthalmologist.

Artificial intelligence can also perhaps assist in better image capture, such as assisted autofocus and identification of landmarks,[63] although this technology is yet to be explored.

The possibility of harnessing information from other sources and incorporating the same in the AI process is also tenable. Images from OCT may well be used in the future to better define the conversion of stage 2 to stage 3, wherein the breach of internal limiting membrane (ILM) by the neovascular tissue may be better delineated.

It is also to be seen whether these AI programs can utilize the nonimaging-related information (birth weight, gestation age, weight gain, etc.) and synthesize the same with the information from the fundus images and better predict the future of these eyes.

Finally, for a novice ophthalmologist and perhaps even for an expert, this tool can well be a good virtual teacher helping to hone one's skills at precisely labeling the disease and predicting the future course.

### ■ CONCLUSION

- ROP is a disease of newborn initiated by low gestational age at birth and low birth weight and modulated by a plethora of factors. Less than optimum neonatal care during crucial periods is responsible for increasing the risk of vision-threatening stages of ROP. The window of opportunity to detect and treat the vision-threatening stages is narrow and needs expert retinal evaluation at periodic intervals, thus posing a tremendous burden on the healthcare system.

- The disease-defining parameters such as plus disease, location of the disease (zone), and staging are all subject to some degree of ambiguity. Notable of these is the identification of plus disease wherein significant differences exist even among experts.
- Digital imaging of the fundus in ROP using wide-angle handheld cameras has helped in several ways, including documentation, seeking second opinion, teleophthalmology, education and, now, processing with AI, thus effectively replacing the role of ophthalmologist at certain steps in the management of at-risk infants.
- Computer-based image analyses have progressed from "feature extraction" to self-learning ANNs such as deep learning that seem to holistically evaluate the fundus picture and come to conclusions, although the processing may not be evident (black box).
- Deep learning is heavily dependent on the amount of data that is used to train the network. Hence, use of pretrained networks, augmentation of images, and transfer learning are tools that enhance the competence of the network that is designed for diagnosis of ROP.
- Current studies have shown that the programs have the ability to identify the following: Presence or absence of ROP, plus disease, zone I disease, grades of severity of disease guiding urgent referral where needed, and nongradable images and help in preliminary screening of images. The networks are able to automatically grade the images in the order of severity scale for plus disease, although the labeling is done as ordinals with no specification of severity (no plus, preplus, and plus).
    - Using probability values and deep learning networks, investigators have come up with "vascular severity score"—a continuous score ranging from 0 to 9. This is likely to replace the present grading system of plus disease, which divides it into three discrete artificially divided segments. With this, ROP specialists have accepted that plus disease is a continuum.
    - Investigations have shown the following associations with vascular severity score:
        - Higher the stage of disease, greater the score, irrespective of the zones of involvement
        - Higher score seen in zone I (for stages 1–3) compared to similar stages in zone II
        - More the circumferential extent of stage 3 disease, higher the score. This applies to both zones I and II.
        - For the same amount of the circumferential extent of stage 3 disease (number of clock hours), the score was higher in zone I compared to zone II.
    - Limitations for the use of deep learning include:
        - Acceptance

- Integration of the network processing into the routine practice
- Differences in populations across the globe with respect to patient profile, disease profile, etc. Data trained on one population may not work on another population.
- Issues of liability
- Compulsory need for digital imaging

## REFERENCES

1. McCarthy J, Minsky ML, Rochester N, Shannon CE. A proposal for the Dartmouth summer research project on artificial intelligence, August 31, 1955. AI Magazine. 2006;27:12-4.
2. Samuel AL. Some studies in machine learning using the game of checkers. IBM J Res Dev. 1967;11:601-17.
3. LeCun Y, Bengio Y, Hinton G. Deep learning. Nature. 2015;521(7553):436-44.
4. Lakhani P, Sundaram B. Deep learning at chest radiography: automated classification of pulmonary tuberculosis by using convolutional neural networks. Radiology. 2017;284(2):574-82.
5. Zheng C, Johnson TV, Garg A, Boland MV. Artificial intelligence in glaucoma. Curr Opin Ophthalmol. 2019;30(2):97-103.
6. Romond K, Alam M, Kravets S, Sisternes L, Leng T, Lim JI, et al. Imaging and artificial intelligence for progression of age-related macular degeneration. Exp Biol Med (Maywood). 2021;246(20):2159-69.
7. Ferrara D, Newton EM, Lee AY. Artificial intelligence-based predictions in neovascular age-related macular degeneration. Curr Opin Ophthalmol. 2021;32(5):389-96.
8. Mohan S, Gaur R, Raman R. Using artificial intelligence in diabetic retinopathy. IHOPE J Ophthalmol. 2022;1:71-8.
9. Foote KD. The history of machine learning and its convergent trajectory towards AI. In: Carta S (Ed). Machine Learning and the City: Applications in Architecture and Urban Design. Hoboken, NJ: Wiley Online Library; 2022. pp. 129-42. [Chapter 7].
10. Weiss S, Kulikowski CA, Safir A. Glaucoma consultation by computer. Comput Biol Med. 1978;8:25-40.
11. Bakkar N, Kovalik T, Lorenzini I, Spangler S, Lacoste A, Sponaugle K, et al. Artificial intelligence in neurodegenerative disease research: use of IBM Watson to identify additional RNA-binding proteins altered in amyotrophic lateral sclerosis. Acta Neuropathol. 2018;135(2):227-47.
12. Kaul V, Enslin S, Gross SA. History of artificial intelligence in medicine. Gastrointest Endosc. 2020;92:807-12.
13. Löwel S, Singer W. Selection of intrinsic horizontal connections in the visual cortex by correlated neuronal activity. Science. 1992;255(5041):209-12.
14. Azad R, Gilbert C, Gangwe AB, Zhao P, Wu WC, Sarbajna P, et al. Retinopathy of prematurity: how to prevent the third epidemics in developing countries. Asia Pac J Ophthalmol (Phila). 2020;9(5):440-8.
15. Hartnett ME. Advances in understanding and management of retinopathy of prematurity. Surv Ophthalmol. 2017;62(3):257-76.
16. Chiang MF, Quinn GE, Fielder AR, Ostmo SR, Chan RVP, Berrocal A, et al. International classification of retinopathy of prematurity, third edition. Ophthalmology. 2021;128(10):e51-68.

17. Haines L, Fielder AR, Scrivener R, Wilkinson AR, Pollock JI, Royal College of Paediatrics and Child Health, et al. Retinopathy of prematurity in the UK I: the organisation of services for screening and treatment. Eye (Lond). 2002;16(1):33-8.
18. Vinekar A, Jayadev C, Dogra M, Shetty B. Improving follow-up of infants during retinopathy of prematurity screening in rural areas. Indian Pediatr. 2016;53(Suppl. 2):S151-4.
19. Vinekar A, Dogra M, Azad RV, Gilbert C, Gopal L, Trese M. The changing scenario of retinopathy of prematurity in middle and low income countries: unique solutions for unique problems. Indian J Ophthalmol. 2019;67(6):717-9.
20. Vinekar A, Bhende P. Innovations in technology and service delivery to improve retinopathy of prematurity care. Community Eye Health. 2017;30(99):S20-2.
21. Gawande A, Kuhlmann-Krieg S. Complications: A Surgeon's Notes on an Imperfect Science. USA: Picador; 2003.
22. Campbell JP, Ryan MC, Lore E, Tian P, Ostmo S, Jonas K, et al. Diagnostic discrepancies in retinopathy of prematurity classification. Ophthalmology. 2016;123(8):1795-801.
23. Fleck BW, Williams C, Juszczak E, Cocker K, Stenson BJ, Darlow BA, et al. An international comparison of retinopathy of prematurity grading performance within the Benefits of Oxygen Saturation Targeting II trials. Eye (Lond). 2018;32(1):74-80.
24. Abràmoff MD, Lavin PT, Birch M, Shah N, Folk JC. Pivotal trial of an autonomous AI-based diagnostic system for detection of diabetic retinopathy in primary care offices. NPJ Digit Med. 2018;1:39.
25. Burlina PM, Joshi N, Pekala M, Pacheco KD, Freund DE, Bressler NM. Automated grading of age-related macular degeneration from color fundus images using deep convolutional neural networks. JAMA Ophthalmol. 2017;135(11):1170-6.
26. Anegondi N, Gao SS, Steffen V, Spaide RF, Sadda SR, Holz FG, et al. Deep learning to predict geographic atrophy area and growth rate from multimodal imaging. Ophthalmol Retina. 2022:S2468-6530(22)00426-2.
27. Schlegl T, Waldstein SM, Bogunovic H, Endstraßer F, Sadeghipour A, Philip AM, et al. Fully automated detection and quantification of macular fluid in OCT using deep learning. Ophthalmology. 2018;125(4):549-58.
28. Park SJ, Ko T, Park CK, Kim YC, Choi IY. Deep learning model based on 3D optical coherence tomography images for the automated detection of pathologic myopia. Diagnostics (Basel). 2022;12(3):742.
29. Vinekar A, Gilbert C, Dogra M, Kurian M, Shainesh G, Shetty B, et al. The KIDROP model of combining strategies for providing retinopathy of prematurity screening in underserved areas in India using wide-field imaging, tele-medicine, non-physician graders and smart phone reporting. Indian J Ophthalmol. 2014;62(1):41-9.
30. Vinekar A, Jayadev C, Mangalesh S, Shetty B, Vidyasagar D. Role of tele-medicine in retinopathy of prematurity screening in rural outreach centers in India—a report of 20,214 imaging sessions in the KIDROP program. Semin Fetal Neonatal Med. 2015;20(5):335-45.
31. Schwartz SD, Harrison SA, Ferrone PJ, Trese MT. Telemedical evaluation and management of retinopathy of prematurity using a fiberoptic digital fundus camera. Ophthalmology. 2000;107(1):25-8.
32. Campbell JP, Ataer-Cansizoglu E, Bolon-Canedo V, Bozkurt A, Erdogmus D, Kalpathy-Cramer J, et al. Expert diagnosis of plus disease in retinopathy of prematurity from computer-based image analysis. JAMA Ophthalmol. 2016;134(6):651-7.

33. Wittenberg LA, Jonsson NJ, Chan RVP, Chiang MF. Computer-based image analysis for plus disease diagnosis in retinopathy of prematurity. J Pediatr Ophthalmol Strabismus. 2012;49(1):11-9 [quiz 10, 20].
34. Campbell JP, Kalpathy-Cramer J, Erdogmus D, Tian P, Kedarisetti D, Moleta C, et al. Plus disease in retinopathy of prematurity: a continuous spectrum of vascular abnormality as a basis of diagnostic variability. Ophthalmology. 2016;123(11):2338-44.
35. Heneghan C, Flynn J, O'Keefe M, Cahill M. Characterization of changes in blood vessel width and tortuosity in retinopathy of prematurity using image analysis. Med Image Anal. 2002;6(4):407-29.
36. Gelman R, Martinez-Perez ME, Vanderveen DK, Moskowitz A, Fulton AB. Diagnosis of plus disease in retinopathy of prematurity using retinal image multiscale analysis. Invest Ophthalmol Vis Sci. 2005;46(12):4734-8. [Erratum in: Invest Ophthalmol Vis Sci. 2007;48(12):5359].
37. Wallace DK, Zhao Z, Freedman SF. A pilot study using "ROPtool" to quantify plus disease in retinopathy of prematurity. J AAPOS. 2007;11(4):381-7.
38. Rabinowitz MP, Grunwald JE, Karp KA, Quinn GE, Ying GS, Mills MD. Progression to severe retinopathy predicted by retinal vessel diameter between 31 and 34 weeks of postconception age. Arch Ophthalmol. 2007;125(11):1495-500.
39. Wilson CM, Cocker KD, Moseley MJ, Paterson C, Clay ST, Schulenburg WE, et al. Computerized analysis of retinal vessel width and tortuosity in premature infants. Invest Ophthalmol Vis Sci. 2008;49(8):3577-85.
40. Johnston SC, Wallace DK, Freedman SF, Yanovitch TL, Zhao Z. Tortuosity of arterioles and venules in quantifying plus disease. J AAPOS. 2009;13(2):181-5.
41. Chiang MF, Gelman R, Jiang L, Martinez-Perez ME, Du YE, Flynn JT. Plus disease in retinopathy of prematurity: an analysis of diagnostic performance. Trans Am Ophthalmol Soc. 2007;105:73-84 [discussion 84-5].
42. Worrall DE, Wilson CM, Brostow GJ. Automated retinopathy of prematurity case detection with convolutional neural networks. Deep Learning and Data Labeling for Medical Applications. DLMIA LABELS, Athens, Greece, 2016. Lecture Notes in Computer Science, vol 10008. Springer, Cham. pp. 68-76.
43. Wang J, Ju R, Chen Y, Zhang L, Hu J, Wu Y, et al. Automated retinopathy of prematurity screening using deep neural networks. EBioMedicine. 2018;35:361-8.
44. Hu J, Chen Y, Zhong J, Ju R, Yi Z. Automated analysis for retinopathy of prematurity by deep neural networks. IEEE Trans Med Imaging. 2019;38(1):269-79.
45. Zhao J, Lei B, Wu Z, Zhang Y, Li Y, Wang L, et al. A deep learning framework for identifying zone I in RetCam images. IEEE Access. 2019;7:103530-7.
46. Huang YP, Vadloori S, Chu HC, Kang EYC, Wu WC, Kusaka S, et al. Deep learning models for automated diagnosis of retinopathy of prematurity in preterm infants. Electronics. 2020;9:1444.
47. Tong Y, Lu W, Deng QQ, Chen C, Shen Y. Automated identification of retinopathy of prematurity by image-based deep learning. Eye Vis (Lond). 2020;7:40.
48. Vijayalakshmi C, Sakthivel P, Vinekar A. Automated detection and classification of telemedical retinopathy of prematurity images. Telemed J E Health. 2020;26(3):354-8.
49. Chen JS, Coyner AS, Ostmo S, Sonmez K, Bajimaya S, Pradhan E, et al. Deep learning for the diagnosis of stage in retinopathy of prematurity: accuracy and generalizability across populations and cameras. Ophthalmol Retina. 2021;5(10):1027-35.

50. Agrawal R, Kulkarni S, Walambe R, Kotecha K. Assistive framework for automatic detection of all the zones in retinopathy of prematurity using deep learning. J Digit Imaging. 2021;34(4):932-47.
51. Brown JM, Campbell JP, Beers A, Chang K, Ostmo S, Chan RVP, et al. Automated diagnosis of plus disease in retinopathy of prematurity using deep convolutional neural networks. JAMA Ophthalmol. 2018;136(7):803-10.
52. Nisha KL, Sreelekha G, Sathidevi PS, Mohanachandran P, Vinekar A. A computer-aided diagnosis system for plus disease in retinopathy of prematurity with structure adaptive segmentation and vessel based features. Comput Med Imaging Graph. 2019;74:72-94.
53. Ramachandran S, Niyas P, Vinekar A, John R. A deep learning framework for the detection of Plus disease in retinal fundus images of preterm infants. Biocybern Biomed Eng. 2021;41:362-75.
54. Ramachandran S, Strisciuglio N, Vinekar A, John R, Azzopardi G. U-COSFIRE filters for vessel tortuosity quantification with application to automated diagnosis of retinopathy of prematurity. Neural Comput Appl. 2020;32:12453-68.
55. Campbell JP, Chiang MF, Chen JS, Moshfeghi DM, Nudleman E, Ruambivoonsuk P, et al. Artificial intelligence for retinopathy of prematurity: validation of a vascular severity scale against international expert diagnosis. Ophthalmology. 2022;129(7):e69-76.
56. Choi RY, Brown JM, Kalpathy-Cramer J, Chan RVP, Ostmo S, Chiang MF, et al. Variability in plus disease identified using a deep learning-based retinopathy of prematurity severity scale. Ophthalmol Retina. 2020;4(10):1016-21.
57. Campbell JP, Kim SJ, Brown JM, Ostmo S, Chan RVP, Kalpathy-Cramer J, et al. Evaluation of a deep learning-derived quantitative retinopathy of prematurity severity scale. Ophthalmology. 2021;128(7):1070-6.
58. Gupta K, Campbell JP, Taylor S, Brown JM, Ostmo S, Chan RVP, et al. A quantitative severity scale for retinopathy of prematurity using deep learning to monitor disease regression after treatment. JAMA Ophthalmol. 2019;137(9):1029-36.
59. Coyner AS, Swan R, Brown JM, Kalpathy-Cramer J, Kim SJ, Campbell JP, et al. Deep learning for image quality assessment of fundus images in retinopathy of prematurity. AMIA Annu Symp Proc. 2018;2018:1224-32.
60. Campbell JP, Singh P, Redd TK, Brown JM, Shah PK, Subramanian P, et al. Applications of artificial intelligence for retinopathy of prematurity screening. Pediatrics. 2021;147(3):e2020016618.
61. Coyner AS, Oh MA, Shah PK, Singh P, Ostmo S, Valikodath NG, et al. External validation of a retinopathy of prematurity screening model using artificial intelligence in 3 low- and middle-income populations. JAMA Ophthalmol. 2022;140(8):791-8.
62. Nisha KL, Ganapathy S, Puthumangalathu Savithri S, Idaguri M, Mohanachandran P, Vinekar A, et al. A novel method to improve inter-clinician variation in the diagnosis of retinopathy of prematurity using machine learning. Curr Eye Res. 2022;48:60-9.
63. Gensure RH, Chiang MF, Campbell JP. Artificial intelligence for retinopathy of prematurity. Curr Opin Ophthalmol. 2020;31(5):312-7.

CHAPTER 11

# Diagnosis of Retinal Detachment by Artificial Intelligence

*Chaitra Jayadev, Aishwarya Joshi*

## ABSTRACT

The advent of deep learning in ophthalmology has been widely exploited to replace more mechanical and high turnover activities of screening a large population for certain diseases. As it deploys various imaging modalities, these images can be processed to give a certain diagnosis for triage and risk stratification. As the prognosis of retinal detachment largely depends upon how early one intervenes, studies have now been undertaken to help with the timely diagnosis of this condition. Various architectural forms of convolutional neural network are now being put to use to "teach" machines how to detect retinal detachments and many other retinal diseases such as diabetic retinopathy, age-related macular degeneration, and retinopathy of prematurity.

***Keywords:*** Retinal detachment; artificial intelligence; ultrawide-field imaging.

## ■ INTRODUCTION

The use of a computer's "trained" intelligent behavior with minimal human intervention is known as artificial intelligence (AI). It originally started with the development of robots but has been widely applied to other fields, especially in medicine, for the diagnosis, classification, prognostication, and monitoring of various diseases. Ophthalmology being a very visually oriented field, based on pattern recognition, and with ample advanced imaging modalities, is an ideal field for the application of machine-based learning. AI is also of great help to ophthalmologists, with its ability to handle high patient turnover and application in telemedicine.[1] Direct visualization of the vascular and nervous tissue is possible in the retina without any invasive intervention. Even without knowing the age or gender of the subject, a retinal image can help the physician make important diagnoses, some of which can be life- and vision-saving. An added advantage of objectivity and rapidity can be offered by AI-based tools for these retinal images. This chapter will elucidate about the available tools and literature on AI-based diagnosis and follow-up for an important retinal condition called retinal detachment (RD), which if left undetected and untreated can lead to permanent visual debility.

## BASIC LAYOUT AND FUNCTIONING OF ARTIFICIAL INTELLIGENCE SYSTEM

Artificial intelligence is mainly based on image processing via convolutional neural network (CNN). These neural networks are a set of simple algorithms designed to function similar to the human brain in recognizing patterns. These are stacked on top of each other like books on a shelf, and the first layer "receives" the input; the signal is fired or propagated forward through the different layers until it reaches the output layer. This network is "taught" how to read images/data by presenting multiple such preanswered images graded by experts in the field. Its accuracy increases with the number of images or amount of data offered to it as it self-corrects its own interpretations.[2] The images are processed pixel by pixel, with each pixel tied to an input layer neuron which gets activated depending upon the brightness of the pixel. The amount of signal received by this input layer neuron is directly proportional to the intensity of the brightness and is not just a simple on-and-off mechanism. These responses are collected and processed by the subsequent layers, and the required output is obtained **(Fig. 1)**.[2] Retinal images have been used for diagnoses by machine learning systems for several diseases such as diabetic retinopathy (DR),[3-6] age-related macular degeneration (AMD),[7-11] retinal tears and RD,[12-14] and retinopathy of prematurity (ROP).[15] Some other studies have been able to diagnose diabetic macular edema,[16] and even predict the progression of wet and dry AMD.[17-23]

## DEVELOPMENT OF ARTIFICIAL INTELLIGENCE FOR RETINAL DETACHMENT DETECTION

A fundus photo is a suitable imaging modality that can be used for visual evaluation by the machine learning system. Taking into consideration the

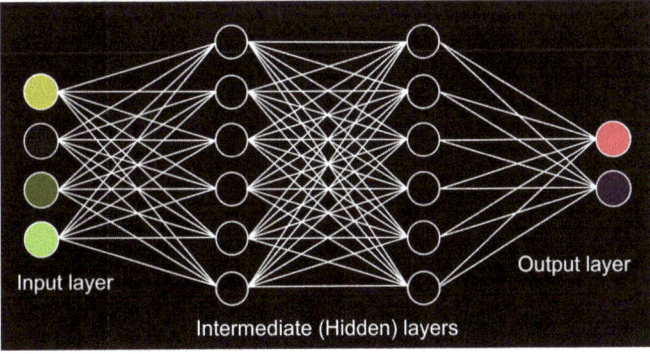

**Fig. 1:** Basic structure of a convolutional neural network.

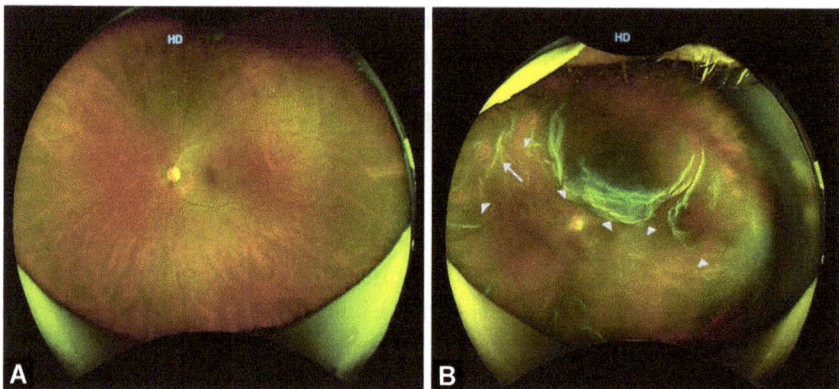

**Figs. 2A and B:** Ultrawide field image of (A) normal retina and (B) rhegmatogenous retinal detachment (white arrowheads), with the corresponding retinal break (white arrow).

extent of retina that needs to be assessed to rule out even the smallest or the most peripheral breaks and detachments right up to the extreme periphery, it warrants the use of ultrawide field imaging modalities **(Figs. 2A and B)**. A quick, nonmydriatic fundus camera, capable of imaging up to ora serrata without the requirement for montaging, would be ideal.[24]

Thousands of images from such a system need to be first selected based on their quality and manually classified before being fed into the system. After poor-quality images are excluded, the rest are standardized in terms of size and pixels and then processed by the system to give a diagnosis.[12] This diagnosis is then validated with that of retinal experts, and the right answer is fed back into the system. The system corrects itself by a method of "backpropagation" and accordingly modifies the intermediate layers to "learn" to give the right answer known as "cost-minimization." After multiple such corrections, the accuracy of this AI system starts shifting more and more toward perfection. By the time 300 such training images are processed, the accuracy of interpreting some standard, prediagnosed images available on MNIST (Modified National Institute of Standards and Technology) collection of digital training images increases to >96%.[25] One such form of AI which is useful for image analysis is the CNN as it is capable of deconstruction and recognition of images. Research is on to combine multiple such CNNs to make one robust system capable of recognizing multiple conditions.[26]

## ■ FRAMEWORK OF CASCADED DEEP LEARNING SYSTEM

InceptionResNetV2 is a machine learning system with an architecture, which is a combination of two previous CNNs: Residual network and inception network.[14] This first model only identifies an RD in the input messages and the second model classifies it into "macula-off or macula-on" RD. A heat map of the fundus photo is used to know the areas where the AI is focusing on.

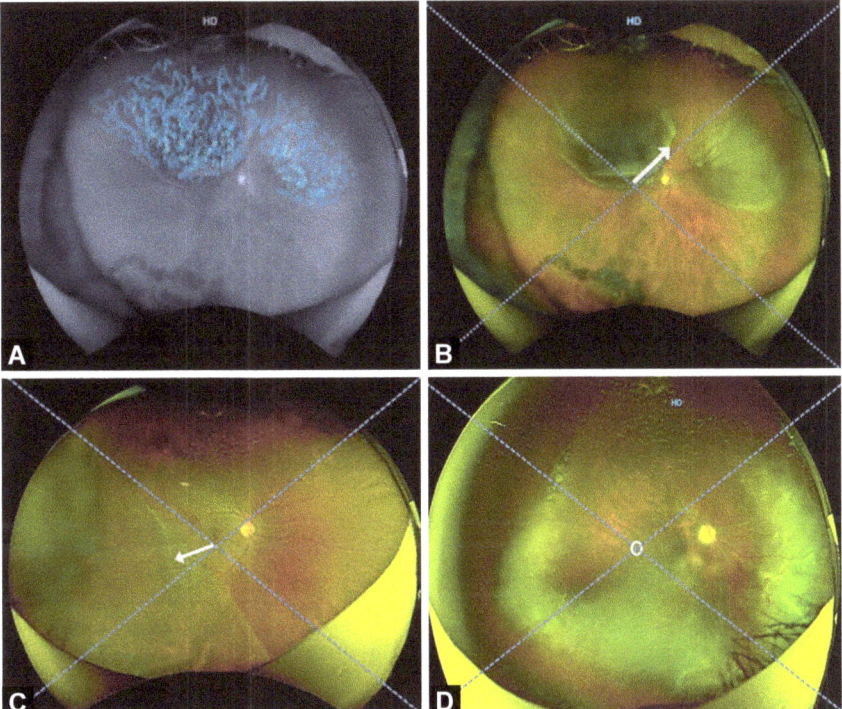

**Figs. 3A to D:** Indicative images of an algorithm showing (A) heatmap in retinal detachment. (B) The arrow toward the area of retinal detachment is generated automatically based on the highlighted region in the heatmap. The arrow in (C) and circle in (D) are used to instruct patients in preoperative posturing to reduce the progression of retinal detachment.

A saliency map technique compares the output of CNN with the brightness of a pixel so that the machine focuses on the most significant pixels. The image is divided into quadrants by dotted lines placed diagonally. The hot areas are suggestive of an RD, and an arrow from the center of the photo to the center of the RD in the respective quadrant is used to denote the direction in which head positioning has to be maintained to prevent further progression of the RD **(Figs. 3A to D)**. Besides InceptionResNetV2, other CNN architectures being used are InceptionV3, ResNet50, and VGG16, with InceptionResNetV2 having the most success in detecting notable peripheral retinal lesions (NPRLs) such as lattice degenerations and retinal holes as it has the most layers.[13] It can also predict the urgency with which the intervention needs to be planned and gives an indication of the prognosis **(Flowchart 1)**.

## ■ LIMITATIONS

Cost remains a significant factor for the development of these algorithms and for the high-resolution widefield imaging modalities.[27] There is limited

**Flowchart 1:** Basic layout of InceptionResNetV2 architecture of a convolutional neural network.

Ultrawide field images are fed into the system for processing

1st step: At the first step, the images are classified into RD versus nonRD

2nd step

Additionally, some systems divide the image into quadrants and an arrow to indicate the preoperative posturing to prevent further progression

At the second step, the images are classified into macula involving versus nonmacula involving to triage for need of emergency intervention

(RD: retinal detachment)

availability of these expensive devices to better "train" the algorithms. Currently, there is more research and emphasis on AI for high-prevalence conditions such as DR, AMD, and ROP, than for RD. AI, available now, is only capable of diagnosing specific diseases and unable to detect the presence of other concurrent or coexisting conditions. Being an image-based application, its role is limited and accuracy is questionable in cases where there are artifacts or media opacities such as cataract, vitreous hemorrhage, posterior capsular opacity, or vitritis **(Figs. 4A to D)**. This can give false readings, known as "garbage in, garbage out" phenomenon. It may even falsely label laser marks or any local pigmentation as significant lesions.[13]

The currently available teaching images are from a few sources and may not be representative of all demographics.[12-14] Also, the use of two-dimensional images which lack stereoscopy makes it difficult to assess elevated lesions such as retinal traction near the NPRLs.[5] The system may miss subtle lesions like retinal holes within the lattices. Even widefield imaging devices do not capture the entire retina and hence increase the chances of AI programs missing very peripheral lesions.[13] Since machine or the AI-based diagnosis misses the human touch and empathy, acceptance by the patient and society may take time. However, a study evaluating AI-based DR screening in an endocrinology clinic found that 96% of the patients were either satisfied

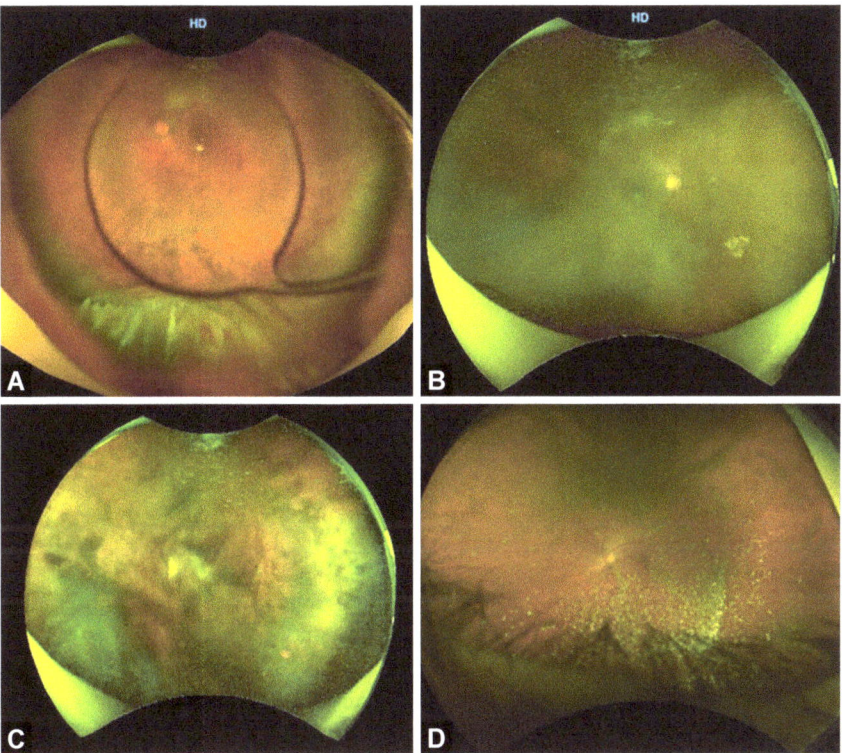

**Figs. 4A to D:** Potential artifacts and media opacities that can compromise the accuracy of an algorithm. (A) Intraocular lens; (B) Cataract haze; (C) Vitreous hemorrhage; (D) Asteroid hyalosis and eyelashes.

or very satisfied with the AI model.[28] Approval from various regulatory authorities can be challenging and fraught with medicolegal issues.[5]

With the current AI models only being able to pick up RD, it would be of added benefit if future models would incorporate a scoring system into the algorithm, which can assess the retina more comprehensively. Taking into consideration risk factors such as age, gender, refractive error, symptomatology, history of trauma, or any recent surgical procedure could help to locate predisposing lesions and predict their progression into an RD. The prediction, in turn, will help plan follow-up visits, prompt diagnosis, and timely intervention.

## ■ CONCLUSION

The use of AI for the diagnosis of RD does not require much knowledge or skill and has a short learning curve, making it easy for technicians to use. Being automated and fast, it enables quick screening with mydriasis, especially in centers with a high patient load. Those with suspected RD on AI screening can be subjected to a detailed dilated fundus examination by the physician and can help save the patient from visual morbidity, and can also be used to motivate and mobilize them for early intervention. Being image-based, triaging of patients who actually need intervention is possible or if there is a diagnostic dilemma, it can be sent to the appropriate specialist for confirmation, thus playing a role in telemedicine.

## ■ REFERENCES

1. Hamet P, Tremblay J. Artificial intelligence in medicine. Metabolism. 2017;69S:S36-40.
2. Ahmad BU, Kim JE, Rahimy E. Fundamentals of artificial intelligence for ophthalmologists. Curr Opin Ophthalmol. 2020;31:303-11.
3. Gulshan V, Peng L, Coram M, Stumpe MC, Wu D, Narayanaswamy A, et al. Development and validation of a deep learning algorithm for detection of diabetic retinopathy in retinal fundus photographs. JAMA. 2016;316:2402-10.
4. Gargeya R, Leng T. Automated identification of diabetic retinopathy using deep learning. Ophthalmology. 2017;124:962-9.
5. Ting DSW, Cheung CY, Lim G, Tan GSW, Quang ND, Gan A, et al. Development and validation of a deep learning system for diabetic retinopathy and related eye diseases using retinal images from multiethnic populations with diabetes. JAMA. 2017;318:2211-23.
6. Ramachandran N, Hong SC, Sime MJ, Wilson GA. Diabetic retinopathy screening using deep neural network. Clin Exp Ophthalmol. 2018;46:412-6.
7. Burlina PM, Joshi N, Pekala M, Pacheco KD, Freund DE, Bressler NM. Automated grading of age-related macular degeneration from color fundus images using deep convolutional neural networks. JAMA Ophthalmol. 2017;135:1170-6.
8. Grassmann F, Mengelkamp J, Brandl C, Harsch S, Zimmermann ME, Linkohr B, et al. A deep learning algorithm for prediction of age-related eye disease study severity scale for age-related macular degeneration from color fundus photography. Ophthalmology. 2018;125:1410-20.
9. Treder M, Lauermann JL, Eter N. Deep learning-based detection and classification of geographic atrophy using a deep convolutional neural network classifier. Graefes Arch Clin Exp Ophthalmol. 2018;256:2053-60.
10. Matsuba S, Tabuchi H, Ohsugi H, Enno H, Ishitobi N, Masumoto H, et al. Accuracy of ultra-wide-field fundus ophthalmoscopy-assisted deep learning, a machine-learning technology, for detecting age-related macular degeneration. Int Ophthalmol. 2019;39:1269-75.
11. Keel S, Li Z, Scheetz J, Robman L, Phung J, Makeyeva G, et al. Development and validation of a deep-learning algorithm for the detection of neovascular age-related macular degeneration from colour fundus photographs. Clin Exp Ophthalmol. 2019;47:1009-18.
12. Ohsugi H, Tabuchi H, Enno H, Ishitobi N. Accuracy of deep learning, a machine-learning technology, using ultra-wide-field fundus ophthalmoscopy for detecting rhegmatogenous retinal detachment. Sci Rep. 2017;7:9425.
13. Li Z, Guo C, Nie D, Lin D, Zhu Y, Chen C, et al. A deep learning system for identifying lattice degeneration and retinal breaks using ultra-widefield fundus images. Ann Transl Med. 2019;7:618.

14. Li Z, Guo C, Nie D, Lin D, Zhu Y, Chen C, et al. Deep learning for detecting retinal detachment and discerning macular status using ultra-widefield fundus images. Commun Biol. 2020;3:15.
15. Coyner AS, Swan R, Brown JM, Kalpathy-Cramer J, Kim SJ, Campbell JP, et al. Deep learning for image quality assessment of fundus images in retinopathy of prematurity. AMIA Annu Symp Proc. 2018;2018:1224-32.
16. ElTanboly A, Ismail M, Shalaby A, Switala A, El-Baz A, Schaal S, et al. A computer-aided diagnostic system for detecting diabetic retinopathy in optical coherence tomography images. Med Phys. 2017;44:914-23.
17. Schmidt-Erfurth U, Bogunovic H, Sadeghipour A, Schlegl T, Langs G, Gerendas BS, et al. Machine learning to analyze the prognostic value of current imaging biomarkers in neovascular age-related macular degeneration. Ophthalmol Retina. 2018;2:24-30.
18. Seebock P, Waldstein SM, Klimscha S, Bogunovic H, Schlegl T, Gerendas BS, et al. Unsupervised identification of disease marker candidates in retinal OCT imaging data. IEEE Trans Med Imaging. 2019;38:1037-47.
19. Bogunovic H, Waldstein SM, Schlegl T, Langs G, Sadeghipour A, Liu X, et al. Prediction of anti-VEGF treatment requirements in neovascular AMD using a machine learning approach. Invest Ophthalmol Vis Sci. 2017;58:3240-8.
20. Prahs P, Radeck V, Mayer C, Cvetkov Y, Cvetkova N, Helbig H, et al. OCT-based deep learning algorithm for the evaluation of treatment indication with anti-vascular endothelial growth factor medications. Graefes Arch Clin Exp Ophthalmol. 2018;256:91-8.
21. Aslam TM, Zaki HR, Mahmood S, Ali ZC, Ahmad NA, Thorell MR, et al. Use of a neural net to model the impact of optical coherence tomography abnormalities on vision in age-related macular degeneration. Am J Ophthalmol. 2018;185:94-100.
22. Schmidt-Erfurth U, Waldstein SM, Klimscha S, Sadeghipour A, Hu X, Gerendas BS, et al. Prediction of individual disease conversion in early AMD using artificial intelligence. Invest Ophthalmol Vis Sci. 2018;59:3199-208.
23. Bogunovic H, Montuoro A, Baratsits M, Karantonis MG, Waldstein SM, Schlanitz F, et al. Machine learning of the progression of intermediate age-related macular degeneration based on OCT imaging. Invest Ophthalmol Vis Sci. 2017;58(6):BIO141-50.
24. Nagiel A, Lalane RA, Sadda SR, Schwartz SD. Ultra-widefield fundus imaging: a review of clinical applications and future trends. Retina. 2016;36:660.
25. LeCun Y, Cortes C, Burges CJC. The MNIST database. [online] Available from: http://yann.lecun.com/exdb/mnist/. [Last accessed February, 2023].
26. Dharmaraj. (2022). Convolutional neural networks (CNN) — architecture explained. [online] Available from https://medium.com/@draj0718/convolutional-neural-networks-cnn-architectures-explained-716fb197b243. [Last accessed February, 2023].
27. Keane PA, Topol EJ. With an eye to AI and autonomous diagnosis. NPJ Digit Med. 2018;1:40.
28. Keel S, Lee PY, Scheetz J, Li Z, Kotowicz MA, MacIsaac RJ, et al. Feasibility and patient acceptability of a novel artificial intelligence-based screening model for diabetic retinopathy at endocrinology outpatient services: a pilot study. Sci Rep. 2018;8:4330.

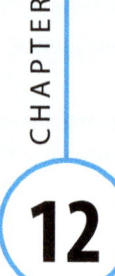

CHAPTER 12

# Artificial Intelligence in Age-related Macular Degeneration

*Brughanya Subramanian, Chitralekha S Devishamani, Parveen Sen, Rajiv Raman*

## ABSTRACT

Life expectancy has increased the burden of providing adequate health facilities by healthcare professionals worldwide. To overcome this problem, artificial intelligence (AI), a branch of computer science that deals with developing algorithms that seek to simulate human intelligence, offers promising solutions. AI is a broad term encompassing multiple components, of which machine learning and deep learning are the two major components. AI is used to diagnose diabetic retinopathy, age-related macular degeneration (AMD), and glaucoma. The other areas explored include retinopathy of prematurity and cataract. This chapter gives an overview of AI, its components, its applicability in AMD, and its limitation.

***Keywords:*** Artificial intelligence; age-related macular degeneration; machine learning; deep learning; neural network; convolution neural network.

## ■ INTRODUCTION

Age-related macular degeneration (AMD) is the leading cause of blindness worldwide in people over the age of 50 years and the third leading cause of blindness overall. As the world population ages, AMD also grows in prevalence, with the estimated cases predicted to reach 288 million by 2040. It substantially affects the quality of life of an individual.[1] Estimates indicate that 10–20% of AMD is the wet form responsible for approximately 90% of severe vision loss. Recent findings from a population-based study from rural India have reported the prevalence of early and late AMD at 2.7% [95% confidence interval (CI), 2.2–3.2] and 0.6% (95% CI, 0.4–0.8), respectively.[2] Three studies done in India reported prevalence rates in the 70 and older age-group as 2, 3.7, and 4.6%, but the number of people in the age-group 70 and older was low (300 in each study).[2-4] The antivascular endothelial growth factor (anti-VEGF) therapy has revolutionized care for patients with neovascular AMD and other neovascular ocular conditions such as retinal vein occlusion (RVO), diabetic macular edema, and retinopathy of prematurity (ROP). It has dramatically improved the visual outcome and quality of life of millions worldwide.[5]

An enormous interest has emerged among the medical fraternity due to the introduction and application of artificial intelligence (AI) in medical services. AI is utilized in many healthcare infrastructures, including hospitals, clinical laboratories, and research facilities. AI enables computers to function independently and intelligently to perform tasks usually done by humans. It involves machine learning (ML) incorporating various algorithms known as neural networks that allow these computers to learn and edit from the provided datasets and subsequently make accurate predictions. An integration of ophthalmology and AI-based techniques is utilized for various purposes such as automatic screening,[6] decision support system for primary clinics,[7] automatic disease severity classification,[8] and treatment optimization.[9] AI/ML-based algorithms have made progress in recent times in diseases such as diabetic retinopathy (DR),[10,11] AMD,[12,13] glaucoma,[14] cataract,[15] ROP,[16] and RVO.[17] AI in ophthalmology has focused mainly on the field of retina since it involves a significant number of images to diagnose a condition.[8,18]

Artificial intelligence tools have also been increasingly developed for AMD. With increased access to big data and analytics and advancements in the neural network approach, computers have learned the combinations and permutations of essential features.[19] This chapter gives an overview of the utilization of AI to analyze various aspects of AMD from detection to treatment.

## ■ BACKGROUND OF ARTIFICIAL INTELLIGENCE

The phrase "artificial intelligence" was first given by John McCarthy in 1955.[20] AI is used to accomplish tasks using advanced computer-based systems with minimal human involvement. AI encompasses two significant components: ML and deep learning (DL).

In ophthalmology, AI began with the traditional ML technique, also called "supervised learning," as described by Ruamviboonsuk et al.[21] The ML system requires the technician to label the clinical features and severity in the images to help AI develop an algorithm to classify images based on the loaded data. DL, also referred to as "unsupervised learning," is the new AI program, and as the name suggests, this system does not require labeling from the technician. DL works on the principle of deep neural networks modeled after the human brain to recognize a pattern.

Deep learning "self-learns" the pointing features to classify disease and its severity using the whole image with their clinical diagnosis. Convolution neural networks (CNN) and massive training artificial neural networks (MTANN) are two types of DL programs. CNN and MTANN, just like the human brain, consist of multiple interconnected layers of neurons designed to simulate "thinking." Input is fed into the first layer, whose output serves as an input for the next layer. The analysis from each layer is transmitted to the network until the outcome is produced. For an image-based diagnosis, a CNN algorithm teaches itself by analyzing pixel or voxel intensities in a labeled training set of expert-graded images and then provides a diagnostic output at the top layer. This process is repeated several times for every image. Once the algorithm optimizes itself, it can work on unknown images.[22] However, the convolution operations are carried within the network in CNN, whereas in MTANN, they are outside the network.[23]

## ■ ROLE OF ARTIFICIAL INTELLIGENCE IN AGE-RELATED MACULAR DEGENERATION

The role and contribution of AI in AMD are briefed in **Flowchart 1**.

### Initial Detection of Age-related Macular Degeneration

The timely detection of AMD by community eye health practitioners and its distinction from healthy aging is a fundamental first step in preventing vision loss from this condition. AI models could also be helpful as assistive clinical tools for community eye health practitioners for identifying eyes requiring more careful assessment to determine the presence of AMD. AI applications can significantly support patients in rural areas by sharing expert knowledge with limited recourses.[24] AI models for identifying AMD are listed in **Table 1**.

### Screening and Diagnosis of Age-related Macular Degeneration

The AI/ML-based algorithms have progressed in diagnosing AMD **(Table 2)**. Evidence is emerging on developing algorithms for retinal images utilizing

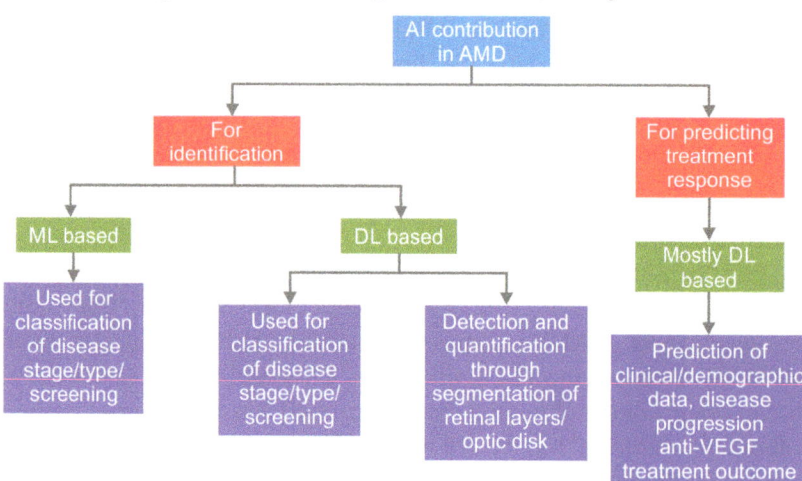

**Flowchart 1:** Hierarchy showing the contribution of artificial intelligence (AI) in age-related macular degeneration (AMD) management.

(DL: deep learning; ML: machine learning; VEGF: vascular endothelial growth factor)

**TABLE 1:** Artificial intelligence (AI) models for detecting age-related macular degeneration (AMD).

| Authors | Objectives | AI models | Results |
|---|---|---|---|
| Ting et al.[9] (2017) | Identify eyes with AMD (based on the presence of numerous medium drusen, ≥1 large drusen, or signs of late AMD) using color fundus photographs | DL based | 93% of fundus photographs were correctly identified for the presence/absence of AMD |
| Jiang et al.[25] (2020) | Two-level classification system using color fundus photographs was programmed for classifying an image as having a macular disease (one of which was AMD), retinal vascular disease, or optic nerve disease | DL based | Achieved an accuracy of 85% |
| Schlegl et al.[26] (2018) | Fully automated detection and quantification of macular fluid using SD-OCT | DL based | The AI model achieved AUC of 0.94 and a mean precision of 0.91. The detection and measurement of subretinal fluid were also highly accurate with an AUC of 0.92 and a mean precision of 0.61 |
| Treder et al.[27] (2018) | Automated detection of exudative AMD in SD-OCT using DL | CNN based | The training accuracy and validation accuracies were 100% |
| Li et al.[28] (2019) | Fully automated detection of retinal disorders by image-based DL | CNN based | The model achieved a prediction accuracy of 98.6%, with a sensitivity of 97.8% and specificity of 99.4% |

(AUC: area under the curve; CNN: convolution neural networks; DL: deep learning; SD-OCT: spectral domain optical coherence tomography)

the ground truth of the grader or the spectral domain optical coherence tomography (SD-OCT) data to diagnose AMD.

With the aging population, there is an urgent clinical need to have a robust DL system to screen these patients for further evaluation in tertiary eye care centers. ML algorithms (AlexNet, GoogLeNet, VGG16, VGG19, ResNet18, ResNet50, and ResNet101) have also been shown to predict visual acuity. Trained neural networks have demonstrated vital accuracy in identifying OCT images of normal and AMD patients, with a sensitivity and specificity

**TABLE 2:** Artificial intelligence (AI) models for diagnosing age-related macular degeneration (AMD).

| Authors | Objectives | AI models | Results |
|---|---|---|---|
| Yoo et al.[29] (2019) | Predict diagnostic accuracy of DL model using SD-OCT and color fundus photograph images in AMD subjects | CNN based | • DL using OCT alone showed AUC of 0.906 and 82.6% accuracy rate DL using fundus photographs exhibited AUC of 0.914 and 83.5% accuracy rate<br>• Combined usage of the fundus photographs with OCT increased the diagnostic power with AUC of 0.969 and 90.5% accuracy rate |
| Fraccaro et al.[30] (2015) | Combining macular clinical signs and patient characteristics for AMD diagnosis: An ML approach | Support vector machines (SVM), AdaBoost, random forest | In terms of AUC, random forests, logistic regression, and AdaBoost showed a mean performance of 0.92, followed by SVM and decision trees (0.90) |
| Hassan et al.[31] (2018) | • Multilayered deep structure tensor<br>• Delaunay triangulation and morphing-based automated diagnosis of dry and wet AMD | CNN based | The proposed model achieved a mean accuracy of 95.27% for extracting retinal and choroidal layers, mean dice coefficient of 0.90 for extracting fluid pathology, and the overall accuracy of 96.07% for maculopathy diagnosis |

(AUC: area under the curve; CNN: convolution neural networks; DL: deep learning; ML: machine learning; SD-OCT: spectral domain optical coherence tomography)

of 92.64% in regular patients and 93.69% in AMD patients.[32] In diagnosing exudative AMD, AI models achieved 91 and 95.5% accuracy in predicting the necessity for injection treatment.[33] The DeepSeeNet program performed better than retina specialists in accuracy (0.671 vs. 0.599), sensitivity (0.590 vs. 0.512), and specificity (0.930 vs. 0.916) in classifying eyes based on the

**TABLE 3:** Artificial intelligence (AI) models for predicting conversion of dry age-related macular degeneration (AMD) to wet AMD.

| Authors | Objectives | AI models | Results |
|---|---|---|---|
| Yim et al.[34] (2020) | Predicting conversion to wet AMD using DL in SD-OCT images | DL segmentation | This model showed an AUC of 0.886 |
| Schmidt-Erfurth et al.[35] (2018) | Prediction of individual disease conversion using SD-OCT in early AMD using AI | CNN based | The model differentiated converting versus nonconverting eyes with a performance of 0.68 and 0.80 for CNV and GA, respectively |

(AUC: area under the curve; CNN: convolution neural networks; CNV: choroidal neovascularization; DL: deep learning; GA: geographic atrophy; SD-OCT: spectral domain optical coherence tomography)

age-related eye disease study (AREDS) severity score.[36] Looking at the literature, it is evident that AI is an excellent tool for diagnosing AMD.

## Predicting Conversion of Dry Age-related Macular Degeneration to Wet Age-related Macular Degeneration

Deep learning describes algorithms that process and analyze data (e.g., images) in a hierarchical manner with artificial neural networks inspired by brain organization.[37] The utilization of DL-based algorithms significantly increased the prediction of AMD progression **(Table 3)**. Researchers use only imaging biomarkers, while few combine them with sociodemographic factors.[38]

## Predicting Response to Anti-vascular Endothelial Growth Factor Treatment and Progression of Age-related Macular Degeneration

Predicting the outcome of intravitreal anti-VEGF injection from baseline data in low-resource settings might help triage the urgency of treatment. In the past decade, intravitreal anti-VEGF drugs have significantly improved the outcomes of eyes with AMD.[39] Predicting how a patient might respond to treatment and how frequently retreatment may be required would enable clinicians to plan treatment schedules more appropriately, mitigating unwanted side effects and financial costs by reducing unnecessary monitoring visits.[40] ML classifiers can predict treatment demand and assist in establishing patient-specific treatment plans. ML approaches are built based on different ML algorithms, such as AdaBoost.R2, gradient boosting,

**TABLE 4:** Artificial intelligence (AI) models for predicting antivascular endothelial growth factor (anti-VEGF) treatment response and progression of age-related macular degeneration (AMD).

| Authors | Objectives | AI models | Results |
| --- | --- | --- | --- |
| Bogunović et al.[41] (2017) | Prediction of anti-VEGF treatment requirements in neovascular AMD using an ML approach | CNN based (random forest classifier) | Classification of low and high treatment requirement subgroups demonstrated an AUC of 0.7 and 0.77, respectively |
| Russakoff et al.[42] (2019) | Deep learning (DL) for prediction of AMD progression | CNN based (AMDnet, VGG16) | AMDnet achieved an AUC of 0.89 at the B-scan level and 0.91 for volumes. VGG16 with preprocessing achieved AUC of 0.82 for B-scans and 0.87 for volumes. VGG16 without preprocessing achieved AUC of 0.66 for B-scans and 0.69 for volumes |
| Banerjee et al.[43] (2020) | A DL approach for prognosis of AMD using SD-OCT imaging biomarkers | RNN based (random forest classifier) | The proposed RNN model achieved high accuracy (0.96 AUC-ROC) and outperformed the traditional random forest model trained |

(AUC: area under the curve; CNN: convolution neural networks; ML: machine learning; RNN: recurrent neural network; ROC: receiver operating characteristic; SD-OCT: spectral domain optical coherence tomography)

random forests, extremely randomized trees, and Lasso, that are currently being used.[44] These methods predict the long-term demand for anti-VEGF treatment using the information from the initial visits. The predictive models rely on features from image segmentation methods and, therefore, have to be accurately extracted.[45] The AI models used to predict the anti-VEGF response and AMD progression are listed in **Table 4**.

## ■ CHALLENGES WITH ARTIFICIAL INTELLIGENCE

Despite the high level of accuracy of AI-based algorithms, specific challenges are required to be addressed. First, the data used is not from a heterogeneous group of the population. Applying the same images to population groups can result in erroneous results. Hence, diversifying the dataset regarding ethnicities may help resolve the issue.[9] Second, the AI tool learns from what is presented to it. Hence, if the dataset is small or not representative of the real-time population, it is likely to produce inaccurate results. Third, there is a fear that AI might de-skill physicians in decision-making and forming opinions in the future. Fourth, AI does not consider human nature's psychological and social aspects, which a skilled physician would typically think. Fifth, most currently used AI machines can simultaneously monitor only a single disease. Switching between different AI for various illnesses is not feasible for physicians, especially at the community level, where resources are already scarce. Last, the lack of infrastructure for implementing the AI system is a significant issue, especially in developing countries where the internet supply is limited.[22]

## CONCLUSION

The development of AI tools to tackle challenges in the management of AMD is rapidly increasing. Promising AI models are being developed to assist clinicians in the initial detection of AMD and early identification of possible neovascular AMD. Similarly, AI systems are being trained to enhance disease risk stratification, which could enable more tailored and precise monitoring of patients at risk of developing vision-threatening late AMD complications. Alongside the development of AI-based clinical support tools, AI techniques even have the potential to accelerate new treatment discoveries in AMD.[46] Despite the challenges, AI has shown promising results in expanding ophthalmic healthcare facilities. It can reduce the barriers to accessing the ophthalmic healthcare systems and prevent avoidable blindness. AI is on the brink of bringing a paradigm shift in the ongoing clinical practice and services in the future, and AI does not intend to replace the human race.

## REFERENCES

1. Wong WL, Su X, Li X, Cheung CMG, Klein R, Cheng CY, et al. Global prevalence of age-related macular degeneration and disease burden projection for 2020 and 2040: a systematic review and meta-analysis. Lancet Glob Health. 2014;2:e106-16.
2. Nirmalan PK, Katz J, Robin AL, Tielsch JM, Namperumalsamy P, Kim R, et al. Prevalence of vitreoretinal disorders in a rural population of Southern India: the Aravind Comprehensive Eye Study. Arch Ophthalmol. 2004;122:581-6.
3. Krishnaiah S, Das T, Nirmalan PK, Nutheti R, Shamanna BR, Rao GN, et al. Risk factors for age-related macular degeneration: findings from the Andhra Pradesh eye disease study in South India. Invest Ophthalmol Vis Sci. 2005;46(12):4442-9.
4. Gupta SK, Murthy GVS, Morrison N, Price GM, Dherani M, John N, et al. Prevalence of early and late age-related macular degeneration in a rural population in northern India: the INDEYE feasibility study. Invest Ophthalmol Vis Sci. 2007;48(3):1007-11.
5. Miller JW, D'Anieri LL, Husain D, Miller JB, Vavvas DG. Age-related macular degeneration (AMD): a view to the future. J Clin Med. 2021;10(5):1124.
6. Fiszman M, Chapman WW, Aronsky D, Evans RS, Haug PJ. Automatic detection of acute bacterial pneumonia from chest X-ray reports. J Am Med Inform Assoc. 2000;7:593-604.

7. Dekker A, Vinod S, Holloway L, Oberije C, George A, Goozee G, et al. Rapid learning in practice: a lung cancer survival decision support system in routine patient care data. Radiother Oncol. 2014;113:47-53.
8. Ting DSW, Pasquale LR, Peng L, Campbell JP, Lee AY, Raman R, et al. Artificial intelligence and deep learning in ophthalmology. Br J Ophthalmol. 2019;103:167-75.
9. Ting DSW, Cheung CYL, Lim G, Tan GSW, Quang ND, Gan A, et al. Development and validation of a deep learning system for diabetic retinopathy and related eye diseases using retinal images from multiethnic populations with diabetes. JAMA. 2017;318:2211-23.
10. Gulshan V, Peng L, Coram M, Stumpe MC, Wu D, Narayanaswamy A, et al. Development and validation of a deep learning algorithm for detection of diabetic retinopathy in retinal fundus photographs. JAMA. 2016;316:2402-10.
11. Lee CS, Tyring AJ, Deruyter NP, Wu Y, Rokem A, Lee AY. Deep-learning based, automated segmentation of macular edema in optical coherence tomography. Biomed Opt Express. 2017;8(7):3440-8.
12. Burlina PM, Joshi N, Pekala M, Pacheco KD, Freund DE, Bressler NM. Automated grading of age-related macular degeneration from color fundus images using deep convolutional neural networks. JAMA Ophthalmol. 2017;135(11):1170-6.
13. Grassmann F, Mengelkamp J, Brandl C, Harsch S, Zimmermann ME, Linkohr B, et al. A deep learning algorithm for prediction of age-related eye disease study severity scale for age-related macular degeneration from color fundus photography. Ophthalmology. 2018;125(9):1410-20.
14. Li Z, He Y, Keel S, Meng W, Chang RT, He M. Efficacy of a deep learning system for detecting glaucomatous optic neuropathy based on color fundus photographs. Ophthalmology. 2018;125(8):1199-206.
15. Gao X, Lin S, Wong TY. Automatic feature learning to grade nuclear cataracts based on deep learning. IEEE Trans Biomed Eng. 2015;62(11):2693-701.
16. Brown JM, Campbell JP, Beers A, Chang K, Ostmo S, Chan RVP, et al. Automated diagnosis of plus disease in retinopathy of prematurity using deep convolutional neural networks. JAMA Ophthalmol. 2018;136(7):803-10.
17. Nagasato D, Tabuchi H, Masumoto H, Enno H, Ishitobi N, Kameoka M, et al. Automated detection of a nonperfusion area caused by retinal vein occlusion in optical coherence tomography angiography images using deep learning. PLoS One. 2019;14(11):e0223965.
18. Padhy SK, Takkar B, Chawla R, Kumar A. Artificial intelligence in diabetic retinopathy: a natural step to the future. Indian J Ophthalmol. 2019;67(7):1004-9.
19. Abràmoff MD. Image processing. In: Schachat AP, Wilkinson CP, Hinton DR, Sadda SR, Wiedemann P (Eds). Ryan's Retina, 6th edition. Amsterdam: Elsevier; 2017. pp. 196-223.
20. McCarthy J, Minsky ML, Rochester N, Shannon CE. A proposal for the Dartmouth summer research project on artificial intelligence. AI Magazine. 2006;27(4):12.
21. Ruamviboonsuk P, Cheung CY, Zhang X, Raman R, Park SJ, Ting DSW. Artificial intelligence in ophthalmology: evolutions in Asia. Asia Pac J Ophthalmol (Phila). 2020;9(2):78-84.
22. Singla E, Ichhpujani P, Kumar S. An overview of artificial intelligence in ophthalmology. Delhi J Ophthalmol. 2020;25:15-19.

23. Kapoor R, Walters SP, Al-Aswad LA. The current state of artificial intelligence in ophthalmology. Surv Ophthalmol. 2019;64(2):233-40.
24. Neely DC, Bray KJ, Huisingh CE, Clark ME, McGwin Jr G, Owsley C. Prevalence of undiagnosed age-related macular degeneration in primary eye care. JAMA Ophthalmol. 2017;135(6):570-5.
25. Jiang P, Dou Q, Shi L. Ophthalmologist-level classification of fundus disease with deep neural networks. Transl Vis Sci Technol. 2020;9(2):39.
26. Schlegl T, Waldstein SM, Bogunovic H, Endstraßer F, Sadeghipour A, Philip AM, et al. Fully automated detection and quantification of macular fluid in OCT using deep learning. Ophthalmology. 2018;125(4):549-58.
27. Treder M, Lauermann JL, Eter N. Automated detection of exudative age-related macular degeneration in spectral domain optical coherence tomography using deep learning. Graefes Arch Clin Exp Ophthalmol. 2018;256(2):259-65.
28. Li F, Chen H, Liu Z, Zhang X, Wu Z. Fully automated detection of retinal disorders by image-based deep learning. Graefes Arch Clin Exp Ophthalmol. 2019;257(3):495-505.
29. Yoo TK, Choi JY, Seo JG, Ramasubramanian B, Selvaperumal S, Kim DW. The possibility of the combination of OCT and fundus images for improving the diagnostic accuracy of deep learning for age-related macular degeneration: a preliminary experiment. Med Biol Eng Comput. 2019;57(3):677-87.
30. Fraccaro P, Nicolo M, Bonetto M, Giacomini M, Weller P, Traverso CE, et al. Combining macula clinical signs and patient characteristics for age-related macular degeneration diagnosis: a machine learning approach. BMC Ophthalmol. 2015;15(1):10.
31. Hassan T, Akram MU, Akhtar M, Khan SA, Yasin U. Multilayered deep structure tensor Delaunay triangulation and morphing based automated diagnosis and 3D presentation of human macula. J Med Syst. 2018;42(11):223.
32. Lee CS, Baughman DM, Lee AY. Deep learning is effective for the classification of OCT images of normal versus age-related macular degeneration. Ophthalmol Retina. 2017;1(4):322-7.
33. Prahs P, Radeck V, Mayer C, Cvetkov Y, Cvetkova N, Helbig H, et al. OCT-based deep learning algorithm for the evaluation of treatment indication with anti-vascular endothelial growth factor medications. Graefes Arch Clin Exp Ophthalmol. 2018;256(1):91-8.
34. Yim J, Chopra R, Spitz T, Winkens J, Obika A, Kelly C, et al. Predicting conversion to wet age-related macular degeneration using deep learning. Nat Med. 2020;26(6):892-9.
35. Schmidt-Erfurth U, Waldstein SM, Klimscha S, Sadeghipour A, Hu X, Gerendas BS, et al. Prediction of individual disease conversion in early AMD using artificial intelligence. Invest Ophthalmol Vis Sci. 2018;59(8):3199-208.
36. Peng Y, Dharssi S, Chen Q, Keenan TD, Agrón E, Wong WT, et al. DeepSeeNet: a deep learning model for automated classification of patient-based age-related macular degeneration severity from color fundus photographs. Ophthalmology. 2019;126(4):565-75.
37. Rampasek L, Goldenberg A. TensorFlow: biology's gateway to deep learning. Cell Syst. 2016;2(1):12-4.
38. Damian I, Nicoară SD. SD-OCT biomarkers and the current status of artificial intelligence in predicting progression from intermediate to advanced AMD. Life (Basel). 2022;12(3):454.

39. Jia H, Lu B, Zhao Z, Yu Y, Wang F, Zhou M, et al. Prediction of the short-term efficacy of anti-VEGF therapy for neovascular age-related macular degeneration using optical coherence tomography angiography. Eye Vis (Lond). 2022;9:16.
40. Fauser S, Lambrou GN. Genetic predictive biomarkers of anti-VEGF treatment response in patients with neovascular age-related macular degeneration. Surv Ophthalmol. 2015;60:138-52.
41. Bogunović H, Montuoro A, Baratsits M, Karantonis MG, Waldstein SM, Schlanitz F, et al. Machine learning of the progression of intermediate age-related macular degeneration based on OCT imaging. Invest Ophthalmol Vis Sci. 2017;58(6):BIO141-50.
42. Russakoff DB, Lamin A, Oakley JD, Dubis AM, Sivaprasad S. Deep learning for prediction of AMD progression: a pilot study. Invest Ophthalmol Vis Sci. 2019;60(2):712-22.
43. Banerjee I, de Sisternes L, Hallak JA, Leng T, Osborne A, Rosenfeld PJ, et al. Prediction of age-related macular degeneration disease using a sequential deep learning approach on longitudinal SD-OCT imaging biomarkers. Sci Rep. 2020;10(1):15434.
44. Rohm M, Tresp V, Müller M, Kern C, Manakov I, Weiss M, et al. Predicting visual acuity by using machine learning in patients treated for neovascular age-related macular degeneration. Ophthalmology. 2018;125(7):1028-36.
45. Bogunovic H, Waldstein SM, Schlegl T, Langs G, Sadeghipour A, Liu X, et al. Prediction of anti-VEGF treatment requirements in neovascular AMD using a machine learning approach. Invest Ophthalmol Vis Sci. 2017;58:3240-8.
46. Kumar H, Goh KL, Guymer RH, Wu Z. A clinical perspective on the expanding role of artificial intelligence in age-related macular degeneration. Clin Exp Optom. 2022;105(7):674-9.

# CHAPTER 13

# Multimodal Imaging in Macular Diseases

*Giridhar Anantharaman, Kiran Chandran*

## ABSTRACT

The field of retinal imaging has undergone significant advancements over the past decade. Multimodal imaging, i.e., employing a combination of different imaging modalities, is becoming essential in the modern clinical practice to arrive at a correct diagnosis. This has benefitted ophthalmologists in the diagnosis and treatment of eye disorders and, most importantly, the patients. In this chapter, we describe the impact of a multimodal imaging approach in describing common macular disorders as well as their ability to differentiate simulating conditions.

***Keywords:*** Multimodal imaging; spectral-domain optical coherence tomography; fundus autofluorescence; fundus fluorescein angiography; indocyanine green angiography; optical coherence tomography angiography.

## ■ INTRODUCTION

Retinal and fundal imaging facilitates the identification and documentation of morphologic and pathologic features not visible to the clinician on biomicroscopy. In recent years, the use of different, established, and novel imaging techniques provided detailed insight into several retinal diseases. In day-to-day ophthalmic practice, it is becoming uncommon for clinicians to rely on a single imaging modality to determine the diagnosis and initiate a management plan. We see more than one technique being employed for a given clinical situation. Common imaging modalities include color fundus photography, near-infrared reflectance (NIR), fundus autofluorescence (FAF),[1,2] dye-based angiography including fundus fluorescein angiography (FFA) indocyanine green angiography (ICGA), scanning laser ophthalmoscopy with and without adaptive optics, optical coherence tomography (OCT),[3] and OCT angiography (OCTA).[4]

This method, now commonly termed "*multimodal imaging,*" is becoming increasingly used in the scientific literature to describe the approach to diagnose a single retinal disease by combining different imaging modalities. It can be defined as the use of more than one complementary technological system that is used to acquire images, concurrently or in a short period of time, for the purpose of diagnosis, prognostication, management, and monitoring of disease. Some of the commonly performed multimodal imaging tests for diagnosing a variety of macular diseases have been briefly outlined in **Table 1**.

The different imaging modalities, when analyzed together, can increase the diagnostic sensitivity and specificity. It is important for the treating physician to understand the utility benefits and pitfalls of each imaging modality to avoid unnecessary testing and increased health care costs for the patient.

Some of the clinical situations where application of a multimodal imaging approach enhances the evaluation and understanding of the condition are detailed below.

**TABLE 1:** Common multimodal imaging modalities.

| Modality | Description |
|---|---|
| Colored fundus photography | • Broad spectrum of illumination without the use of filters<br>• Color image of the fundus, traditionally 30° or 50° field of view; widefield color fundus photography (Optos p200 system provides image capture with a 200° field of view)[5]<br>• Provides real color representation of disease. Best correlates with clinical ophthalmoscopy |
| Near-infrared reflectance | • Uses near-infrared region of electromagnetic spectrum (700–2,500 nm)<br>• Minimally absorbed by media opacities, neurosensory retinal layers, and macular luteal pigments. Penetrates more easily through the optical media<br>• Since the wavelength used is barely visible, this technique is well tolerated by patients<br>• Provides information on deeper structures such as RPE and choroid |
| Multicolor imaging | • Based on confocal scanning ophthalmoscopy<br>• Simultaneously acquires three reflectance images of the retina using three individual lasers of different wavelengths: blue (488 nm), green (515 nm), and infrared (820 nm)<br>• Penetrates the tissue to different depths, simultaneously capturing and depicting information originating from different retinal structures<br>• The infrared reflectance (IR) image visualizes structures at the level of the outer retina and choroid. The green reflectance (GR) images retinal blood vessels, hemorrhages, and exudates. The blue reflectance (BR) particularly provides details of inner retina and the vitreoretinal interface such as epiretinal membranes, retinal nerve fiber layer (RNFL) thinning, and macular pigment changes<br>• The information from these three images is integrated to form a composite multicolor image |

*Contd...*

*Contd...*

| Modality | Description |
|---|---|
| Optical coherence tomography (OCT) | • Utilizes principle of low coherence interferometry to produce cross-sectional images of the retina with histopathological grade resolution<br>• Initial algorithms based on time-domain OCT technology had limited speed (400 A-scans) and resolution (10–15 μm)<br>• Spectral-domain OCT (SD-OCT) technology provides greater speed (20,000–70,000 A-scans) and better resolution (5–6 μm)<br>• More recently, with swept-source OCT technology, augmented-depth visualization became possible. OCT has become the gold-standard imaging modality to assess macular edema and its response to treatment and can localize the level of retinal loss and atrophy<br>• In conventional SD-OCT imaging systems, it is possible to image the choroid—enhanced depth imaging (EDI), which enables an overall assessment of the choroid and the choroidoscleral interface[6] |
| Fundus autofluorescence (FAF) | • Noninvasive imaging technique that indirectly evaluates the functions of the outer retina and RPE<br>• Excitation and emission filters in traditional fundus-based or SLO cameras are used to capture the inherent fluorescent characteristics of ocular tissues<br>• FAF excitation wavelength may vary from 300 to 600 nm, and emission filters are typically >500 nm<br>• Analyze RPE function and specifically lipofuscin, a by-product of photoreceptor outer segments metabolism<br>• The absence of RPE lipofuscin, due to atrophy, shows a severely reduced signal, appearing dark<br>• Two types of FAF imaging techniques, namely short-wave FAF (SW-FAF) and near-infrared reflectance FAF (NIR-FAF). The former originates from the lipofuscin pigment of the RPE, while the latter originates from the melanin pigment of both the choroid and the RPE.[7] Of these, SW-FAF is more commonly used[8] |
| Dye-based angiography | • Can be performed using a flood-illuminated fundus camera incorporating band-pass excitation and emission filters or using SLO devices that can achieve better resolution and contrast<br>• Circulating dye molecules absorb the light and emit light of a different wavelength<br>• A barrier filter blocks any reflected light so that the images capture only light emitted from the dye<br>• FFA is used for visualization of retinal vessel integrity, perfusion, and leakage<br>• ICG has a greater binding affinity to plasma proteins than fluorescein dye, leaks minimally from the choriocapillaris, and provides improved visualization of the choroidal vasculature |

*Contd...*

*Contd...*

| Modality | Description |
|---|---|
| OCT angiography | - Noninvasive<br>- Employs motion contrast to detect blood flow and acquires three-dimensional volumetric information of the retina and choroid to provide high-resolution, depth-resolved segmentation of these microscopic vascular layers<br>- Identification of the microvascular morphology of neovascular lesions in AMD and their response to therapy<br>- Analysis of the deep retinal capillary plexus in retinal vascular disease to assess for ischemia is also expedited with OCT angiography |

(AMD: age-related macular degeneration; FFA: fundus fluorescein angiography; ICG: indocyanine green; RPE: retinal pigment epithelium; SLO: scanning laser ophthalmoscopy)

# MULTIMODAL IMAGING IN COMMON MACULAR DISEASES

## Central Serous Chorioretinopathy

Central serous chorioretinopathy (CSCR) is a disease characterized by the presence of a serous detachment of the neurosensory retina in the macula. In clinical practice, CSCR has a wide range of presentation. Multimodal imaging helps in differentiating acute from chronic CSCR and also CSCR from CSCR-like diseases.

The various multimodal imaging techniques, which include spectral-domain OCT (SD-OCT), FAF, FFA, and ICGA, play a very important role in the diagnosis, classification, prognosis, and management of CSCR **(Figs. 1 and 2)**. OCT is the single most important diagnostic modality in the diagnosis of CSCR.

The various features seen in SD-OCT depending on the stage of the disease include:
- Serous macular detachment (SMD)
- Hyperreflective foci within the SMD.[9] This is an indication of a larger duration of SMD and early signs of chronicity.
- Outer retinal abnormalities include focal ellipsoid loss, focal external limiting membrane (ELM) loss, thinning, and irregularity of the retinal pigment epithelium (RPE). All these are signs of chronic CSCR.
- *Retinal pigment epithelial detachment (PED):* Serous PED in CSCR is seen in 50-100% of eyes.[10] Sometimes, a small discontinuity in the RPE over the PED would be visible, and this is described as an RPE rip **(Figs. 3A to C)**.
- *Choroid:* Multimodal imaging using the enhanced depth imaging (EDI) mode in SD-OCT demonstrates the increased thickness of the

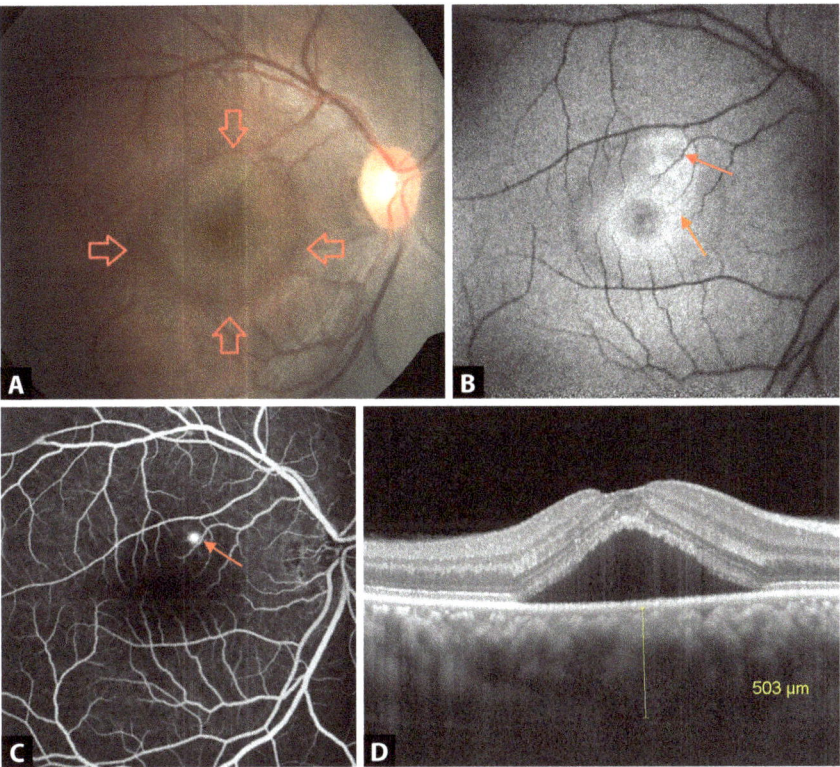

**Figs. 1A to D:** Multimodal imaging in a case of acute central serous chorioretinopathy (CSCR). (A) Color fundus photograph of right eye of a 32-year-old male showing serous macular detachment (SMD) (red open arrows); (B) fundus autofluorescence (FAF) showing hypoautofluorescence border corresponding to the area of SMD with hyperautofluorescence centrally (orange arrow) with hypoautofluorescent lesion (red arrow); (C) inkblot pattern of leak on fundus fluorescein angiography (FFA) (red arrow) that corresponds to hypoautofluorecent lesion (red arrow) on FAF; (D) spectral-domain optical coherence tomography (SD-OCT) with enhanced depth imaging shows uniform hyporeflective space between the outer segment of photoreceptors and retinal pigment epithelium (RPE) suggestive of subretinal fluid; dilated choroidal vessels with increased choroidal thickness (pachychoroid) is also seen.

choroid in the affected and fellow eyes of CSCR. Based on various studies, 395 μm can be used as a value to diagnose thick choroid or pachychoroid.[11] Increase in choroidal thickness could be a uniform increase involving all layers or just an enlargement of vessels in Haller's layer with atrophy or thinning of the inner choroid and overlying RPE.

Fundus autofluorescence is an important investigation tool in CSCR along with SD-OCT. SD-OCT tells about the stage of activity of the disease and is very useful for follow-up, while FAF gives useful information about functional damage to the RPE and outer retina and, therefore, is an important prognostic indicator. The signs on FAF are as follows:

- *Hypoautofluorescence in acute CSCR*: In acute CSCR, a decreased FAF is seen in the area corresponding to the SMD. This is due to the fluid blocking the normal autofluorescence.

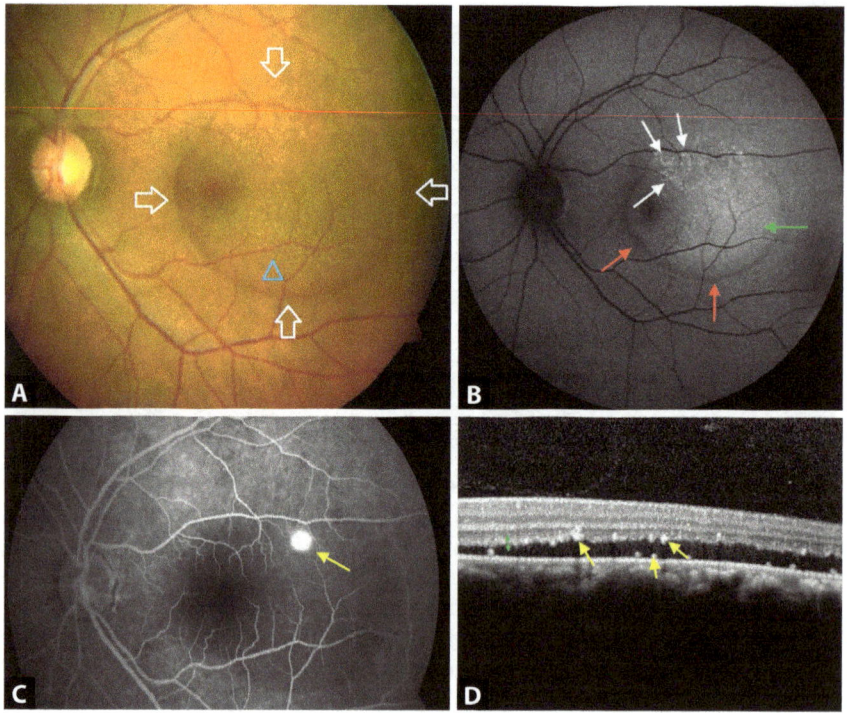

Chronic central serous chorioretinopathy (CSR)

**Figs. 2A to D:** Multimodal imaging in chronic and recurrent chronic serous chorioretinopathy (CSCR). (A to D) Chronic CSCR: (A) Color fundus photograph of left eye of a 38-year-old male showing a large oval area of serous macular detachment (SMD) extending to midperiphery (white open arrows) with yellowish white deposits seen within it (blue arrowhead); (B) Fundus autofluorescence (FAF) shows a grainy or coarse region (white arrows) of increased autofluorescence (AF) (speckled pattern) with a more uniform hyper-AF temporally (green arrow) bordered by a circumferential hypo-AF rim (red arrow) corresponding to the area of SMD clinically. This pattern is seen with longer duration of SMD; (C) Fundus fluorescein angiography (FFA) shows an inkblot leak superotemporally (yellow arrow); (D) Spectral-domain optical coherence tomography (SD-OCT) shows subretinal fluid (SRF) which is serous; outer segment elongation (green double arrow) and subretinal hyperreflective dots (yellow arrows) appear and increase in number with disease duration; (E to I) Chronic recurrent central serous retinopathy (CSR).

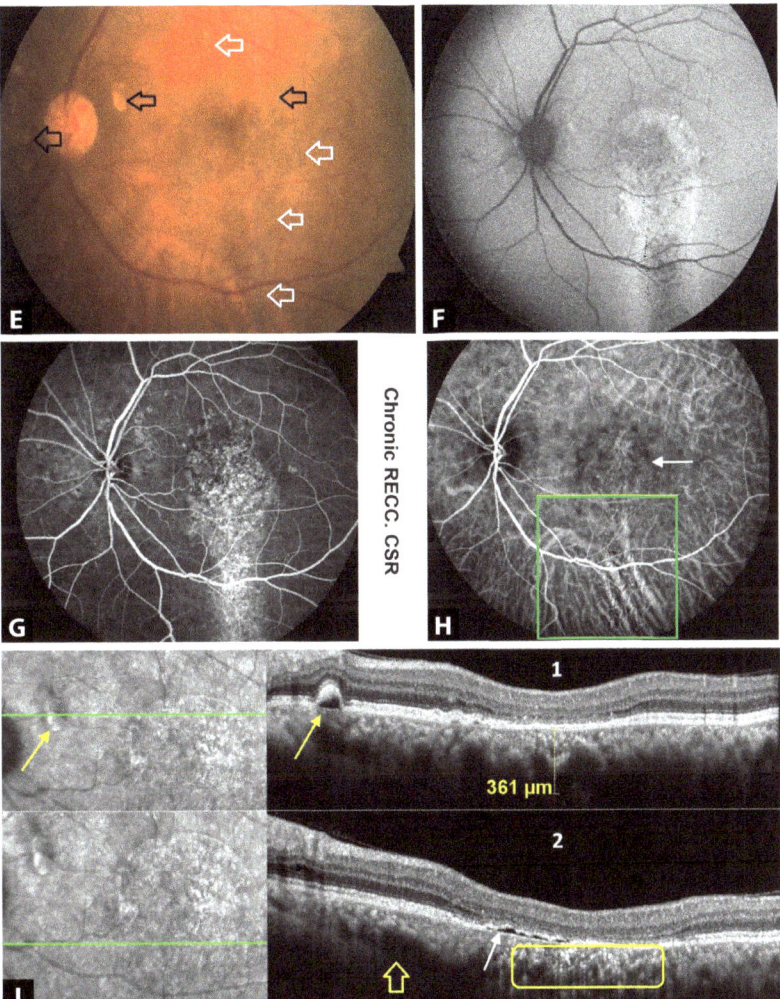

**Figs. 2G to I:** Multimodal imaging in chronic and recurrent chronic serous chorioretinopathy (CSCR). (E) Color fundus photograph of the left eye of a 67-year-old male, showing retinal pigment epithelium (RPE) atrophy at posterior pole and nasal to disk (black open arrows), and inferiorly extending RPE track lesion (white open arrows) caused by gravitating SRF; (F) FAF shows downward leading swathe of decreased auto-AF surrounded by hyper-AF rim, originating from posterior pole and extending below the level of the inferior arcade (descending tract). This hypo-AF occurs as RPE cells get damaged in the pathway of fluid over time; (G) FFA showing mottled hyperfluorescence in midphase signifying window defects suggestive of RPE atrophy; (H) Indocyanine green angiography in midphase shows an irregular area of hyperfluorescence at the macula (white arrow) with dilated choroidal vessels inferiorly (green box) along the gravitational tract; (I) SD-OCT sections at macula show downward bowing suggestive of collapse of inner into outer retina with disruption of all outer retinal bands—external limiting membrane, ellipsoid, and interdigitation zones, with irregularity and slight elevation of RPE (white arrow), a small pigment epithelial detachment (yellow arrow), choroidal hyperreflective dots (yellow box), and dilated choroidal vessels suggestive of pachyvessels (yellow open arrow).

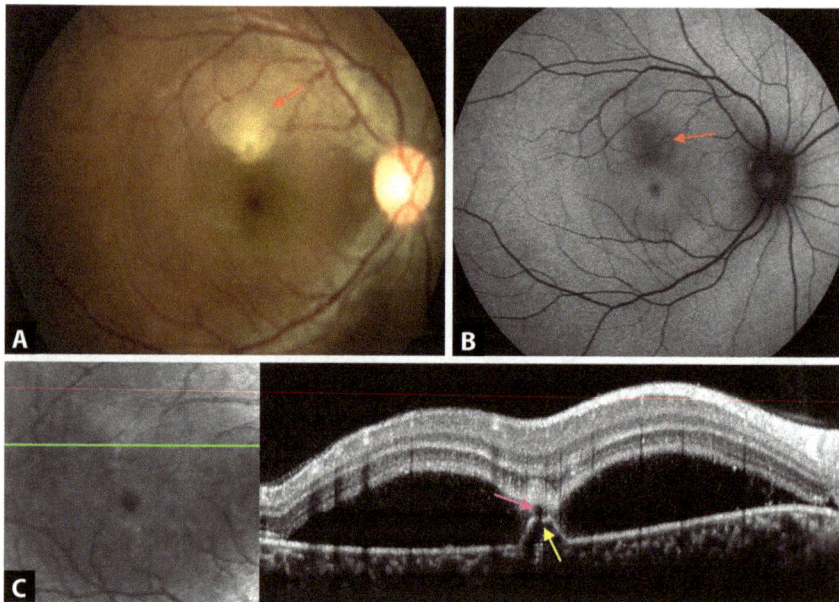

**Figs. 3A to C:** Multimodal imaging in a case of central serous chorioretinopathy showing retinal pigment epithelial (RPE) rip. (A) Color fundus photograph showing serous macular detachment (SMD) with an yellowish lesion above fovea (red arrow); (B) Fundus autofluorescence (FAF) showing a hypoautofluorescent border with inner hyperautofluorescence corresponding to SMD with hypoautofluorescence corresponding to the subretinal lesion (red arrow); (C) Spectral-domain optical coherence tomography (SD-OCT) demonstrating microrip in RPE corresponding to area of leak (yellow arrow) with subretinal hyperreflectivity overlying it; between it, a hyporeflective cavitation called "vacuole sign" can be seen (pink arrow).

- *Hyperautofluorescence*: As an acute episode of CSCR recovers, focal areas of hyperautofluorescence may appear, which are due to fluorophores accumulated in the outer segment of the photoreceptor. Presence of a normal OCT with hyperautofluorescence is an indication of the previous episode of CSCR, and this has clinical significance in the management of CSCR.
- *Pattern of significantly decreased autofluorescence*: Descending tracts of decreased autofluorescence are pathognomonic of chronic CSCR. However, it has recently been observed in masquerades of CSCR such as polypoidal choroidal vasculopathy (PCV).
- *FAF changes in asymptomatic fellow eyes*: Presence of patches of abnormal autofluorescence in fellow asymptomatic eyes with increased autofluorescence for fresh lesions and decreased autofluorescence for older lesions is an indication of the past episodes of CSCR.

Fundus fluorescein angiography is used to exclude the presence of other pathologies that produce serous retinal detachments as well as to confirm the diagnosis.

- *Features in acute CSCR*: There are two leak patterns on FFA:[12]
  - *Inkblot:* Pinpoint leak in the early phase, which concentrically enlarges in the late phase
  - *Smoke stack (10-15%):* Leak gradually increases from a pinpoint, ascends, and expands in a mushroom cloud configuration.
- *Features in chronic CSCR*: Diffuse RPE window defect and patchy hyperfluorescence due to RPE atrophy.

Indocyanine green angiography helps demonstrate choroidal vascular changes. There is a delay in choroidal filling in the early phase with hypofluorescence due to choriocapillaris nonperfusion. In midphase, there is choroidal hyperpermeability (seen as zones of hyperfluorescence). This hyperfluorescence slowly fades in the late phase.[12]

## Subretinal Hyperreflective Material in Central Serous Chorioretinopathy

Subretinal fibrin in CSCR was first reported by Gass.[13] This condition has been reported to be more prevalent in pregnant women[14] or in those with a history of steroid intake.[15] Although CSCR classically presents with a clear subretinal fluid (SRF) on OCT, subretinal deposits may be seen that appear hyperreflective on OCT, described as subretinal hyperreflective material (SHRM).[16,17] The composition of the SHRM is not clearly understood. It is likely to be deposition of products from leaking fluid over the photoreceptors, classically composed of fibrin.[18]

The OCT features in CSCR associated with fibrin have been reported before,[19-21] with the "dipping or sagging sign" being the most common finding reported. It is described as dipping of the neurosensory retina over the area of fibrin and PED, with the fibrin acting like an adhesive in between the PED and the neurosensory retina.

The presence of a hyporeflective vacuole amid the hyperreflective fibrin adjacent to RPE detachment probably indicates the site of constant fluid egress and is an important sign of disease activity. On FFA, hyporeflective vacuole was seen to correspond to the location of RPE leak. The vacuole probably depicts the site of active flow of clear fluid within the fibrin. This clear fluid would probably be responsible for the "vacuole" appearance surrounding the fibrin hyperreflectivity.[22]

The multimodal imaging features in fibrin CSCR are shown in **Figures 4A to D**.

## Masquerades of Central Serous Chorioretinopathy

### Polypoidal Choroidal Vasculopathy

The typical form of PCV poses little diagnostic challenge; certain atypical forms which present with small PEDs and only an SMD can masquerade

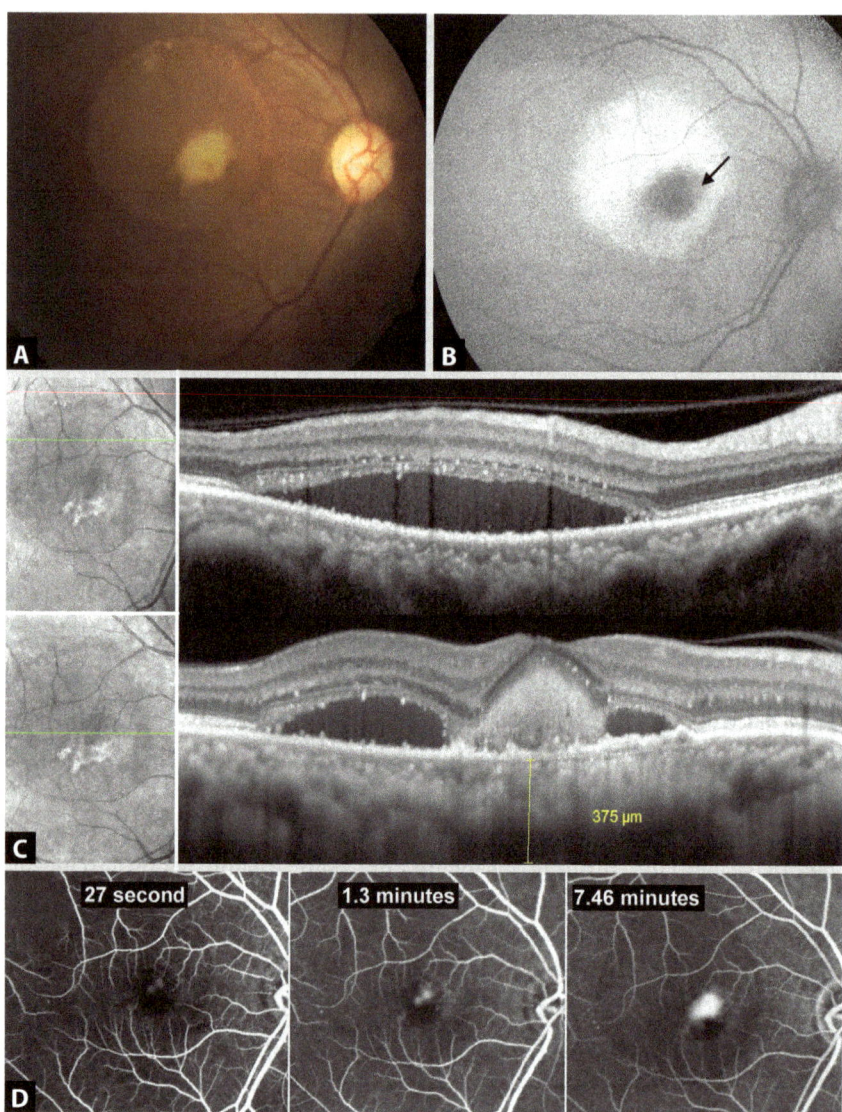

**Figs. 4A to D:** Multimodal imaging in fibrin central serous chorioretinopathy. (A) Color fundus photography of the right eye of a 41-year-old male showing neurosensory detachment (NSD) at the macula with a subretinal yellowish lesion involving the fovea, suggestive of fibrin; (B) Fundus autofluorescence (FAF) demonstrates hyperautofluorescence corresponding to NSD and hypoautofluorescence (black arrow) corresponding to the subretinal lesion; (C) Spectral-domain optical coherence tomography (SD-OCT) shows subretinal fluid with dense subretinal hyperreflective material (fibrin) at the fovea and double-layer sign; hyperreflective dots can be seen overlying the photoreceptors and on enhanced depth imaging pachychoroid with few dilated vessels in Haller's layer is noted; (D) Fundus fluorescein angiography (FFA) demonstrating leak within the subretinal lesion.

as CSCR.[23,24] PCV has also been seen in eyes with a history of long-standing CSCR, and these were described to be solitary, located at the margin or near the atrophic retina.[25] It is still uncertain whether CSCR and PCV can coexist in the same patient or if CSCR transforms into PCV with time.[25,26]

Indocyanine green angiography is particularly helpful in identifying small polypoidal lesions and branching vascular network (BVN) in the early phase. It not only differentiates the two conditions but also helps localize the area of treatment. The polyps show a high flow signal as a ring at the periphery of the lesion on OCTA due to intrinsic low flow and high velocity at the periphery of the lesion.

The coexistence of CSCR and PCV was picked up on multimodal imaging using SD-OCT, FFA, and ICGA as shown in **Figures 5A and B**.

## Type 1 Macular Neovascularization in CSCR

Type 1 MNV can present as an SMD mimicking CSCR. The double-layer sign (i.e., separation of the irregularly elevated RPE from the inner layer of Bruch's membrane), which has been described in some eyes with pachychoroid,[27] is also a characteristic of type 1 MNV. **Figures 6A to F** show the characteristic multimodal imaging features which help in differentiating CSCR and type 1 MNV.

## Best Vitelliform Macular Dystrophy

Best vitelliform macular dystrophy (BVMD) presents with a bilateral, egg yolk-like round lesion affecting the macula.[28] Subretinal deposits are seen as hyperreflective structures on OCT; however, in few cases, the deposits can be replaced by a clear fluid, thus simulating a serous retinal detachment of CSCR. The classical "pseudohypopyon" may not be visible, and ancillary tests such as FAF, FFA, and electrooculogram (EOG) may be necessary. Typical imaging characteristics of BVMD in the vitelliruptive stage mimicking CSCR are illustrated in **Figures 7A to C**.

## Neovascular Age-related Macular Degeneration

Neovascular age-related macular degeneration (nAMD) is one of the advanced stages of age-related macular degeneration (AMD), which is associated with the presence of new and fragile vessels beneath the retina.[29]

Based on the OCT and FFA characteristics, macular neovascularization (MNV) has been divided into three types:
1. *Type 1 MNV*: Neovascular membrane is present below the RPE.
2. *Type 2 MNV*: Neovascular membrane is present in the subretinal space (above the RPE).[30,31]

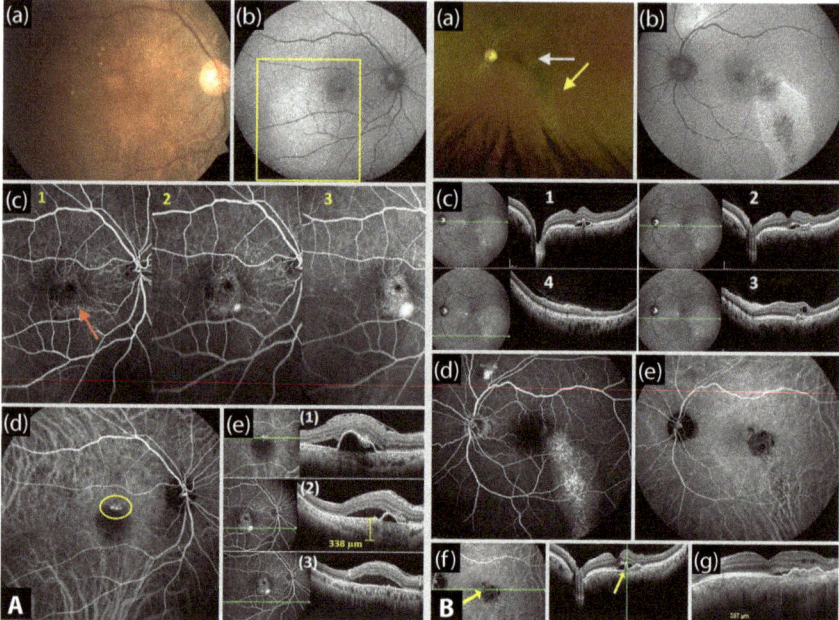

**Figs. 5A and B:** Multimodal imaging of polypoidal choroidal vasculopathy (PCV) masquerading with central serous chorioretinopathy (CSCR). (A) PCV mimicking acute CSCR: (a) Color fundus photograph of the right eye of a 68-year-old female showing few orange nodular lesions at fovea with scattered drusen at posterior pole and neurosensory detachment at macula; (b) Fundus autofluorescence (FAF) showing the extent of hyperautofluorescence, temporal to fovea extending to below the inferior arcade (yellow box); (c) Fundus fluorescein angiography (FFA) showing inkblot pattern leak (red arrow); pooling can be seen at the macula; (d) Indocyanine green angiography (ICGA) demonstrating multiple nodular hyperfluorescent lesions superior to fovea suggestive of polyps (circled yellow); (e) Spectral-domain optical coherence tomography (SD-OCT) shows subretinal fluid in all sections, notched pigment epithelial detachment (PED) through polyp (ICGA + OCT; section 1), and serous PED through the CSCR leak (FFA + OCT; section 2); (B) PCV mimicking chronic CSCR: (a) Color fundus photograph of the left eye of a 54-year-old male showing an orange nodular lesion (white arrow) at the fovea with an inferiorly extending retinal pigment epithelium (RPE) track lesion (yellow arrow); (b) FAF shows mixed hyper- (outer) and hypo (inner)- autofluorescence starting from temporal to fovea to below the inferior arcade of the gravitational tract lesion suggestive of chronicity of CSCR; (c) SD-OCT showing tall peaked PED with subretinal fluid (SRF) at the fovea (section 1), double-layer sign (section 2), intraretinal fluid (section 3), and retinal thinning with loss of outer retinal bands across the tract lesion (section 4); (d) FFA showing mottled hyperfluorescence in midphase corresponding to areas of window defects caused by RPE defects; (e) ICGA demonstrating a single nodular polyp at fovea with dilated choroidal vessels along the RPE tract lesion; (f) ICGA and OCT through the fovea showing tall peaked PED corresponding to the exact location of the polyp (yellow arrow); (g) enhanced depth OCT imaging showing pachychoroid. Although the findings appear like CSCR clinically, multimodal imaging confirmed features of PCV.

Multimodal Imaging in Macular Diseases

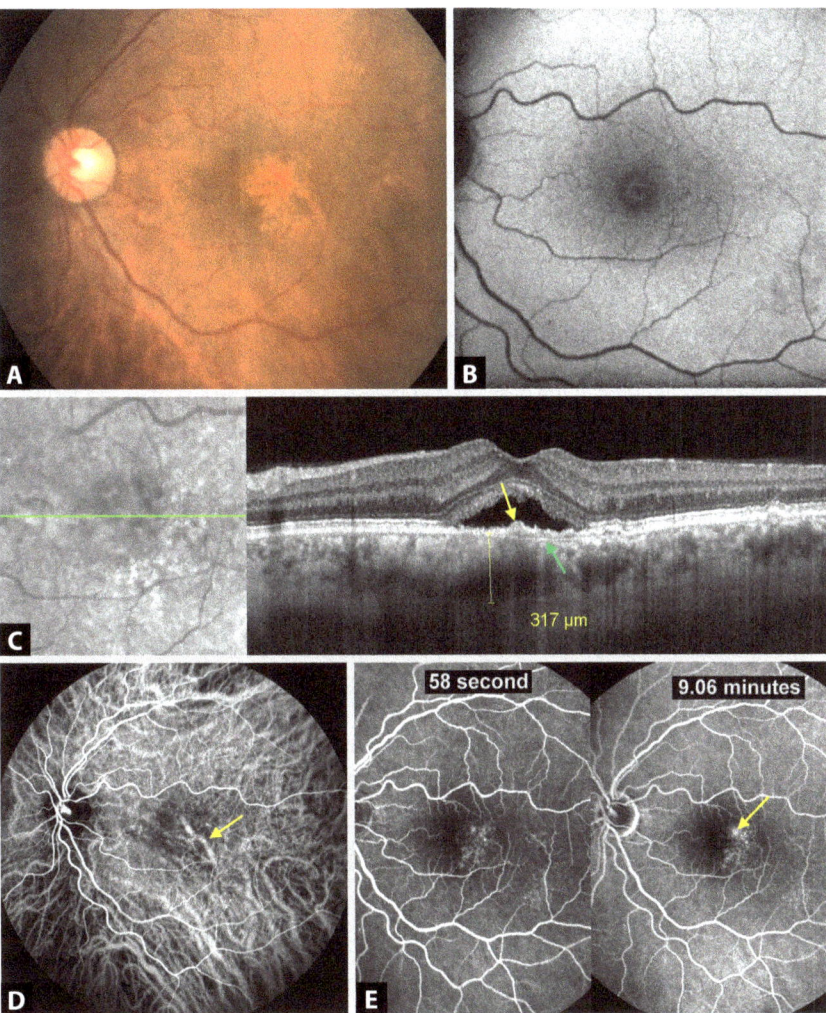

**Figs. 6A to E:** Type 1 macular neovascularization (MNV) mimicking central serous chorioretinopathy. (A) Color fundus photograph of the right eye of a 57-year-old male showing retinal pigment epithelium (RPE) changes with dark orange prominence of underlying choroidal vessels at the macula; (B) Fundus autofluorescence (FAF) shows patchy hyperautofluorescence at the macula (predominantly temporal to fovea); (C) Spectral-domain optical coherence tomography (SD-OCT) reveals subretinal fluid with a subtle double-layer sign (seen between yellow and green arrows) with dilated choroidal vessels in the Haller's layer suggestive of pachyvessels; (D) Indocyanine green angiography (ICGA) shows hyperfluorescence of prominent dilated choroidal vessels at the macula (yellow arrow); (E) Fundus fluorescein angiography (FFA) demonstrates a suspicious leak (late phase, yellow arrow) surrounded by stippled hyperfluorescence at macula which is inconclusive.

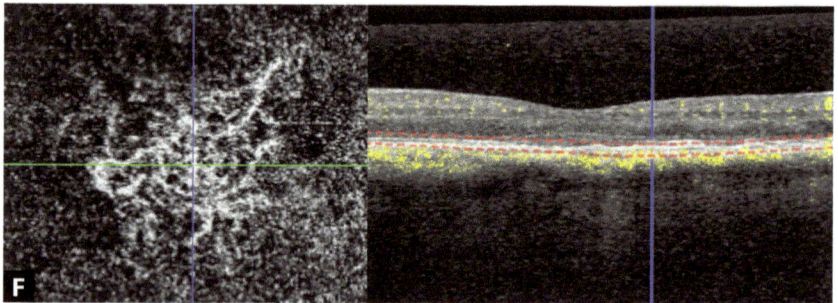

**Fig. 6F:** Type 1 macular neovascularization (MNV) mimicking central serous chorioretinopathy. (F) Optical coherence tomography (OCT) angiography shows sub-RPE entangled network at the level of double-layer sign with flow signals suggestive of active type 1 neovascularization.

3. *Type 3 MNV or retinal angiomatous proliferation (RAP):* Yannuzzi et al. used a three-stage sequence to describe the evolution of RAP as:[32]
    a. *Stage 1:* Intraretinal neovascularization (IRN): Capillaries that originate from the deep capillary plexus in the paramacular area proliferate within the retina.
    b. *Stage 2:* Subretinal neovascularization (SRN): IRN extends deeper into the subretinal space, past the photoreceptor layer, resulting in SRN.
    c. *Stage 3:* Choroidal neovascularization (CNV) with a vascularized PED and a retinal choroidal anastomosis

**Table 2** details the various characteristics of multimodal imaging that help to differentiate between the types of macular/choroidal neovascularizations.

The multimodal imaging characteristics in types 1, 2, and 3 MNV are shown in **Figures 8 and 9**.

## Why is it Important to Differentiate between the Types of Neovascularization?

Identification of the correct subtype of MNV using multimodal imaging helps prognosticate the visual outcome, plan follow-up, and predict the course of the fellow eye.

Retinal angiomatous proliferation has a strong predilection toward being bilateral. 80% of fellow eyes will show activation after 1 year and 100% before 3 years in comparison to 43% reported in cases of types 1 and 2 MNV within 5 years of one eye being involved.

Retinal angiomatous proliferation tends to have a poor visual prognosis owing to its high vasculogenic potential and exudative nature. The disease shows a rapid progression than types 1 and 2 MNV.[33]

Type 1 MNV usually shows a slower growth and has lesser propensity to geographical atrophy and subretinal fibrosis than type 2 MNV and, therefore, is associated with a better visual outcome.[34]

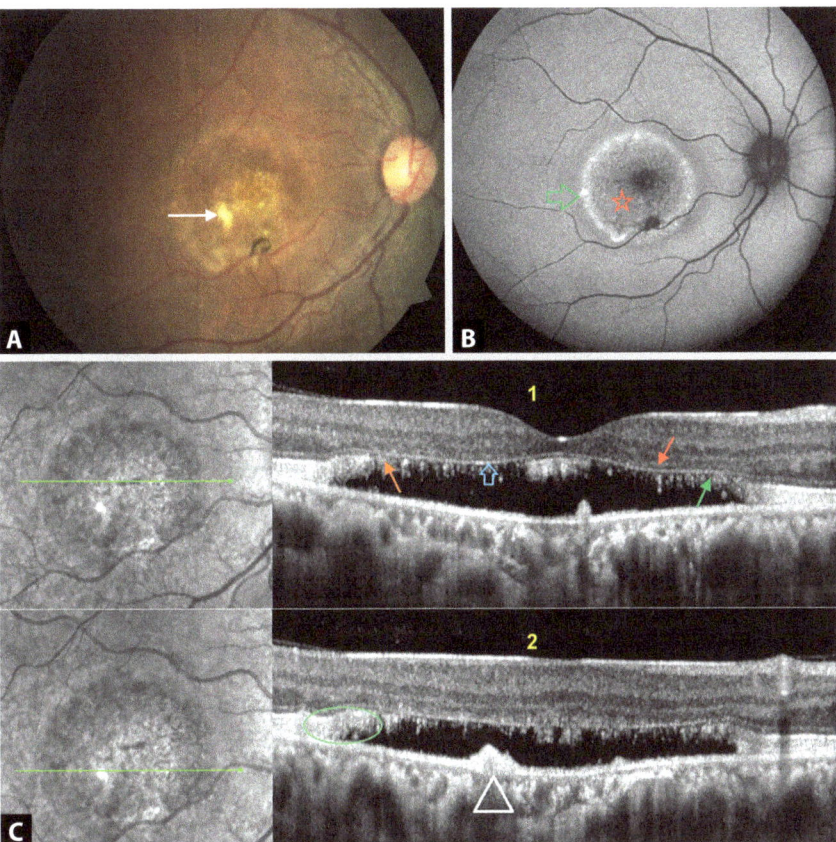

**Figs. 7A to C:** Multimodal imaging of best vitelliform macular dystrophy (BVMD) mimicking central serous chorioretinopathy (CSCR). (A) Color fundus photograph of the right eye of a 55-year-old male showing vitelliruptive stage of BVMD. The subretinal tissue at the center of the dome-shaped lesion (white arrow) corresponds to hyperreflective mounds at the level of outer-hyperreflective layer retinal pigment epithelium (RPE)/Bruch complex; (B) Fundus autofluorescence (FAF) demonstrates a mottled pattern of hyper/hypoautofluorescence (red star) surrounded by a rim of hyperautofluorescence (green open arrow; the outer rim corresponds to yellowish vitelliruptive material seen clinically); (C) Spectral-domain optical coherence tomography (SD-OCT) shows subretinal fluid; outer segment is discontinuous/fragmented (orange arrows; section 1); outer nuclear layer is attenuated and less clearly discernible (red arrow); external limiting membrane is intact (blue open arrow); subretinal mound overlying RPE–Bruch complex is also seen (white arrowhead; section 2); the outer hyperautofluorescence on FAF (green arrow) corresponds on SD-OCT to the homogeneous material between outer segment and RPE–Bruch complex (circled green).

## Non-neovascular Age-related Macular Degeneration

Advances in multimodal imaging have improved our understanding of the clinical features, prognosis, and various subtypes of non-neovascular age-related macular degeneration (nnAMD). For decades, color photography

**TABLE 2:** Comparison of types 1, 2, and 3 macular neovascularization (MNV) on multimodal imaging.

| Particulars | Type 1 MNV | Type 2 MNV | Type 3 MNV/RAP |
|---|---|---|---|
| **SD-OCT:** | | | |
| • Subretinal hyperreflectivity | Not usually seen | Present | May be seen |
| • Fibrovascular PED | Common | Usually absent | Either PED or FVPED; PEDs have a trapezoid configuration with discontinuity at roof |
| • SRF | Common | Common | Common |
| • IRF | Usually absent | Common | Common |
| • DLS | Common | Less common | Not seen |
| **FFA:** | Occult MNV | Classic MNV | Usually similar to occult or minimally classic MNV. May show focal intraretinal hyperfluorescence |
| • Phase and characteristic leak pattern<br>• Borders | • FVPED: May hyperfluorescence in early or mid-phase; often has stippled appearance<br>• LLUS: Late hyperfluorescence only; often has stippled appearance<br>• FVPED: Maybe poorly or well demarcated<br>• LLUS: Poorly defined | Early intense hyperfluorescence (especially at perimeter of MNV); lacy pattern may be seen<br><br>Well-defined; intense fuzzy leakage in late phase; there may be a hypofluorescent rim due to blocked fluorescence from hemorrhage | |
| ICGA | Not diagnostic; helps delineate the extent of occult MNV; three morphological variants: Hot spot, plaque, or mixed | Not diagnostic; no specific finding and not very useful to differentiate between types 1 and 2 MNV | Diagnostic in most cases<br>• Hot spot in mid and/or late frames (usually center of PED)<br>• Hairpin loop (perfusing retinal arteriole and draining venule) may be seen |
| OCTA | Diagnostic: Sensitive in picking up network at the level of flat irregular PED or DLS | Sensitive in detecting MNV, especially at the level of subretinal hyperreflectivity | Sensitive in stages 1 and 2 but not through large PED seen in stage 3 |

(DLS: double-layer sign; FFA: fundus fluorescein angiography; FVPED: fibrovascular pigment epithelial detachment; ICGA: indocyanine green angiography; IRF: intraretinal fluid; LLUS: late leakage of undetermined source; OCTA: optical coherence tomography angiography; PED: pigment epithelial detachment; RAP: retinal angiomatous proliferation; SD-OCT: spectral-domain optical coherence tomography; SRF: subretinal fluid) alone was used to assess drusen and RPE abnormalities. Over the years, SD-OCT, along with FAF, has emerged as a multimodal imaging tool to diagnose, classify, and prognosticate nnAMD. The various manifestations of nnAMD are described below.

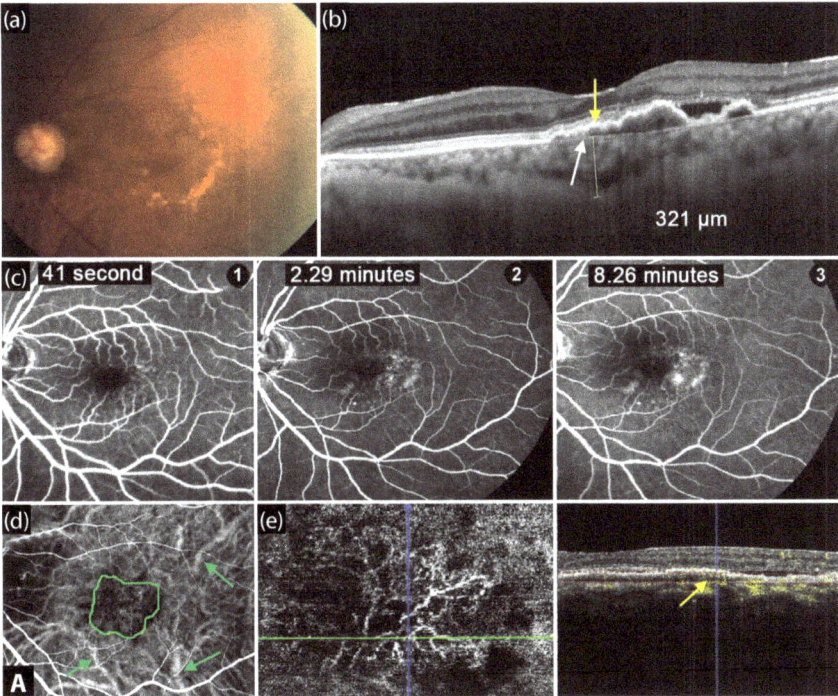

**Fig. 8A:** Multimodal imaging of (A) type 1 macular neovascularization (MNV) and (B) type 2 MNV. (A) Type 1 MNV: (a) Color fundus photograph of the left eye of a 66-year-old woman with retinal pigment epithelium (RPE) abnormalities at the macula with a yellowish-gray lesion inferiorly suggestive of MNV; (b) Spectral-domain optical coherence tomography (SD-OCT) shows subretinal fluid with shallow irregular elevation of RPE (yellow arrow) leading to its separation from Bruch's membrane (white arrow), with the gap between them showing moderate reflectivity (double-layer sign; this region is indicative of an abnormal vascular network); there is increased subfoveal choroidal thickness with dilatation of Haller's layer on enhanced depth imaging; (c) Early, mid, and late frames of fundus fluorescein angiography (FFA) showing stippled hyperfluorescence but no well-defined leakage; (d) Indocyanine green angiography (ICGA) shows dilated choroidal vessels at macula (green arrows) with an area of hyperfluorescence at fovea (encircled green) corresponding to a suspicious abnormal vascular network; (e) Optical coherence tomography angiography (OCTA) avascular complex slab shows a neovascular complex at the sub-RPE level with flow signals (yellow arrow) and with vessels radiating from one side of the lesion in a characteristic *"sea-fan" pattern*; note the absence of a feeder vessel. OCTA was diagnostic in this case. The above multimodal imaging characteristics are typical of pachychoroid neovasculopathy.

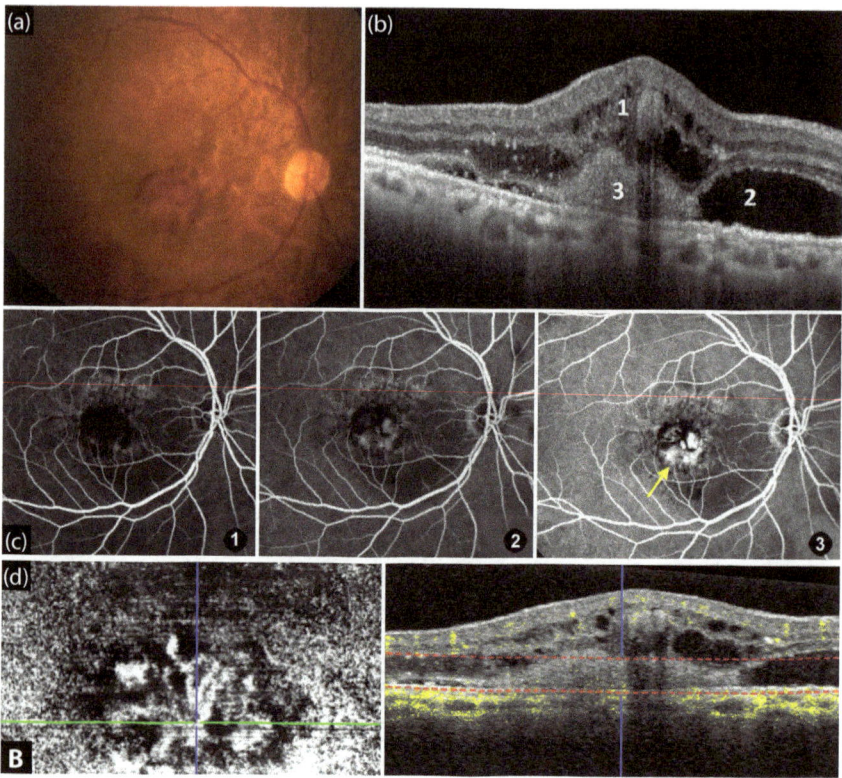

**Fig. 8B:** Multimodal imaging of (A) type 1 macular neovascularization (MNV) and (B) type 2 MNV. (B) Type 2 MNV: (a) Color fundus photograph showing a circular reddish-orange lesion of one-half disk diameter size at the macula with hemorrhages surrounding it and exudates inferiorly; (b) SD-OCT demonstrating subretinal hyperreflectivity at fovea (numbered 3) along with intraretinal (numbered 1) and subretinal (numbered 2) fluid. The lesions are entirely located above RPE, indicating type 2 MNV; (c) FFA showing a well-defined lacy hyperfluorescent lesion from the early phase (numbered 1), which increases in size and intensity in mid (numbered 2) to late (numbered 3, yellow arrow) phases suggestive of leakage of type 2 MNV. The surrounding hypofluorescence is due to blocked fluorescence from hemorrhages; (d) OCTA avascular complex slab showing a well-defined circular network at the level of subretinal hyperreflectivity which is radiating in all directions in a medusa head configuration with a perilesional halo suggesting an active MNV.

## Drusen

Multimodal imaging using a combination of color photography, FAF, IR, and SD-OCT is useful to define the various types of drusenoid lesions seen in nnAMD.

- Hard (small) drusen, by definition, are <63 µm in color photography and are seen as small yellowish white lesions scattered in the macula. SD-OCT defines these lesions as small hyperreflective sub-RPE lesions with corresponding elevation of the RPE.

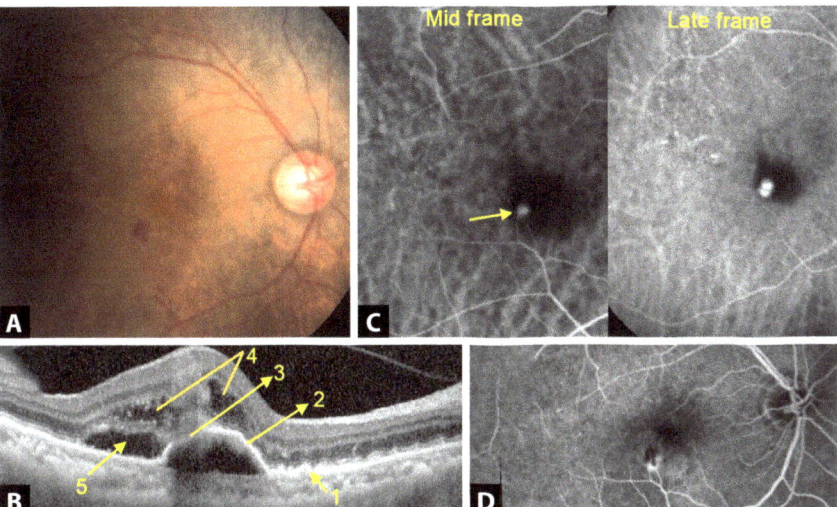

**Figs. 9A to D:** Multimodal imaging in retinal angiomatous proliferation (RAP). (A) Color fundus photograph of the right eye of an 86-year-old woman showing subretinal hemorrhage inferotemporal to fovea with serous macular detachment and drusen at macula; (B) spectral-domain optical coherence tomography (SD-OCT) demonstrates reticular pseudodrusen (labeled 1), pigment epithelial detachment (labeled 2) with disruption at its apex (labeled 3), intraretinal fluid (labeled 4), subretinal fluid (labeled 5), and inner retinal hyperreflective dots; (C) indocyanine green angiography (ICGA) early (1.3 minutes) and late (8.49 minutes) phases shows a hot spot at the central apical disruption of pigment epithelial detachment (PED), characteristic of RAP (yellow arrow); (D) Fundus fluorescein angiography (FFA) shows point hyperfluorescence inferiorly with staining of regions corresponding to PED.

- Soft drusen are large drusen over 125 μm in size in color photography and are seen as deep yellow lesions. SD-OCT defines these lesions as focal elevations of the RPE, which are sometimes confluent **(Figs. 10A and B)**. FAF demonstrates hyperautofluorescence due to high lipofuscin content. Large drusen are high-risk biomarkers for the development of geographic atrophy (GA) and MNV.
- *Reticular pseudodrusen (RPD):* Subretinal deposits and RPD are seen as faint lesions on color photography distributed more temporal to the fovea. They are best illustrated with NIR and FAF. It is important to recognize RPD as they predispose to type 3 MNV and GA. **Figure 11A** demonstrates the multimodal imaging characteristics of RPD.
- Cuticular drusen are less common. They are otherwise basal laminar drusen. They are small (50-75 μm) in size[35] and are seen in clusters with a characteristic starry sky pattern in FFA. SD-OCT demonstrates a characteristic "sawtooth pattern." Cuticular lesions can also predispose to advanced AMD, including GA. **Figure 11B** demonstrates the multimodal imaging characteristics of cuticular drusen.

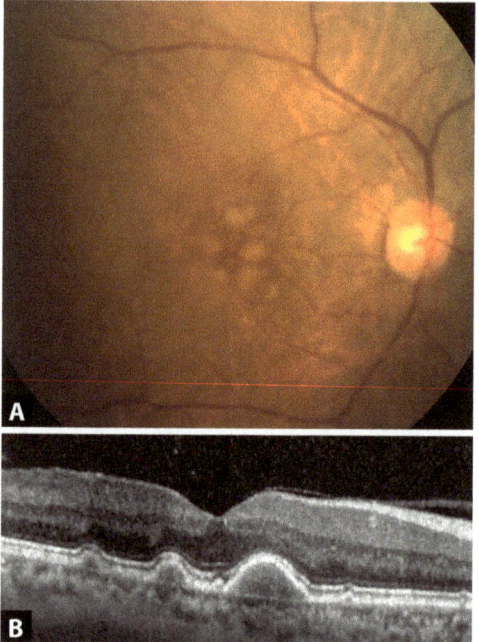

**Figs. 10A and B:** Multimodal imaging of soft drusen. (A) Color fundus photograph of the right eye showing large soft drusen with less clearly defined edges; (B) The corresponding spectral-domain optical coherence tomography (SD-OCT) shows elevation of retinal pigment epithelium (RPE) from Bruch's membrane, with medium-to-high hyperreflectivity located under the RPE.

## Drusenoid Pigment Epithelial Detachment

Color photography defines a drusenoid PED as a reasonably large, well-defined yellowish subretinal lesion, and this could be confused with a confluent soft drusen. SD-OCT is diagnostic with a characteristic smooth elevation of the RPE with underlying uniform hyperreflective material. There will be no associated intraretinal fluid or SRF which are hallmarks of neovascularization.[36] **Figures 12A to C** demonstrate the multimodal imaging evolution of a drusenoid PED.

## Geographic Atrophy

Geographic atrophy is currently defined as a late stage of nnAMD[37] and is characterized by an area of RPE and choriocapillaris loss with baring of the choroidal vessels and measuring >175 μm in diameter.[38] Color fundus photography was the gold standard in identifying GA, but quantitative capability is limited. However, with the advent of multimodal imaging, FAF and SD-OCT are the gold standard for defining, classifying, and quantifying GA.[39] More recently, classification of atrophy in late AMD has been proposed by Classification of Atrophy Meetings (CAM) based on the anatomic layers affected on SD-OCT, which divided into complete and incomplete RPE and outer retinal atrophy.[40] In **Figures 13A to C**, progressive outer retinal and RPE changes on OCT are shown along with late nnAMD changes on FAF.

Multimodal Imaging in Macular Diseases

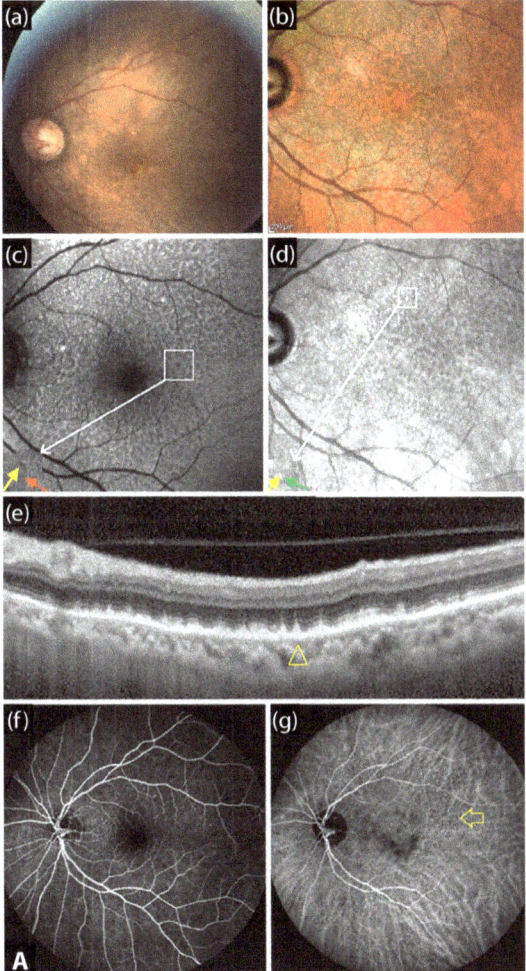

**Fig. 11A:** Multimodal imaging in (A) reticular pseudodrusen (RPD) and (B) basal laminar drusen (BLD). (A) RPD: (a) Color fundus photograph of the left eye of an 86-year-old woman showing macular retinal pigment epithelium (RPE) lesions in an interlacing pattern; (b) Multicolor imaging showing a yellowish-green reticular pattern of RPD. Some RPD have a target appearance characterized by a more intense yellowish/greenish core surrounded by a decreased intensity; (c) Fundus autofluorescence (FAF) showing RPD as hypoautofluorescent dots (inset: yellow arrow) surrounded by a faint hyperautofluorescent halo (inset: red arrow). Several RPD have an isoautofluorescent core, responsible for the "target aspect"; (d) Infrared imaging showing RPD as small lesions clustered in a reticular pattern and a variable target aspect, with an isoreflective core (inset: yellow arrow) surrounded by hyporeflective halo (inset: green arrow); (e) Spectral-domain optical coherence tomography (SD-OCT) showing RPD as discrete accumulation of hyperreflective spike-like material above the RPE in the subretinal space (yellow arrowhead); (f) Fundus fluorescein angiography (FFA) showing a patchy choroidal filling, but RPD is more or less silent; (g) Indocyanine green angiography (ICGA) midphase showing a reticular pattern corresponding to RPD seen as hypoautofluorescent dots (yellow open arrow).

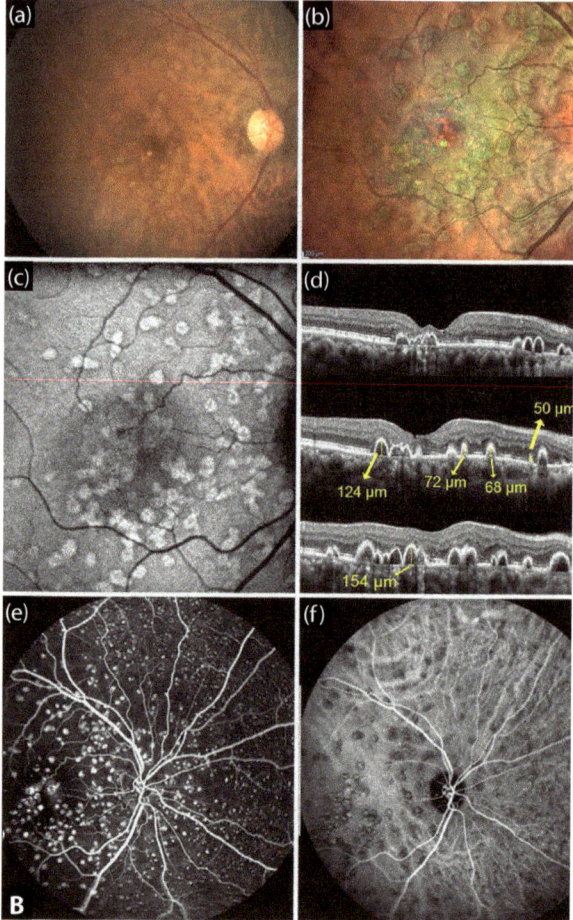

**Fig. 11B:** Multimodal imaging in (A) reticular pseudodrusen (RPD) and (B) basal laminar drusen (BLD). (B) BLD: (a) Color fundus photograph of the right eye of a 68-year-old male with counting finger at 2 m distance vision showing circular, multiple, well-demarcated but, occasionally, coalescent lesions suggestive of multiple retina pigment epithelial detachments (RPEDs) in the macula, posterior pole, midperiphery, and periphery; (b) Multicolor photo showing circular elevated lesions suggestive of pigment epithelial detachment (PED), which appear greenish with an orange outer rim and the central macula demonstrating a bright orange appearance due to enhanced visualization of underlying bright orange choroidal vessels as a result of retinal pigment epithelial atrophy; (c) FAF shows ring-pattern lesions (outnumbering those seen clinically) with a hyperautofluorescent circle and hypoautofluorescent center. This pattern is the result of central RPE erosion from triangular elevations of the RPE-basal lamina; (d) SD-OCT shows multiple RPEDs; some are pointed (the smaller PEDs), while others are dome-shaped (larger PEDs); RPEDs have steep sides and hyporeflective content with RPE atrophy at the peak with backscattering (yellow arrow). Additionally, in this case, subfoveal coalescent PEDs along with RPE and photoreceptor disintegration can also be seen; (e) FFA shows hyperfluorescent lesions in a characteristic starry sky appearance; staining in the macula is also seen, which is due to loss of the outer retinal layers; (f) ICGA shows central hyperfluorescence surrounded by hypofluorescence.

## Acquired Vitelliform Lesion

Acquired vitelliform lesions (AVLs) are defined as an accumulation of organized yellowish material in the subretinal space at the foveal center. The hyperreflective material is supposed to be lipofuscin and melanolipofuscin from dissociated RPE cells.[41] AVLs are usually associated with the presence of different types of drusen, including RPD.[42] When seen in isolation, they have to be distinguished from adult-onset foveomacular dystrophy (AOFVD), which is usually bilateral. **Figures 14A to F** show the multimodal imaging in AVL and AOFVD.

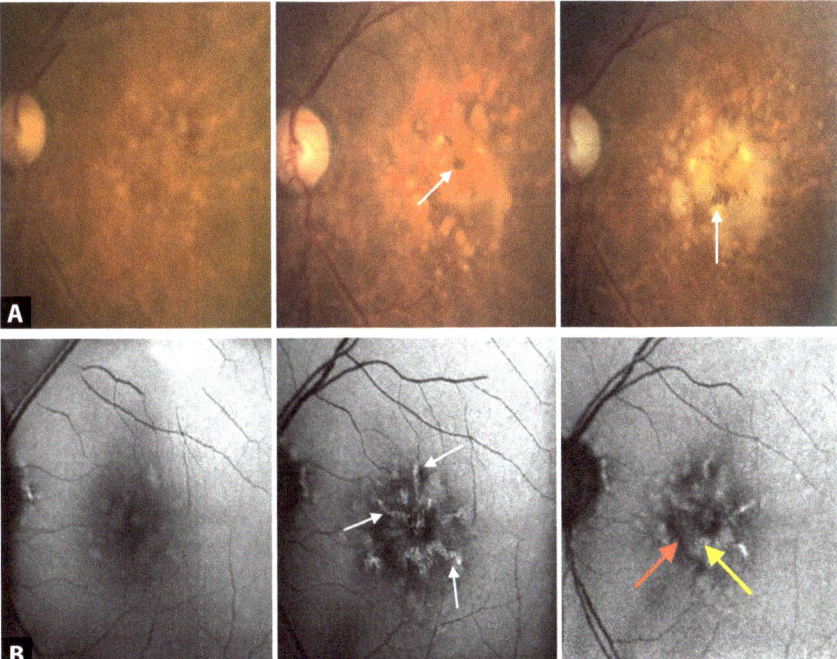

**Figs. 12A and B:** Multimodal imaging of drusenoid pigment epithelial detachment (PED) evolution in a 60-year-old man. (A) Color fundus photograph of the left eye (at presentation) shows an elevated yellow macular lesion with scalloped borders consistent with a drusenoid PED and surrounded by multiple soft drusen. Reddish-brown pigmentation on the surface of PED showing stellate distribution may be seen (white arrow). Subsequent follow-ups, 5 and 8 years later, show increase in size of PED and formation of a full-fledged drusenoid PED; (B) Fundus autofluorescence (FAF) shows an evenly distributed circular mild increase of the FAF signal (yellow arrow) surrounded by a well-defined, hypoautofluorescent halo (red arrow) delineating the entire border of the lesion (more prominent in the second and third follow-ups). The pigment on the surface of the PED appears hyperautofluorescent on FAF (white arrows).

## Multimodal Imaging in Macular Diseases

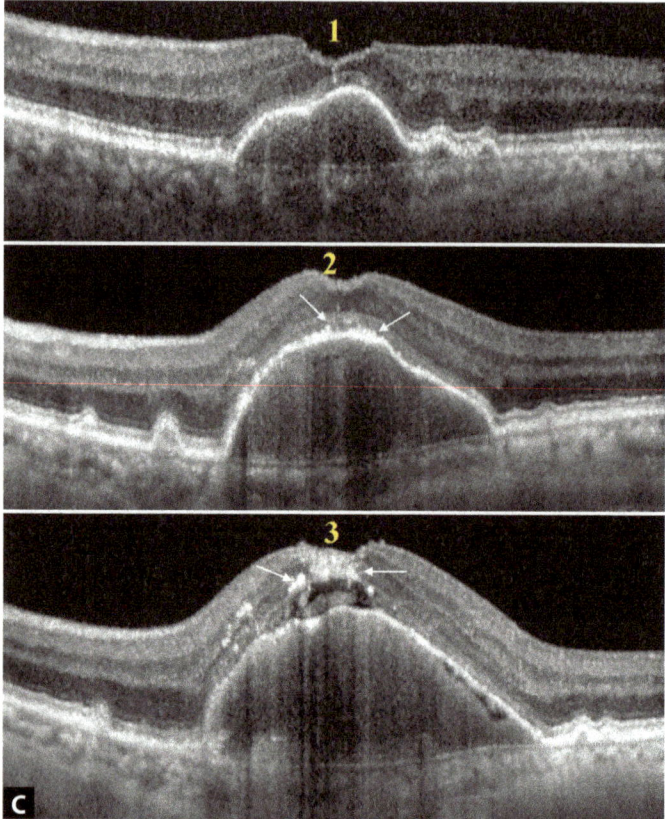

**Fig. 12C:** Multimodal imaging of drusenoid pigment epithelial detachment (PED) evolution in a 60-year-old man. (C) The pigment on the surface of the PED is hyperreflective with posterior shadowing on spectral-domain optical coherence tomography (SD-OCT) (white arrows, section 2). There is an increase in height of PED in subsequent follow-ups with multiple isoreflective dots at the apex of PED. These dots probably represent debris originating from passage of drusen material into the subretinal space through defects in the retinal pigment epithelium (RPE) above the drusen, a phenomenon termed *"drusen ooze"* (section 3; white arrows).

## Multimodal Imaging Biomarkers of Non-neovascular Age-related Macular Degeneration

The poor prognostic indicators for progression to advanced AMD include:
- Reduced subfoveal choroidal thickness[43]
- Presence of RPD,[44] soft drusen, and drusenoid PED
- Presence of the following features in drusenoid PED:
    - Moderate internal reflectivity[45]
    - Hyperreflective foci over the roof of PED
- Patches of hypoautofluorescence on FAF suggestive of RPE atrophy
- Patches of outer retinal atrophy on SD-OCT[46]

Multimodal Imaging in Macular Diseases

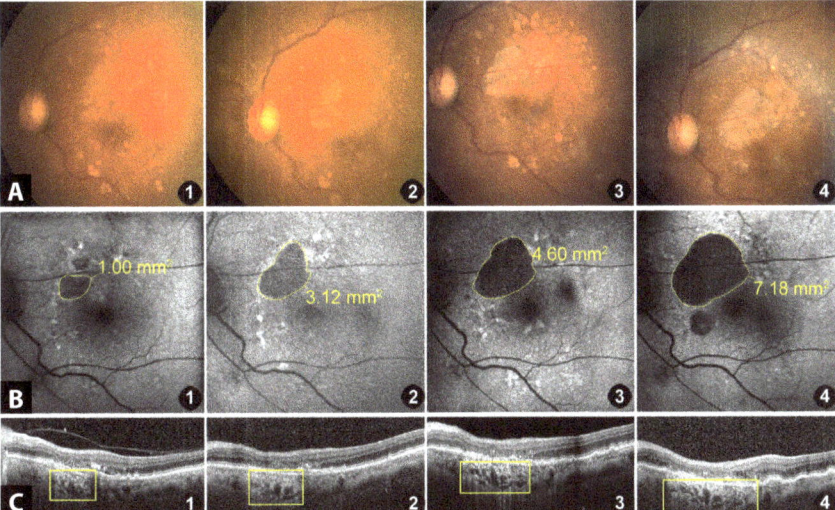

**Figs. 13A to C:** Multimodal imaging of progression of retinal pigment epithelial and outer retinal atrophy in a case of age-related macular degeneration. (A) Color fundus photograph of the left eye of a 72-year-old male showing a well-delineated oval area of hypopigmentation which is progressively increasing in size over the course of 8-year follow-up (labeled 1–4). Numerous drusen can be seen scattered across the posterior pole, between the arcades and nasal to disk; (B) Fundus autofluorescence (FAF) imaging illustrating the progression of atrophy area over time, which is segmented for its quantification (yellow outline). During a follow-up period of 8 years, the atrophic area increased to seven times the size from the baseline (labeled 1–4). The enlargement of atrophy predominantly takes place in areas where there is a high FAF intensity in the perilesional zone at baseline; (C) Spectral-domain optical coherence tomography (SD-OCT) shows thinning and progression in loss of outer retinal layers, including photoreceptor loss and thinning of retinal pigment epithelium (RPE). The region of hypertransmission in the choroid (indicated by a yellow box) is seen increasing at each follow-up (labeled 1–4).

## Polypoidal Choroidal Vasculopathy

Polypoidal choroidal vasculopathy is a distinct clinical entity characterized by subretinal polypoidal lesions along with BVN. The multimodal imaging features of PCV are as follows:
- *SD-OCT*:
    - Thumb-shaped PED/sharp-peaked PED that denotes polyp
    - Notched PED which signifies the polypoidal lesion at the margin of PED
    - Double-layer sign (DLS) on SD-OCT is a shallow and irregular elevation of RPE from the underlying Bruch's membrane. The space between the two layers shows moderate hyperreflectivity and is seen in 91.43-93.75% cases of PCV.
- IGCA is diagnostic with the presence of focal nodular hyperfluorescence appearing within the first 6 minutes of dye injection (well appreciated

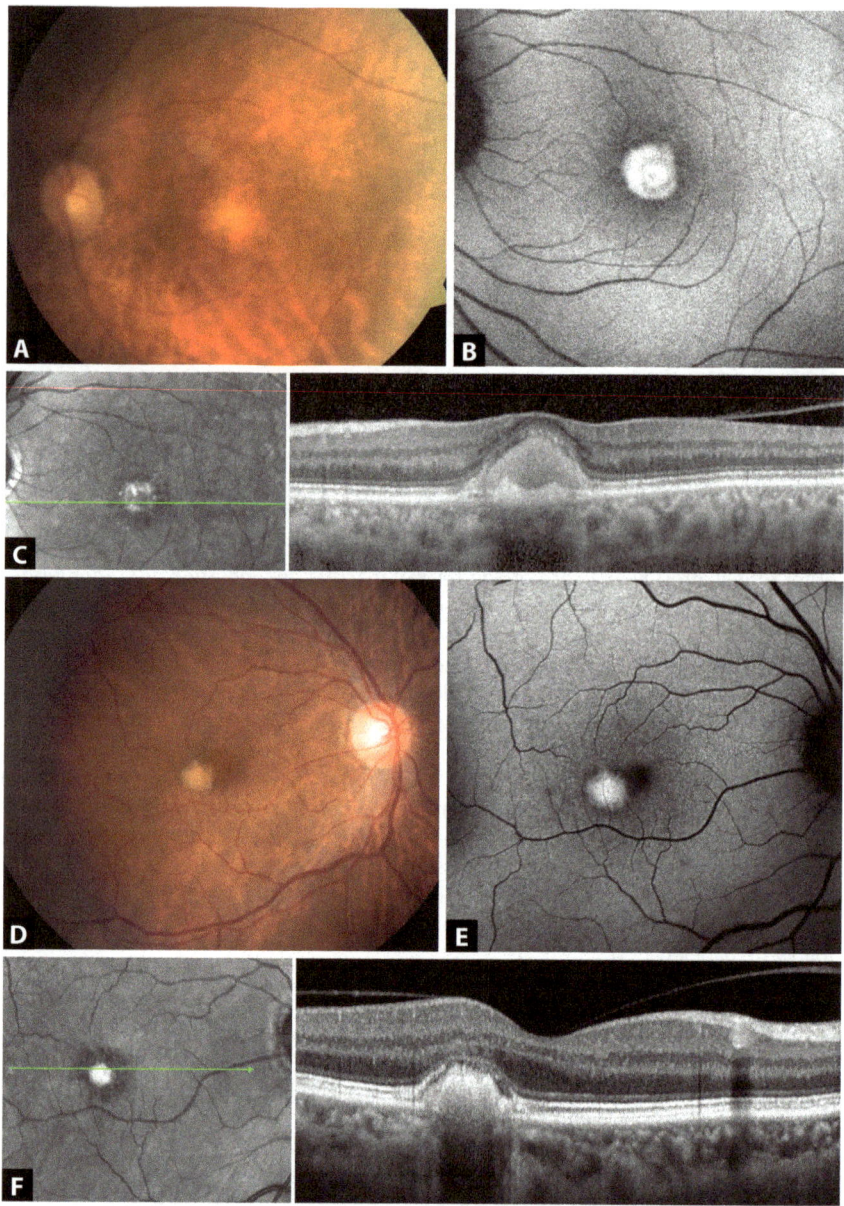

**Figs. 14A to F:** Multimodal imaging in adult-onset foveomacular vitelliform dystrophy (AOFVD) and acquired vitelliform lesion (AVL). Color fundus photographs of a 58-year-old and a 72-year-old male with AOFVD and AVL showing a circular yellowish lesion at the fovea (A) and temporal to the fovea (D), respectively. Fundus autofluorescence shows a uniform circular hyperautofluorescent signal corresponding to the vitelliform lesions (B and E). Spectral-domain optical coherence tomography (SD-OCT) through fovea shows an accumulation of subretinal hyperreflective material with a dome-shaped configuration (C and F). The key differentiating feature between these two entities is the eccentric location of AVL as opposed to the foveal location of AOFVD.

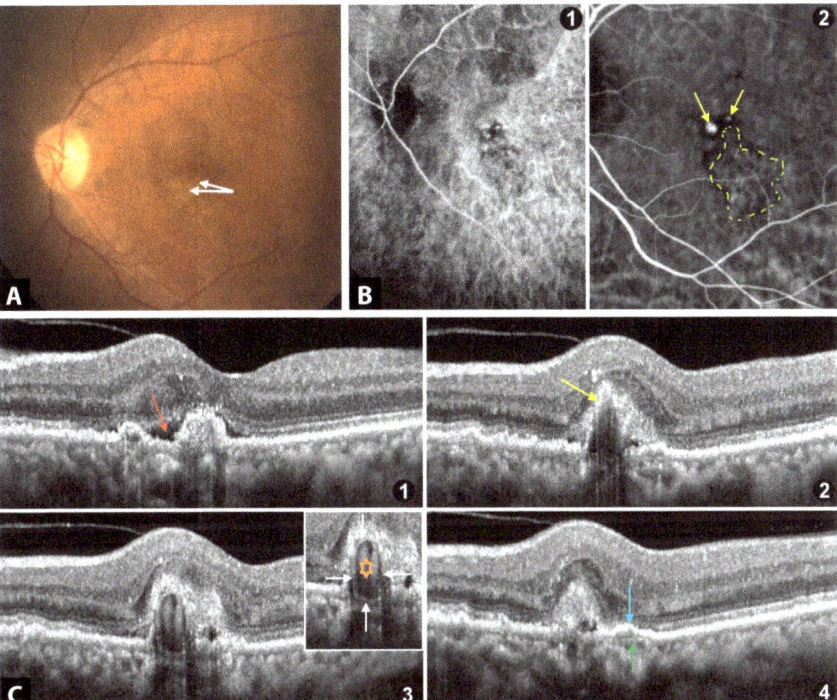

**Figs. 15A to C:** Multimodal imaging of polypoidal choroidal vasculopathy (PCV). (A) Color fundus photograph of the left eye of a 69-year-old male showing multiple orange–red nodular lesions at the macula (white arrows) with surrounding serous macular detachment and retinal pigment epithelium (RPE) changes; (B) Early (labeled 1) and mid (labeled 2) phases of indocyanine green angiography (ICGA) showing multiple nodular hyperfluorescent lesions (yellow arrows) surrounded by a rim of hypofluorescence (indicating fluid) at fovea increasing in intensity suggestive of polyps; surrounding it inferiorly is an abnormal vascular network (delineated in green) in the absence of feeder vessel suggestive of interconnecting channels; (C) Spectral-domain optical coherence tomography (SD-OCT) sections taken through macula show subretinal fluid (labeled 1, red arrow), tall peaked pigment epithelial detachment (PED) (labeled 2, yellow arrow), moderate hyperreflective ring (white arrows) surrounding an area of hyporeflectivity (orange asterisks) located underneath the PED—called *"bubble sign"* (labeled 3, probably representing the lumen of the polypoidal lesion; it is attached to the posterior surface of RPE and corresponds in a location with the polypoidal lesion seen on ICGA) and *"double-layer sign"* (labeled 4) due to separation of RPE (blue arrow) from the Bruch's membrane (green arrow).

on dynamic/video ICGA). It is the gold standard to detect polyps in PCV. ICGA has multiple features in PCV, but the focal nodular hyperfluorescence appearing scattered in the macula or in cluster is diagnostic. The DLS corresponds to the abnormal vascular network in ICGA. The DLS may end in a thumb-shaped or notched PED harboring the polypoidal detachment.

**Figures 15A to C** illustrate the salient multimodal imaging characteristics of PCV.

## ■ CONCLUSION

Identifying the characteristic multimodal imaging features of macular diseases helps the clinician in diagnosis, prognostication, and management of these diseases.

## ■ ACKNOWLEDGMENTS

I would like to acknowledge the help and assistance of fellows in the department of vitreoretina—Drs Mahak Bhandary, Vineet Shah, Sachin Desai, and Jiz Mary Santhosh as well as Mr Murukan Velayudhan (administrative officer and my secretary) in preparing the manuscript.

## ■ REFERENCES

1. Yannuzzi LA, Ober MD, Slakter JS, Spaide RF, Fisher YL, Flower RW, et al. Ophthalmic fundus imaging: today and beyond. Am J Ophthalmol. 2004;137(3):511-24.
2. Schmitz-Valckenberg S, Holz FG, Bird AC, Spaide RF. Fundus autofluorescence imaging: review and perspectives. Retina. 2008;28(3):385-409.
3. Bhende M, Shetty S, Parthasarathy MK, Ramya S. Optical coherence tomography: a guide to interpretation of common macular diseases. Indian J Ophthalmol. 2018;66(1):20-35.
4. Chalam KV, Sambhav K. Optical coherence tomography angiography in retinal diseases. J Ophthalmic Vis Res. 2016;11(1):84-92.
5. Witmer MT, Kiss S. Wide-field imaging of the retina. Surv Ophthalmol. 2013;58:143-54.
6. Spaide RF, Koizumi H, Pozzoni MC. Enhanced depth imaging spectral-domain optical coherence tomography. Am J Ophthalmol. 2008;146:496-500.
7. Kim SK, Kim SW, Oh J, Huh K. Near-infrared and short-wavelength autofluorescence in resolved central serous chorioretinopathy: association with outer retinal layer abnormalities. Am J Ophthalmol. 2013;156:157-64.e2.
8. Ayata A, Tatlipinar S, Kar T, Unal M, Ersanli D, Bilge AH. Near-infrared and short-wavelength autofluorescence imaging in central serous chorioretinopathy. Br J Ophthalmol. 2009;93:79-82.
9. Kon Y, Iida T, Maruko I, Saito M. The optical coherence tomography-ophthalmoscope for examination of central serous chorioretinopathy with precipitates. Retina. 2008;28:864-9.
10. Daruich A, Matet A, Dirani A, Bousquet E, Zhao M, Farman N, et al. Central serous chorioretinopathy: recent findings and new physiopathology hypothesis. Prog Retin Eye Res. 2015;48:82-118.
11. Lehmann M, Bousquet E, Beydoun T, Behar-Cohen F. PACHYCHOROID: an inherited condition? Retina. 2015;35:10-6.
12. Das S, Das D. Central serous chorioretinopathy (CSCR). Sci J Med Vis Res Foun. 2017;XXXV:10-20.
13. Gass JD. Stereoscopic Atlas of Macular Diseases. St Louis, MO: CV Mosby; 1987. pp. 56-7.
14. Gass JD. Central serous chorioretinopathy and white subretinal exudation during pregnancy. Arch Ophthalmol. 1991;109:677-81.

15. Bouzas EA, Karadimas P, Pournaras CJ. Central serous chorioretinopathy and glucocorticoids. Surv Ophthalmol. 2002;47:431-48.
16. Landa G, Barnett JA, Garcia PMT, Tai KW, Rosen RB. Quantitative and qualitative spectral domain optical coherence tomography analysis of subretinal deposits in patients with acute central serous retinopathy. Ophthalmologica. 2013;230:62-8.
17. Maruko I, Iida T, Ojima A, Sekiryu T. Subretinal dot-like precipitates and yellow material in central serous chorioretinopathy. Retina. 2011;31:759-65.
18. Ie D, Yannuzzi LA, Spaide RF, Rabb MF, Blair NP, Daily MJ. Subretinal exudative deposits in central serous chorioretinopathy. Br J Ophthalmol. 1993;77:349-53.
19. Fujimoto H, Gomi F, Wakabayashi T, Sawa M, Tsujikawa M, Tano Y. Morphologic changes in acute central serous chorioretinopathy evaluated by Fourier-domain optical coherence tomography. Ophthalmology. 2008;115:1494-500.
20. Hussain N, Baskar A, Ram LM, Das T. Optical coherence tomographic pattern of fluorescein angiographic leakage site in acute central serous chorioretinopathy. Clin Exp Opthalmol. 2006;34:137-40.
21. Saxena S, Sinha N, Sharma S. Three-dimensional imaging by spectral domain optical coherence tomography in central serous chorioretinopathy with fibrin. J Ocul Biol Dis Infor. 2012;4:149-53.
22. Rajesh B, Kaur A, Giridhar A, Gopalakrishnan M. "Vacuole" sign adjacent to retinal pigment epithelial defects on spectral domain optical coherence tomography in central serous chorioretinopathy associated with subretinal fibrin. Retina. 2017;37(2):316-24.
23. Moorthy RS, Lyon AT, Rabb MF, Spaide RF, Yannuzzi LA, Jampol LM. Idiopathic polypoidal choroidal vasculopathy of the macula. Ophthalmology. 1998;105:1380-5.
24. Yannuzzi L, Ciardella A, Spaide R, Rabb M, Freund K, Orlock DA. The expanding clinical spectrum of idiopathic polypoidal choroidal vasculopathy (IPCV). In: Retinal Pigment Epithelium and Macular Diseases. Berlin: Springer; 1998. pp. 173-83.
25. Park HS, Kim IT. Clinical characteristics of polypoidal choroidal vasculopathy associated with chronic central serous chorioretionopathy. Korean J Ophthalmol. 2012;26:15-20.
26. Koizumi H, Yamagishi T, Yamazaki T, Kinoshita S. Relationship between clinical characteristics of polypoidal choroidal vasculopathy and choroidal vascular hyperpermeability. Am J Ophthalmol. 2013;155:305-313.e1.
27. Sheth J, Anantharaman G, Chandra S, Sivaprasad S. "Double-layer sign" on spectral domain optical coherence tomography in pachychoroid spectrum disease. Indian J Ophthalmol. 2018;66:1796-801.
28. Boon CJ, Klevering BJ, Leroy BP, Hoyng CB, Keunen JE, den Hollander AI. The spectrum of ocular phenotypes caused by mutations in the BEST1 gene. Prog Retin Eye Res. 2009;28(3):187-205.
29. Gass JD. Pathogenesis of disciform detachment of the neuroepithelium. Am J Ophthalmol. 1967;63(3):1-139.
30. Krishnan T, Ravindran RD, Murthy GVS, Vashist P, Fitzpatrick KE, Thulasiraj RD, et al. Prevalence of early and late age-related macular degeneration in India: the INDEYE Study. Invest Ophthalmol Vis Sci. 2010;51:701-7.
31. Chopdar A, Chakravarthy U, Verma D. Age related macular degeneration. BMJ. 2003;326(7387):485-8.

32. Yannuzzi LA, Negrão S, Iida T, Carvalho C, Rodriguez-Coleman H, Slakter J, et al. Retinal angiomatous proliferation in age-related macular degeneration. Retina. 2001;21(5):416-34.
33. Tsai ASH, Cheung N, Gan ATL, Jaffe GJ, Sivaprasad S, Wong TY, et al. Retinal angiomatous proliferation. Surv Ophthalmol. 2017;62(4):462-92.
34. Gallego-Pinazo R, Monje-Fernández L, García-Marín N, Andreu-Fenoll M, Dolz-Marco R. Implications of the anatomical classification of the neovascular form of age-related macular degeneration. Arch Soc Esp Oftalmol. 2017;92(2):71-7.
35. Balaratnasingam C, Cherepanoff S, Dolz-Marco R, Killingsworth M, Chen FK, Mendis R, et al. Cuticular drusen: clinical phenotypes and natural history defined using multimodal imaging. Ophthalmology. 2018;125:100-18.
36. Roquet W, Roudot-Thoraval F, Coscas G, Soubrane G. Clinical features of drusenoid pigment epithelial detachment in age related macular degeneration. Br J Ophthalmol. 2004;88:638-42.
37. Bressler NM, Bressler SB, Fine SL. Age-related macular degeneration. Surv Ophthalmol. 1988;32:375-413.
38. Freund KB, Sarraf D, Mieler WF, Yannuzzi LA. The Retinal Atlas, 2nd edition. Amsterdam: Elsevier; 2017.
39. Yehoshua Z, Rosenfeld PJ, Gregori G, Feuer WJ, Falcão M, Lujan BJ, et al. Progression of geographic atrophy in age-related macular degeneration imaged with spectral domain optical coherence tomography. Ophthalmology. 2011;118:679-86.
40. Guymer RH, Rosenfeld PJ, Curcio CA, Holz FG, Staurenghi G, Freund KB, et al. Incomplete retinal pigment epithelial and outer retinal atrophy in age-related macular degeneration: Classification of Atrophy Meeting report 4. Ophthalmology. 2020;127:394-409.
41. Balaratnasingam C, Messinger JD, Sloan KR, Yannuzzi LA, Freund KB, Curcio CA. Histologic and optical coherence tomographic correlates in drusenoid pigment epithelium detachment in age-related macular degeneration. Ophthalmology. 2017;124:644-56.
42. Zweifel SA, Spaide RF, Yannuzzi LA. Acquired vitelliform detachment in patients with subretinal drusenoid deposits (reticular pseudodrusen). Retina. 2011;31:229-34.
43. Fleckenstein M, Mitchell P, Freund KB, Sadda S, Holz FG, Brittain C, et al. The progression of geographic atrophy secondary to age-related macular degeneration. Ophthalmology. 2018;125:369-90.
44. Spaide RF. Improving the age-related macular degeneration construct: a new classification system. Retina. 2018;38:891-9.
45. Querques G, Souied EH. Vascularized drusen: slowly progressive type 1 neovascularization mimicking drusenoid retinal pigment epithelium elevation. Retina. 2015;35:2433-9.
46. Ouyang Y, Heussen FM, Hariri A, Keane PA, Sadda SR. Optical coherence tomography-based observation of the natural history of drusenoid lesion in eyes with dry age-related macular degeneration. Ophthalmology. 2013;120:2656-65.

CHAPTER 14

# Recent Advances in Optic Nerve Tumors

*Dipankar Das, Obaidur Rehman, Sakshi Mishra, Madhusmita Mahapatra*

## ABSTRACT

Among the variety of lesions that may affect the optic nerve, tumors are an uncommon entity. A wide array of tumors has been described, out of which optic nerve glioma and nerve sheath meningioma remain the most common primary optic nerve tumors. Suspicion of a secondary tumor may probe a clinician to look in a different direction. The diagnostic modalities in investigation have continuously evolved over the years and so have the management protocols. Immunohistological studies have provided new insights into the existing knowledge of tumor pathology. This chapter discusses the current understanding of optic nerve tumors along with the recent advances in diagnosis and management.

***Keywords:*** Astrocytes; choroidal melanoma; meningioma; metastasis; optic nerve glioma; optic nerve melanocytoma; optic nerve sheath meningioma; primary optic nerve tumors; Rosenthal fibers; secondary optic nerve tumors.

## ■ INTRODUCTION

Optic nerve tumors (ONTs) are rare occurrences and may be classified as primary or secondary tumors. A primary optic nerve tumor (PONT) may arise from the nerve proper or its sheath while a secondary tumor might be a result of infiltration of the nerve from a surrounding malignancy or a distant malignancy. Secondary optic nerve tumors (SONTs) are more frequently encountered than primary tumors.[1] ONTs can have varied presentations and carry a significant risk of visual morbidity. Majority of ONTs are benign with slow progression, but a few may be highly malignant and potentially dangerous if left untreated. For optimum management of a patient, it is imperative for a clinician to remain up to date with evolving investigative modalities and current treatment protocols.

## ■ PRIMARY OPTIC NERVE TUMORS
## Optic Nerve Glioma

Optic nerve glioma (ONG) is a part of the optic pathway glioma (OPG) spectrum, which affects the anterior visual pathway system. When confined to the optic nerve (ON) alone, such tumors are called *ONGs*. They account for 1.5-4% of all orbital tumors,[2] and being the most common PONTs, they constitute 65% of all intrinsic ONTs.[3] They mostly present in the younger age group and have a female preponderance,[2] with the majority diagnosed within the first 10 years of life and nearly 90% within the first two decades.[4] ONGs are low-grade, slow-growing tumors typically, but may rarely turn malignant. The World Health Organization (WHO) recognizes ONGs as low-grade I juvenile pilocytic astrocytomas or grade II diffuse fibrillary astrocytomas.[5] ONGs are sporadic in most cases but may be associated with neurofibromatosis-1 (NF1). Approximately 8-31% of cases with NF1 may develop ONG; however, these patients carry a better prognosis.[4]

### *Pathogenesis*

Optic nerve gliomas mostly arise from astrocytes and rarely from oligo-dendrocytes.[3] Neurofibromin is a tumor suppressor protein that is inactivated in NF1, leading to activation of proto-oncogene retrovirus-associated sequence (RAS). In sporadic cases, the most frequent genetic mutation is *BRAF-KIAA1549* fusion.[6] There is controversy regarding classification of ONGs as some authors argue that mucopolysaccharide accumulation is the cause of ONG enlargement and not tumor mitotic activity; therefore, they consider them a hamartoma and not a true tumor.[7]

### *Presentation*

The presenting features depend on the actual location of the tumor; anterior lesions cause disk edema and signs of neuropathy while disk pallor may be noted in posterior lesions. The most frequent findings encountered at presentation include proptosis (94%), followed by loss of vision, pale optic disk, edema of the optic disk, and squint.[4] Patients typically complain of unilateral protrusion of eye and/or slow, progressive vision loss. Other signs and symptoms may include visual field loss, afferent pupillary defect, decreased ocular motility, headache, and nystagmus. Rarely, venous stasis retinopathy, neovascular glaucoma, anterior segment ischemia, or retinal vascular occlusion may be noted on examination. Features such as severe retro-orbital pain, rapid unilateral or bilateral vision loss, and massive disk swelling and hemorrhages on the ON head may point toward malignant gliomas.

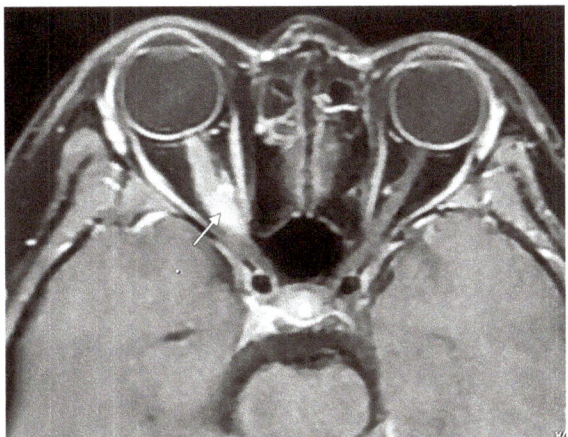

**Fig. 1:** Magnetic resonance imaging (MRI) T1-weighted axial scan of right-sided optic nerve glioma showing enlargement and kinking of optic nerve (white arrow).

## Investigations

Magnetic resonance imaging (MRI) has a superior diagnostic value over computed tomography (CT) scans. The lesion appears hypointense/isointense on T1-weighted scans, and hyperintensity is noted on T2-weighted scans, with contrast enhancement. CT scan in the bone window setting shows enlargement of the optic canal. Fusiform enlargement of the ON is the classical finding in radiology, which is more common in the sporadic variety of ONG. In cases of NF1, thickened ON is visualized with kinking **(Fig. 1)**. Optical coherence tomography (OCT) has been used to study retinal nerve fiber layer (RNFL) thickness in ONGs in children. As vision testing is unreliable and difficult in young children, stationary or hand-held OCT may be used as a surrogate means to evaluate the ON status. Zahavi et al.[8] noted that RNFL thinning on OCT scan was associated with poor visual acuity in children, and worsening of RNFL parameters was associated with visual field loss.

## Histopathological and Immunohistochemical Features

The gross specimen of a resected tumor reveals a smooth, fusiform intradural lesion **(Fig. 2)**. While on cut section, macroscopically, the tumor may have solid, gelatinous, or cystic appearance **(Fig. 3)**. On histopathological examination, elongated, spindle-shaped, pilocytic (hair-like) astrocytes can be seen. Rosenthal fibers (cigar-shaped eosinophilic bodies) surrounded by hyalinized connective tissue can be observed **(Fig. 4)**. Older gliomas appear fibrotic with lipoidal astrocytic proliferations and thick-walled blood vessels, making them difficult to recognize. Rarely, histopathology demonstrates mitotic figures or malignant degeneration. Glial filaments may be stained

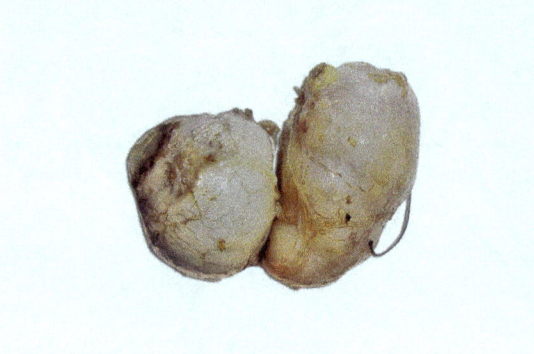

**Fig. 2:** Gross pathology specimen of the enucleated eyeball with an attached enlarged optic nerve. The optic nerve glioma is contained within the dura mater, which appears tan to dusky red from vascular congestion. The lesion is fusiform in shape. The lesion can invade the arachnoid and pia mater and may extend through subdural space.

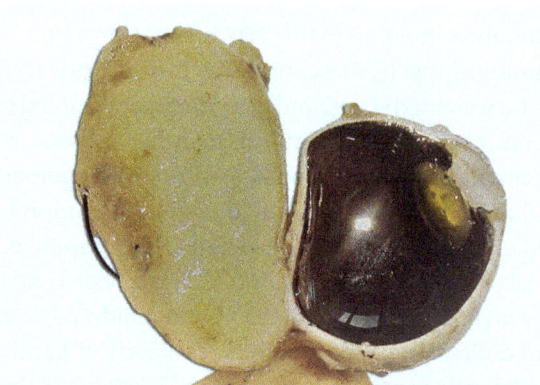

**Fig. 3:** Cut section of enucleated eyeball with optic nerve glioma on gross pathology. A solid, tan-colored mass is seen filling the optic nerve parenchyma.

with glial fibrillary acidic protein (GFAP) stain. Other immunohistochemical markers confirming type-I astrocyte origin include HNK-1, S-100, and vimentin. The two distinctly identified growth patterns are perineural and intraneural, with perineural spread being more common in NF1 cases.

## Management

No standard management protocols exist that may be applied uniformly to all ONG patients. Management strategy has to be patient specific and may vary in different cases. The WHO recommendations state that detailed visual assessment should be done in children with NF1 on a yearly basis till they

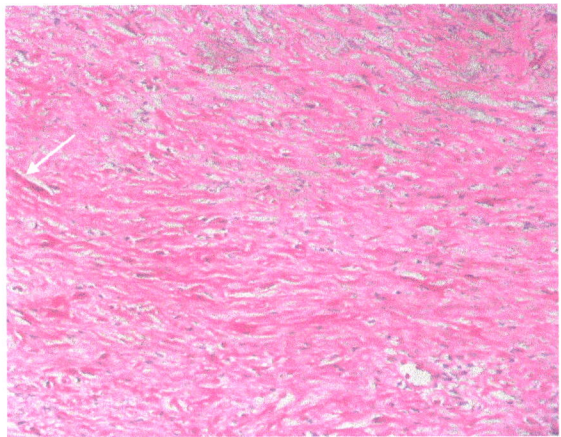

**Fig. 4:** Rosenthal fibers seen on histopathology (white arrow) surrounded by hyalinized connective tissues.

reach 17 years of age while MRI is recommended for those who present with signs of ONG.[9] Those diagnosed with OPG should have a 3-monthly MRI evaluation during infancy and an annual MRI thereafter.[9] ONGs are extremely slow growing and may become stable after a certain point of time, usually not progressing beyond 12 years of age. Patients having good vision and static appearance on radiological imaging can be observed. Intervention may be planned if visual function deterioration and progression of tumor are observed. Chemotherapy is the currently accepted first-line management choice in progressive disease, especially in younger children (<5 years). Different agents being used include carboplatin, vincristine, temozolomide, and vinblastine. The preferred first-line chemotherapy is combined vincristine and carboplatin treatment, which has shown a 70% progression-free survival.[2] Thioguanine, procarbazine, CCNU and vincristine (called TPCV regimen) forms another potential therapeutic combination. As management strategies evolve from broad to specific and with molecular-level targets, several newer agents have been used in recent times in ONGs. Use of antivascular endothelial growth factor (VEGF) agent, bevacizumab, has been associated with stable or regressing lesions, but progression in few cases was noted after discontinuation of therapy.[10,11] Gene therapy has recently gained attention and MEK inhibitors such as refametinib and trametinib, which target MEK/microtubule-associated protein kinase (MAPK)/extracellular signal-regulated kinase (ERK) pathway, may hold promise in the future.

The role of radiotherapy remains controversial in ONGs due to its variable results. Different options include external beam radiotherapy, stereotactic fractionated radiotherapy, and proton beam therapy. The risk of secondary cancers, central nervous system (CNS) side effects, and intellectual disability should be kept in mind. Radiation therapy may be tried in refractory cases as an adjunct treatment.

Previously, surgery was considered as the first line of treatment but with evolution of newer drugs and therapeutic modalities, the management protocols have also shifted to less-invasive treatments. ONGs do not usually progress to involve the optic chiasma or contralateral ON.[12] Surgery is now limited to diagnostic biopsies and debulking in cases of extreme proptosis. Surgical excision through a lateral orbitotomy remains the standard technique, but newer developments, such as ultrasonic aspirator machines used in neurosurgical tumor excision, may provide a safer and more accurate surgical debulking option.

## Malignant Glioma

Malignant glioma is a rare entity, classified as grade III (anaplastic astrocytoma) or grade IV (glioblastoma) tumor by the WHO.[5] It mainly affects the adult population, in contrast to ONG. Presentation includes acute-onset unilateral/bilateral severe pain with vision loss. Common clinical findings are disk edema, disk pallor, or central retinal vein occlusion. A generalized enlargement of the ON is noted on radiological imaging, which may also include the chiasma or optic tract. Histopathological examination has characteristic anaplastic cells. The prognosis is very poor and treatment, including chemotherapy and radiotherapy, is usually unsuccessful.

## Optic Nerve Sheath Meningioma

This tumor arises from the sheath of the ON due to proliferation of meningoepithelial cells. Optic nerve sheath meningiomas (ONSMs) are second-most common ONTs after ONGs. Primary ONSMs arise from the sheath of the ON, while secondary ONSMs arise from the cranial meninges and extend into the orbit. ONSMs are usually benign, and up to 90% are due to extension from the intracranial side (secondary ONSM).[13] ONSMs are usually unilateral with rare bilateral presentation in NF2 patients.[14]

### *Presentation*

Patients classically present in the fourth decade with a triad of vision loss, optic atrophy, and optociliary shunt vessels on fundoscopy.[15] However, this triad presenting in its entirety is rare. Vision loss is common (97%) at presentation in the affected eye, but the degree is variable, with 45% of patients having an acuity of 20/40 or better and 24% having an acuity of counting fingers or worse.[13] Wright et al. described a presenting acuity of "no perception of light" (NLP) in 24% of patients.[16] Proptosis (59%) and strabismus (47%) are other common findings.[13]

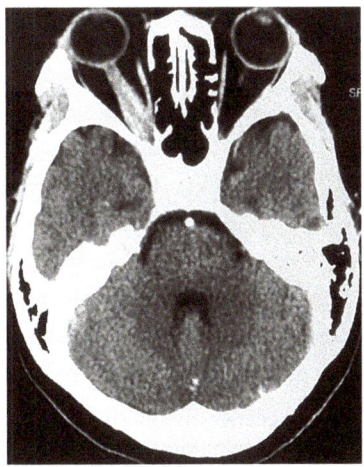

**Fig. 5:** Magnetic resonance imaging (MRI) T1-weighted axial scan showing tram track appearance in optic nerve sheath meningioma of the right optic nerve.

## Investigations

Magnetic resonance imaging is better suited for investigating ONSMs and shows a normal ON parenchyma. Calcification of the sheath leads to the classic "tram track" sign: Hyperintense ON sheath on either side relative to the ON in the center **(Fig. 5)**. Typical radiological findings are tubular expansion of the meninges around the ON (most common), globular enlargement, fusiform enlargement, and focal enlargement of the ON. Multifocal visual-evoked potential (mfVEP) is a newer modality with particular applicability in pediatric population, where MRI scan needs general anesthesia and has its own associated risks.[17-19] mfVEP may guide the need of early intervention in patients.

## Histopathology

On gross and cut-section examinations, an enlarged ON sheath is observed around the nerve **(Figs. 6A and B)**. Histological examination shows meningothelial cap cells, which are mesodermal in origin. Spindle- or oval-shaped cap cells may be seen in concentric whorls along with psammoma bodies (PB), which are hyalinized calcium deposits **(Fig. 7)**. Rarely, mitotic figures or malignant degeneration may be observed. Fluorescein staining can pick up the PB in raw specimen, and author(s) had innovated the staining procedure for rapid diagnosis.[20] Fluorescein staining and histopathological examination may also reveal fibroblastic proliferation **(Figs. 8A to C)**.

## Management

In patients who maintain a central visual acuity of 20/50 or better, conservative management and observation can be employed. Serial visual fields

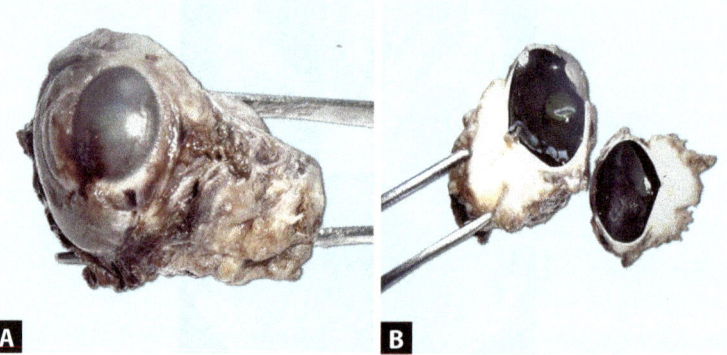

**Figs. 6A and B:** (A) Gross specimen and (B) cut section showing morphology of optic nerve meningioma in an enucleated eye.

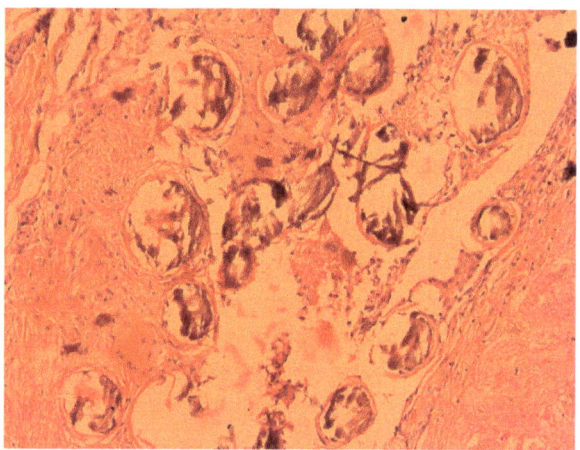

**Fig. 7:** Histopathological section showing spindle- or oval-shaped concentric whorls with calcified psammoma bodies.

and peripapillary RNFL OCT scans can be used for grading the progression. Annual MRI is performed to look for disease progression. Radiation therapy is the first-line accepted treatment for ONSMs. Stereotactic radiotherapy (SRT) is superior to conventional external beam radiotherapy and has promising results. The delivery of radiation in a localized fashion is important and is possible through SRT. The side effects include optic neuropathy, optic atrophy, and radiation-induced retinopathy. An eye dose of >50 Gy predisposes to retinal injury.[21]

Surgical intervention is usually not preferred due to imminent vision loss, but resection may be performed when the risk of intracranial extension and contralateral involvement is high. The introduction and increasing

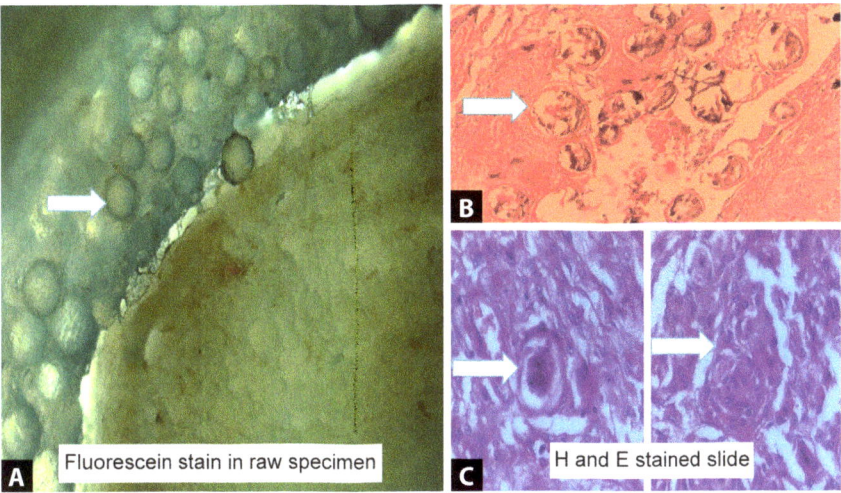

**Figs. 8A to C:** (A) Fluorescein stain in raw specimen of optic nerve sheath meningioma that the author had innovated; (B) Hematoxylin and eosin (H&E)-stained specimen showing fibrocystic component along with psammoma bodies (10×); (C) Magnified view of the same (40×).

applicability of endoscopic endonasal techniques to access lesions in the optic canal and orbit have progressively displaced well-established transcranial approaches.

## Optic Disk Melanocytoma

Melanocytoma is a variant of melanocytic nevus, which is a deeply pigmented lesion occurring mainly in the optic disk with occasional involvement of the adjacent retina or choroid. The tumor has often been confused with malignant melanoma in the past, both clinically and histopathologically. Zimmerman first used the term "melanocytoma" to describe a benign, asymptomatic hamartomatous tumor growth that arises from melanocytes.[22]

### Pathogenesis

Intraocular melanocytoma is a benign, deeply pigmented melanocytic tumor situated eccentrically on the ONH.[23-26] It may be elevated, and it typically extends into the adjacent retina as well as posteriorly into the ON. Melanocytomas may grow slowly; however, malignant transformation to melanoma rarely occurs.[24-28] Primary malignant melanoma of the optic disk is extremely rare with few well-documented cases in the literature.[27-30]

### Presentation

The mean age at diagnosis of optic disk melanocytoma is 50 years with a median age of 52 years and a range of 1–91 years.[24] It appears to have a

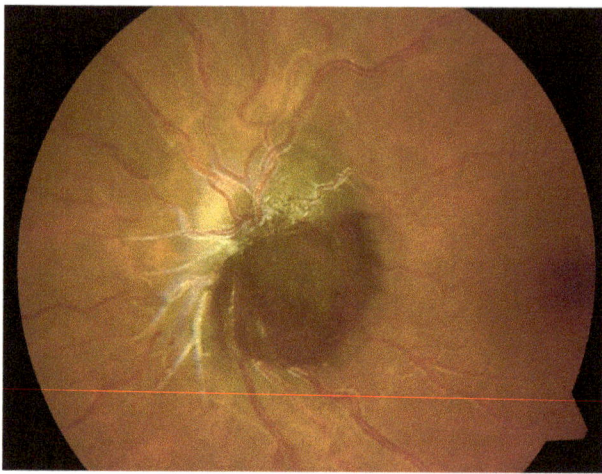

**Fig. 9:** Fundus photograph of left eye showing optic disk melanocytoma with an elevated blackish brown lesion occupying almost the entire optic disk surface and extending over the edges of optic nerve.

slight predilection for females. Melanocytoma is often unilateral but bilateral cases have been rarely reported, usually in children.[31,32] It usually does not compromise visual acuity;[22,24] however, visual symptoms may be attributed to mild exudation with foveal involvement or tumor necrosis.[33,34] Patients can present with severe visual loss secondary to malignant transformation.[24,26,35] An afferent pupillary defect may be noted due to compression of the optic disk fibers by the melanocytoma cells. Fundus examination shows a black to dark brown elevated mass lesion, which can be reddish tinged with feathery edges, occupying the optic disk surface and extending over the edges of ON **(Fig. 9)**. Pigment dispersion in mid and posterior vitreous space may be appreciated. Sometimes, a pigmented lesion may be found but without any peripheral serrations.

## Investigations

Visual field defects that may be observed include enlarged blind spots and nerve fiber bundle defects, including nasal step (10%), relative nerve fiber bundle defect (20%), and arcuate scotoma (20%).[36,37] B-scan ultrasonography (USG) of the involved eye shows a hyperechoic small dome-shaped lesion **(Fig. 10)**. Fundus fluorescein angiography reveals hypofluorescence in all stages without any evidence of late-phase hyperfluorescence of the mass lesion **(Figs. 11A to D)**. On OCT examination, a gradually sloped mass with a thin bright anterior surface and dense posterior shadowing is noted **(Figs. 12A and B)**. The thicker the tumor, the thinner the anterior surface signal.

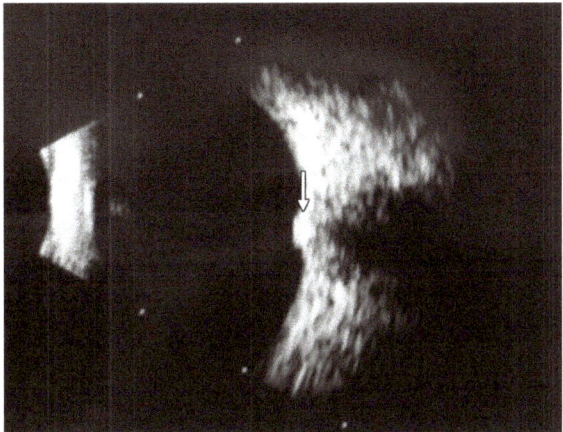

**Fig. 10:** B-scan ultrasonography of the involved eye showing a hyperechoic small dome-shaped lesion (white arrow).

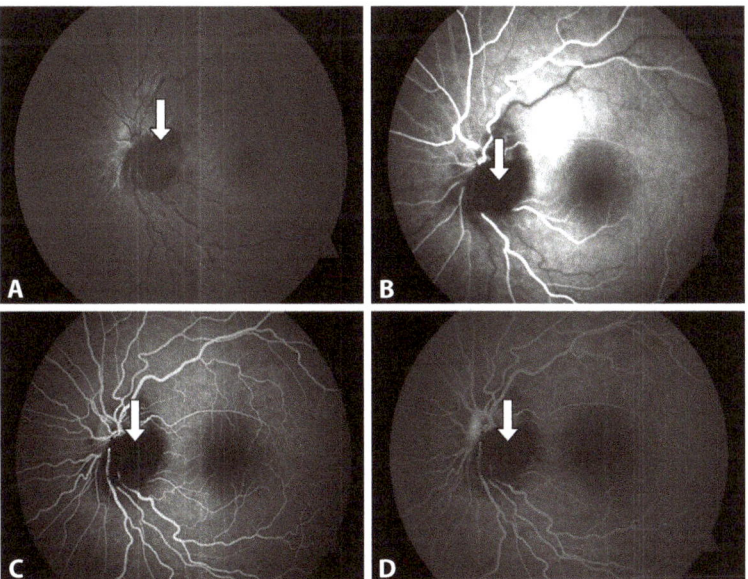

**Figs. 11A to D:** Fundus fluorescein angiography of the left eye showing hypofluorescence in all phases of angiography (white arrows).

## Histopathology

In 54% of cases, the tumor extends beyond disk margin to involve the adjacent choroid. In 30% of patients, it grows into the adjacent retina.[38,39] Histopathology of melanocytoma shows two types of cells **(Fig. 13)**, with type 1 being oval, round cells containing round cytoplasmic melanosomes. The nuclei and nucleoli are small. In type 2 cells, the nevus cell is spindle shaped,

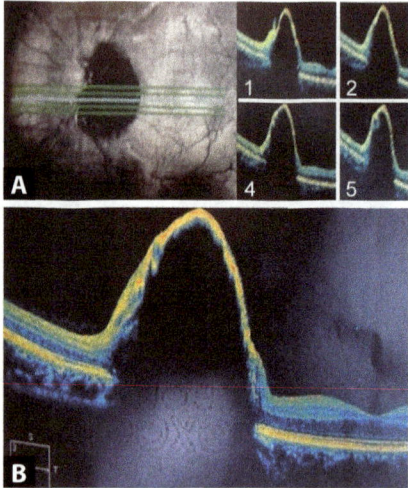

**Figs. 12A and B:** Optical coherence tomography (OCT) scan showing a gradually sloped mass with a thin bright anterior surface and dense posterior shadowing.

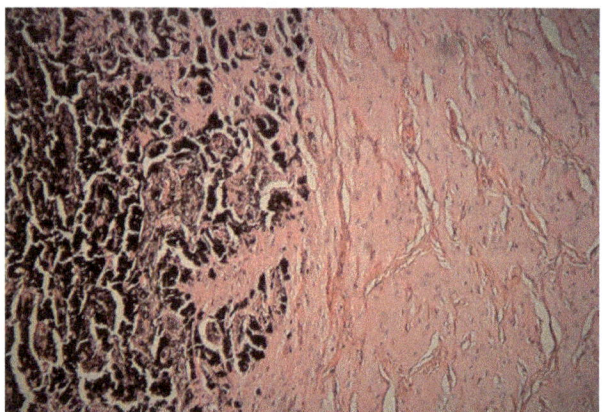

**Fig. 13:** Histopathology of melanocytoma showing oval, round cytoplasmic melanosomes.

with larger nucleoli, rod-shaped melanosomes, and more cytoplasmic organelles.

## Management

As the transformation of optic disk melanocytoma into malignant melanoma is rare, patients can be observed with clinical examination and fundus photography performed annually. No specific treatment is required. However, deterioration of vision and rapid growth suggest malignant transformation and enucleation should be considered.

## Complications

Although optic disk melanocytoma is associated with few local complications, the possible complications based on recent evidence are as follows:[24]
- Vision loss (26%)
- Optic disk edema (25%)
- Retinal edema (16%)
- Localized subretinal fluid (14%)
- Retinal exudation (12%)
- Retinal hemorrhage (5%)
- Vitreous seeds (4%)
- Retinal vein occlusion (3%)

Malignant transformation of ON melanocytoma may be suspected when the following clinical features are noted:
- Moderate visual loss
- Marked elevation (on USG B-scan, OCT, neuroimaging)
- Progressive growth with worsening visual loss

Another rare complication apart from malignant transformation can be ischemic tumor necrosis.

## Differential Diagnosis

Differential diagnoses for ON melanocytoma include the following:
- *Juxtapapillary choroidal melanoma*: Sometimes, it is extended around the posterior termination of Bruch's membrane and invades the sensory retina causing a fibrillary margin similar to melanocytoma and leading to diagnostic confusion.[40,41]
- *Choroidal nevus*: It is a flat or minimally elevated choroidal lesion that remains outside the disk.
- *Hyperplasia of retinal pigment epithelium (RPE)*: The lesion is irregular with evidence of chorioretinal scarring.[22] A history of ocular trauma or inflammation may be noted.
- *Combined hamartoma of retina and RPE*: It does not have a juxtapapillary choroidal component or feathery invasion of the nerve fiber layer of the retina.[38,42]
- *Adenoma of RPE*: It does not show a feathery margin, and yellowish retinal exudation is more likely in these cases.
- *Metastatic melanoma to optic disk*: It is extremely rare and has a tendency to grow more rapidly.
- Peripapillary vitreous hemorrhage

## ■ SECONDARY OPTIC NERVE TUMORS

Secondary optic nerve tumors are more commonly encountered in clinical practice than PONTs. Most intraocular metastatic tumors occur in the uveal tract, and isolated metastasis to the ON is rarely found. Majority of tumors in ON are secondary malignancies.

Four main routes of invasion that are noted include:
1. Direct extension from eye
2. Meninges
3. Adjacent structures
4. Blood-borne metastatic invasion via the ophthalmic artery

The most common points of origin of primary tumor in SONTs[43] are as follows:
- Intraocular tumors (39%)
- Blood-borne (33%)
- Meningeal tumors (20%)
- Adjacent structures (8%)

Most of the metastatic neoplasms that involve the optic disk are carcinomas. Metastasis to the ON can settle in the retrobulbar portion of the nerve when the route of metastasis is hematogenous, where it can simulate retrobulbar neuritis. It can also present anteriorly in the optic disk, where it manifests as an elevated ON head lesion.[43-48] In a decreasing order of frequency, the most common tumors that have been reported to metastasize to the orbit and associated structures are as follows: Breast, lung, genitourinary, and gastrointestinal cancers.[49,50]

## Presentation

If there is no history of cancer and no detectable systemic cancer, then the ophthalmoscopic features must be taken into consideration, and the optic disk swelling must be differentiated from papilledema and other causes of swollen optic disk. Optic disk metastasis is usually unilateral and is characterized by central edema of the disk. In some cases, intensely white, chalky infiltrates are seen that appear on ophthalmoscopy and fluorescein angiography to be relatively avascular. The margins are usually sharply circumscribed with nodules or scallops. Flame-shaped hemorrhages, often multilayered, are observed in the swollen tissue in 42% of the eyes.[50] Clinically, patients present with symptoms of unilateral loss of visual acuity. Pain and exophthalmos are the other possible ocular manifestations. Optic disk metastases are generally the result of direct spread from juxtapapillary choroidal metastasis or hematogenous spread via the posterior ciliary arteries supplying the ON head.[51,52] Blood-borne metastases from leukemias and lymphomas may also occur in the ON. Disk swelling, pallor, and splinter hemorrhages in multiple layers of retina have been seen in patients with secondary metastasis **(Figs. 14A and B)**. Increased intracranial pressure on evaluation has been noted in few patients. Perivascular and discrete tumor invasion could be seen in such cases on histopathological examination **(Figs. 15A to D)**.[53,54]

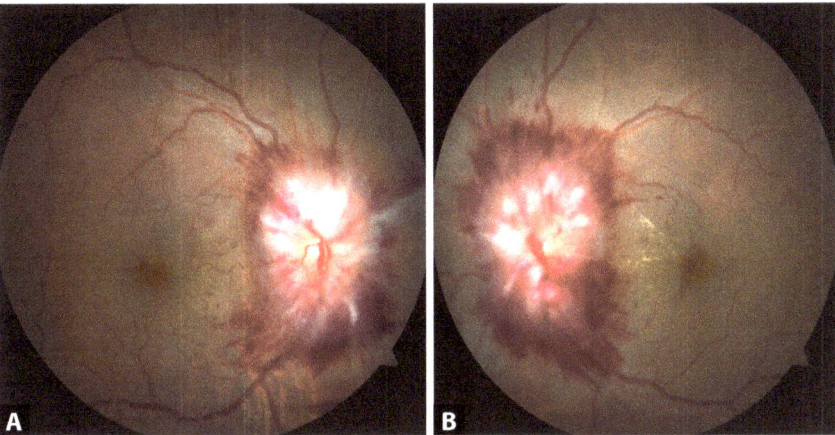

**Figs. 14A and B:** Fundus photograph showing bilateral disk swelling, pallor, and splinter hemorrhages in multiple layers of the retina in secondary metastasis of the optic nerve.

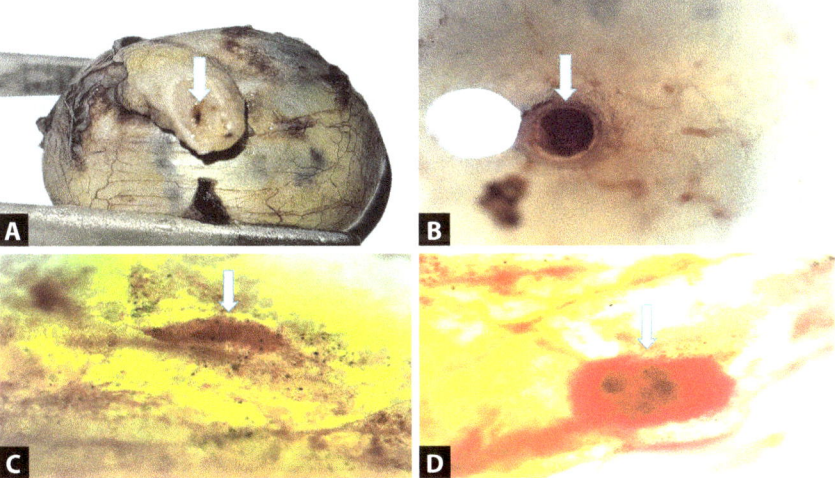

**Figs. 15A to D:** (A) Gross section of the enucleated specimen and histopathological examination (B to D) showing perivascular and discrete tumor invasion in a leukemic eye (white arrows).

In cases of intraocular tumors such as retinoblastoma (RB), the authors have demonstrated pathologic evidence of RB seeds, supported by field emission scanning electron microscopy and Raman spectroscopy in enucleated eyes of 35 out of 59 cases. The metastatic spread of RB seeds to ON was noted in 15 such cases.[55] Metastasis to ON can also be seen in cases of choroidal melanoma on gross examination of the enucleated eye **(Fig. 16)**, and on histopathologic examination, HMB45-positive melanoma cells may be seen **(Fig. 17)**. Rare tumors such as ciliary body medulloepithelioma can also involve optic disk.[56] ON metastasis may occur with primary carcinoma in brain, bone, and anorectum. Such cases have been reported in literature[57]

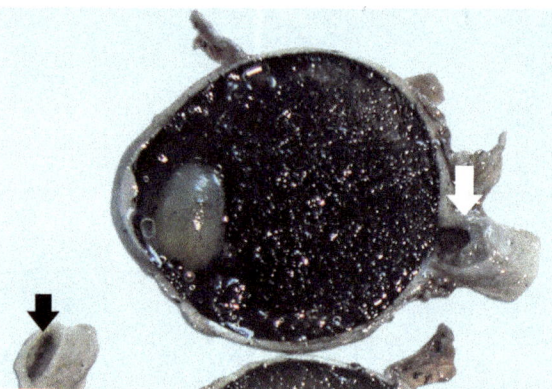

**Fig. 16:** Cut section of enucleated eye showing metastasis to optic nerve in a case of choroidal melanoma (white arrow). Black arrow highlights metastasis in a separately processed optic nerve section.

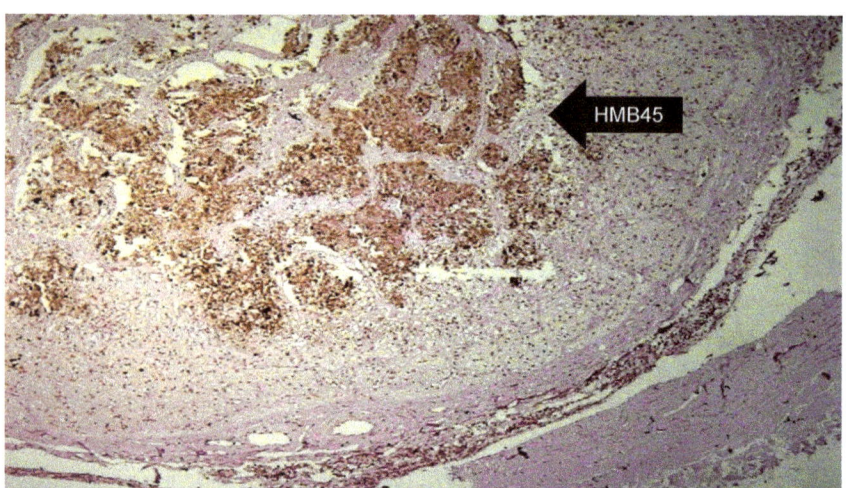

**Fig. 17:** Cut section of optic nerve showing HMB45-positive melanoma cells in immunohistochemistry (black arrow).

with patients reporting diminution of vision and headache and having a clinical picture of infiltrating disk edema **(Figs. 18A and B)**. On further imaging, the underlying primary source of carcinoma can be diagnosed, and appropriate treatment modalities may be given. Bilateral optic disk edema in a patient with primary tumor elsewhere should be evaluated thoroughly to rule out metastasis.

## Differential Diagnosis

Retinitis, exudative retinopathies, occlusive retinal vasculopathies, uveal metastasis, primary retinal tumors, and disciform macular degeneration can all mimic ONTs.[45]

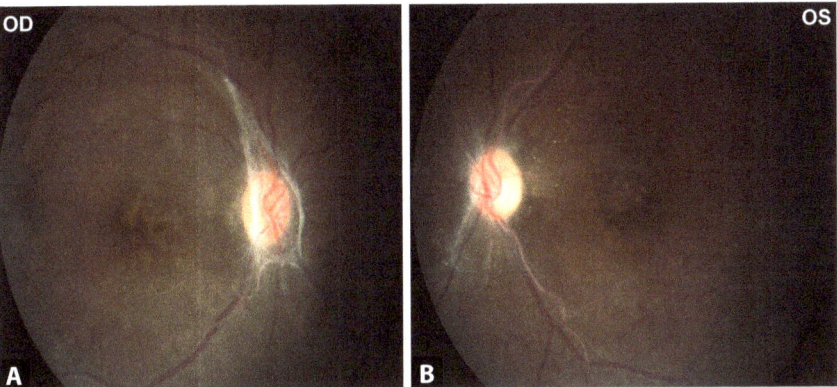

**Figs. 18A and B:** Fundus photographs showing bilateral infiltrating disk edema in a case of secondary metastasis of optic nerve.

## Diagnosis

The combination of severe progressive visual loss and a normal disk appearance in patients with cancer should raise the possibility of ON metastasis.[58] A careful and detailed history of any prior cancer along with meticulous slit-lamp biomicroscopy and ophthalmoscopy is essential for diagnosing a case of intraocular metastasis. Ancillary studies such as USG and fundus fluorescein angiography can be of assistance in diagnosis. Fine needle aspiration with cytologic evaluation of aspirate can be used in difficult-to-diagnose cases to establish the diagnosis. Imaging modalities such as CT scan, MRI, and positron emission tomography (PET) CT scan are beneficial in diagnosing the primary source and grading of metastasis of carcinoma.

## Management

Treatment of the primary source of cancer with appropriate chemotherapy should be initiated, and these patients should undergo external ocular irradiation to the posterior segment and anterior orbit of the affected eye. About 35–40 Gy radiation dose is generally recommended. It should be usually given shortly after the diagnosis of optic disk metastasis. Follow-up in the case of secondary tumors of optic disk is of utmost importance, and these patients should be investigated in detail for other systemic metastases. Combined intrathecal chemotherapy and localized radiotherapy can improve vision in some cases of blood-borne metastasis.[53,54] Although the systemic prognosis for patients with optic disk metastasis is poor, metastasis to the optic disk can lead to severe visual loss if not treated early.[59]

## ■ PARANEOPLASTIC OPTIC NEUROPATHY

Paraneoplastic optic neuropathy (PON) leads to bilateral, progressive loss of vision.[60] ON appearance may be normal or edematous.[59] There may be other clinical signs of paraneoplastic systemic involvement.[60] Small cell carcinoma of lung is most commonly associated with such conditions.[60] Antigen found in PON is collapsin response-mediating protein 5 (CRMP5), expressed in CNS and peripheral nervous system.[60] The other molecule with less specificity that is thought to be associated with PON is CV2 expressed in oligodendroglia.[60]

## ■ MISCELLANEOUS TUMORS

Other miscellaneous intraocular tumors that may involve the ON include:
- Glial tumor of retina: Astrocytic hamartoma
- *Vascular tumors of retina:* Capillary hemangioma, cavernous hemangioma, ON hemangioblastoma, racemose hemangioma
- Combined hamartoma of retina and RPE

An ON cyst may mimic the clinical findings of SONT. Fundus findings in such patients can show fully developed disk edema, gross elevation of ON head with engorged veins, and peripapillary hemorrhages. USG is helpful in clinching the diagnosis of the cystic lesion. Further imaging, such as CT scan of the orbits, also aids in further differentiation. Management in cases of cystic lesions is aspiration of cyst with a 22G lumbar puncture needle.[61]

## ■ CONCLUSION

Optic nerve tumors are a rare diagnosis in Ophthalmology, the secondary variety being more common than the primary variety. A high index of clinical suspicion should be kept in mind while considering a diagnosis of optic nerve tumor. Recent advances in diagnosis and treatment have improved the management outcomes.

## ■ ACKNOWLEDGMENTS

We are thankful to Sri Kanchi Sankara Health and Educational Foundation and Mr Apurba Deka, MSc, for their contributions.

## ■ REFERENCES

1. Christmas NJ, Mead MD, Richardson EP, Albert DM. Secondary optic nerve tumors. Surv Ophthalmol. 1991;36:196-206.
2. Huang M, Patel J, Patel BC. Optic Nerve Glioma. StatPearls. Treasure Island, FL: StatPearls Publishing; 2022.
3. Dutton JJ. Gliomas of the anterior visual pathway. Surv Ophthalmol. 1994;38:427-52.
4. Alkatan H, Alshowaeir D, Alzahem T. Optic nerve: developmental anomalies and common tumors. In: Ferreri FM (Ed). Optic Nerve. London: IntechOpen; 2018.
5. Louis DN, Perry A, Reifenberger G, von Deimling A, Figarella-Branger D, Cavenee WK, et al. The 2016 World Health Organization classification of tumors of the central nervous system: a summary. Acta Neuropathol. 2016;131:803-20.

6. Chen YH, Gutmann DH. The molecular and cell biology of pediatric low-grade gliomas. Oncogene. 2014;33:2019-26.
7. Burnstine MA, Levin LA, Louis DN, Hedley-Whyte ET, Kupsky WJ, Doepner D, et al. Nucleolar organizer regions in optic gliomas. Brain. 1993;116:1465-76.
8. Zahavi A, Toledano H, Cohen R, Sella S, Luckman J, Michowiz S, et al. Use of optical coherence tomography to detect retinal nerve fiber loss in children with optic pathway glioma. Front Neurol. 2018;9:1102.
9. Listernick R, Louis DN, Packer RJ, Gutmann DH. Optic pathway gliomas in children with neurofibromatosis 1: consensus statement from the NF1 Optic Pathway Glioma Task Force. Ann Neurol. 1997;41:143-9.
10. Sylvester CL, Drohan LA, Sergott RC. Optic-nerve gliomas, chiasmal gliomas and neurofibromatosis type 1. Curr Opin Ophthalmol. 2006;17:7-11.
11. Hwang EI, Jakacki RI, Fisher MJ, Kilburn LB, Horn M, Vezina G, et al. Long-term efficacy and toxicity of bevacizumab-based therapy in children with recurrent low-grade gliomas. Pediatr Blood Cancer. 2013;60:776-82.
12. Farazdaghi MK, Katowitz WR, Avery RA. Current treatment of optic nerve gliomas. Curr Opin Ophthalmol. 2019;30:356-63.
13. Dutton JJ. Optic nerve sheath meningiomas. Surv Ophthalmol. 1992;37:167-83.
14. Bosch MM, Wichmann WW, Boltshauser E, Landau K. Optic nerve sheath meningiomas in patients with neurofibromatosis type 2. Arch Ophthalmol. 2006;124:379-85.
15. Frisèn L, Royt WF, Tengroth BM. Optociliary veins, disc pallor and visual loss. A triad of signs indicating spheno-orbital meningioma. Acta Ophthalmol (Copenh). 1973;51:241-9.
16. Wright JE, McNab AA, McDonald WI. Primary optic nerve sheath meningioma. Br J Ophthalmol. 1989;73:960-6.
17. Jayanetti V, Klistorner AI, Graham SL, Dexter M, Flaherty MP, Jones K, et al. Monitoring of optic nerve function in neurofibromatosis 2 children with optic nerve sheath meningiomas using multifocal visual evoked potentials. J Clin Neurosci. 2018;50:262-7.
18. Cahoon GD, Davison TE. Prediction of compliance with MRI procedures among children of ages 3 years to 12 years. Pediatr Radiol. 2014;44:1302-9.
19. Ghassemi AM, Neira V, Ufholz L-A, Barrowman N, Mulla J, Bradbury CL, et al. A systematic review and meta-analysis of acute severe complications of pediatric anesthesia. Paediatr Anaesth. 2015;25:1093-102.
20. Das D, Deka P, Bhattacharjee H, Deshmukh S, Gupta P, Deka A, et al. Fluorescein dye as a novel cost-effective approach for staining raw specimens in ophthalmic pathology. Indian J Ophthalmol. 2020;68:2175-8.
21. Brown GC, Shields JA, Sanborn G, Augsburger JJ, Savino PJ, Schatz NJ. Radiation retinopathy. Ophthalmology. 1982;89:1494-501.
22. Zimmerman LE. Melanocytes, melanocytic nevi, and melanocytomas. Invest Ophthalmol. 1965;4:11-41.
23. Shields JA, Demirci H, Mashayekhi A, Eagle Jr RC, Shields CL. Melanocytoma of the optic disk: a review. Surv Ophthalmol. 2006;51:93-104.
24. Shields JA, Demirci H, Mashayekhi A, Shields CL. Melanocytoma of optic disc in 115 cases: the 2004 Samuel Johnson Memorial Lecture, part 1. Ophthalmology. 2004;111(9):1739-46.

25. Demirci H, Mashayekhi A, Shields CL, Eagle Jr RC, Shields JA. Iris melanocytoma: clinical features and natural course in 47 cases. Am J Ophthalmol. 2005;139(3):468-75.
26. Shields JA, Shields CL, Eagle Jr RC, Lieb WE, Stern S. Malignant melanoma associated with melanocytoma of the optic disc. Ophthalmology. 1990;97(2):225-30.
27. Besada E, Shechtman D, Barr RD. Melanocytoma inducing compressive optic neuropathy: the ocular morbidity potential of an otherwise invariably benign lesion. Optometry. 2002;73:33-8.
28. Lee CS, Bae JH, Jeon IH, Byeon SH, Koh HJ, Lee SC. Melanocytoma of the optic disk in the Korean population. Retina. 2010;30:1714-20.
29. De Potter P, Shields CL, Eagle Jr RC, Shields JA, Lipkowitz JL. Malignant melanoma of the optic nerve. Arch Ophthalmol. 1996;114:608-12.
30. Deveer JA. Juxtapapillary malignant melanoma of the choroid and so-called malignant melanoma of the optic disc; a pathologic study. AMA Arch Ophthalmol. 1954;51:147-60.
31. Erzurum SA, Jampol LM, Territo C, O'Grady R. Primary malignant melanoma of the optic nerve simulating a melanocytoma. Arch Ophthalmol. 1992;110:684-6.
32. Thomas CI, Purnell EW. Ocular melanocytoma. Am J Ophthalmol. 1969;67:79-86.
33. Walsh TJ, Packer S. Bilateral melanocytoma of the optic nerve associated with intracranial meningioma. Ann Ophthalmol. 1971;3:885-8.
34. Shinoda K, Hayasaka S, Nagaki Y, Kadoi C, Kurimoto M, Okada E. Melanocytoma of the left optic nerve head and right retrobulbar optic neuropathy compressed by a tuberculum sellae meningioma. Ophthalmologica. 2000;214:161-3.
35. García-Arumí J, Salvador F, Corcostegui B, Mateo C. Neuroretinitis associated with melanocytoma of the optic disk. Retina. 1994;14:173-6.
36. Archdale TW, Magnus DE. Melanocytoma of the optic disc. J Am Optom Assoc. 1993;64:98-103.
37. Apple DJ, Craythorn JM, Reidy JJ, Steinmetz RL, Brady SE, Bohart WA. Malignant transformation of an optic nerve melanocytoma. Can J Ophthalmol J. 1984;19:320-5.
38. Schachat AP, Shields JA, Fine SL, Sanborn GE, Weingeist TA, Valenzuela RE, et al. Combined hamartomas of the retina and retinal pigment epithelium. Ophthalmology. 1984;91:1609-15.
39. Aghdam KA, Zand A, Sanjari MS. Isolated unilateral infiltrative optic neuropathy in a patient with breast cancer. Turk J Ophthalmol. 2019;49:171-4.
40. Shields CL, Demirci H, Karatza E, Shields JA. Clinical survey of 1643 melanocytic and nonmelanocytic conjunctival tumors. Ophthalmology. 2004;111:1747-54.
41. Loeffler KU, Tecklenborg H. Melanocytoma-like growth of a juxtapapillary malignant melanoma. Retina. 1992;12:29-34.
42. De Potter P, Shields CL, Shields JA, Cater JR, Brady LW. Plaque radiotherapy for juxtapapillary choroidal melanoma. Visual acuity and survival outcome. Arch Ophthalmol. 1996;114:1357-65.
43. Brown GC, Shields JA. Tumors of the optic nerve head. Surv Ophthalmol. 1985;29:239-64.
44. Shields CL, Shields JA, Gross NE, Schwartz GP, Lally SE. Survey of 520 eyes with uveal metastases. Ophthalmology. 1997;104:1265-76.
45. Mack HG, Jakobiec FA. Isolated metastases to the retina or optic nerve. Int Ophthalmol Clin. 1997;37:251-60.

46. Davis WT. Metastatic carcinoma of the optic disk: with report of a case. Arch Ophthalmol. 1932;8:226-37.
47. Norton Jr HJ. Adenocarcinoma metastatic to the distal nerve and optic disc; a stereographic clinicopathologic analysis. Am J Ophthalmol. 1959;47:195-9.
48. Cherington FJ. Metastatic adenocarcinoma of the optic nerve-head and adjacent retina. Br J Ophthalmol. 1961;45:227-30.
49. Parsons JT, Fitzgerald CR, Hood CI, Ellingwood KE, Bova FJ, Million RR. The effects of irradiation on the eye and optic nerve. Int J Radiat Oncol Biol Phys. 1983;9:609-22.
50. Font RL, Ferry AP. Carcinoma metastatic to the eye and orbit III. A clinicopathologic study of 28 cases metastatic to the orbit. Cancer. 1976;38:1326-35.
51. Verma R, Chen KC, Ramkumar HL, Goldbaum MH, Shields CL. Optic nerve head problem. Surv Ophthalmol. 2019;64:579-83.
52. Fox B, Pacheco P, DeMonte F. Carcinoma of the breast metastatic to the optic nerve mimicking an optic nerve sheath meningioma: case report and review of the literature. Skull Base. 2005;15:281-7; discussion 287-9.
53. Allen RA, Straatsma BR. Ocular involvement in leukemia and allied disorders. Arch Ophthalmol. 1961;66:490-508.
54. Kincaid MC, Green WR. Ocular and orbital involvement in leukemia. Surv Ophthalmol. 1983;27:211-32.
55. Das D, Bhattacharjee K, Barman MJ, Bhattacharjee H, Maity S, Bandyopadhyay D, et al. Pathologic evidence of retinoblastoma seeds supported by field emission scanning electron microscopy and Raman spectroscopy. Indian J Ophthalmol. 2021;69:3612-7.
56. Agarwalla I, Das D, Bhattacharjee K, Deka P, Borthakur S, Agarwal B, et al. Blessing in disguise: medulloepithelioma unmasked by incidental trauma. Adv Ophthalmol Vis Syst. 2018;8:234-6.
57. Agarwalla I, Das D, Bhattacharjee H, Kuri G, Mehta B, Garg M, et al. Bilateral metastasis to optic nerve head—interesting case report series. TNOA J Ophthalmic Sci Res. 2021;59:202-4.
58. Cho HK, Park SH, Shin SY. Isolated optic nerve metastasis of breast cancer initially mimicking retrobulbar optic neuritis. Eur J Ophthalmol. 2011;21:513-5.
59. Shields JA, Shields CL, Singh AD. Metastatic neoplasms in the optic disc: the 1999 Bjerrum Lecture: part 2. Arch Ophthalmol. 2000;118:217-24.
60. Cross SA, Solomao DR, Parisi JE, Kryzr TJ, Bradley EA, Mines JA, et al. Paraneoplastic autoimmune optic neuritis with retinitis defined by CRMP-5-IgG. Ann Neurol. 2003;54:38-50.
61. Das D, Deka P, Deka AC, Bhattacharjee K, Bhattacharjee H, Das JK, et al. An unusual case of retrobulbar arachnoid cyst and its management. Orbit. 2009;28:169-71.

# CHAPTER 15

# Choroidal Metastasis

*Kalpita Das, Raghulnadhan Ramanadhane*

## ABSTRACT

Choroidal metastases are one of the most common intraocular malignancies in adults. The most common primary cancers leading to choroidal metastases are breast cancer (47%) and lung cancer (21%). Choroidal metastasis is seen in 2-7% of cancer patients and suggests disseminated disease and poor prognosis. Highly vascular structure of the choroid causes hematogenous dissemination of the tumor emboli and makes it the primary ocular site for metastasis. The treatment of choroidal metastasis mainly depends on the systemic status of the patient and number, location, and laterality of the choroidal tumors. Treatment options include observation in patients with poor systemic status or asymptomatic disease; systemic chemotherapy, immunotherapy, hormone therapy, or whole eye radiotherapy in active disease with other system involvement or when the tumor is multifocal and bilateral; plaque radiotherapy, transpupillary radiotherapy, or photodynamic therapy for active, solitary metastasis; and enucleation for those with blind painful eye.

***Keywords:*** Choroidal metastases; metastasis; ocular oncology; intraocular malignancy; breast cancer; lung cancer; exudative retinal detachment; transpupillary thermotherapy.

## ■ INTRODUCTION

Choroid is considered the most typical site for metastasis among the various ocular structures due to its rich vascular supply. Despite previously being thought of as a rare illness, choroidal metastases are now believed to be the most common intraocular malignancies in the adult population. Approximately 10% of cancer patients on autopsy are found to have ocular metastasis, most commonly to the choroid. Choroidal metastases are very often associated with metastatic diseases in other parts of the body and indicate an advanced and disseminated disease and dismal prognosis.

Perls reported the first instance of choroidal metastasis in 1872.[1] The high-flow choroidal vasculature gives a conduit to metastatic cells to have hematogenous dissemination from distant sites.[2] The choroid provides tumor emboli with a circulatory channel to sequester them and fosters a growth-friendly environment.[3]

Breast cancer (40-47%) and lung cancer (21-29%) are the tumors that most frequently result in choroidal metastases. Bilateral, multiple choroidal metastases are most typically associated with breast cancer, while unilateral, unifocal metastases are commonly found in lung cancer. Other primary cancers that can spread to the choroids include gastrointestinal tract carcinoma (4%), prostate cancer (2%), kidney cancer (2-4%), and skin cancer (2%).[4,5] Tumors from the submandibular gland, thyroid, contralateral choroid, testes, ovaries, urothelial tract, neuroendocrine tumor, and sarcoma are examples of uncommon primary carcinomas that metastasize to the choroid.

The majority of individuals with choroidal metastasis already have systemic cancer when their eye condition is diagnosed. However in 34% of cases, the choroidal metastasis is found before the systemic cancer is identified. Lung cancer (7%), breast cancer (35%), and an unidentified initial tumor location account for 50% of patients with no prior history of cancer.[5]

## ■ CLINICAL FEATURES

Patients with choroidal metastasis usually present with blurred vision in 70-80% of the cases, while the less common presentation being flashes, floaters, field defects, photophobia, and pain (5-10%). However, 9-11% of patients can be asymptomatic, and lesions may be located in the posterior pole and might be unilateral or bilateral, solitary or multifocal. Shields et al., in a series of 479 eyes with choroidal metastasis, reported that choroidal metastases most commonly present as a creamy-yellow subretinal mass (94%) accompanied with subretinal fluid (73%).[4] These lesions are relatively flat with a large basal diameter, and associated serous retinal detachment is usually out of proportion to the size of the tumor **(Figs. 1A and B)**. Rarely, the mass may be orange in color, associated with metastatic renal cell carcinoma, carcinoid tumor, or thyroid cancer (3%), or brown-gray in appearance, commonly associated with metastatic melanoma (3%).[5]

## ■ DIAGNOSIS

History of a primary systemic malignancy, along with typical ophthalmoscopic features of a yellow-white subretinal mass lesion and exudative retinal detachment, usually points toward a diagnosis of choroidal metastasis. However, it can be challenging to diagnose instances without a history of a primary malignancy or unilateral lesions.[5] Differential diagnoses include choroidal melanoma, choroidal hemangioma, choroidal osteoma, choroidal granuloma, choroidal neovascularization with disciform scar, nodular

## Choroidal Metastasis

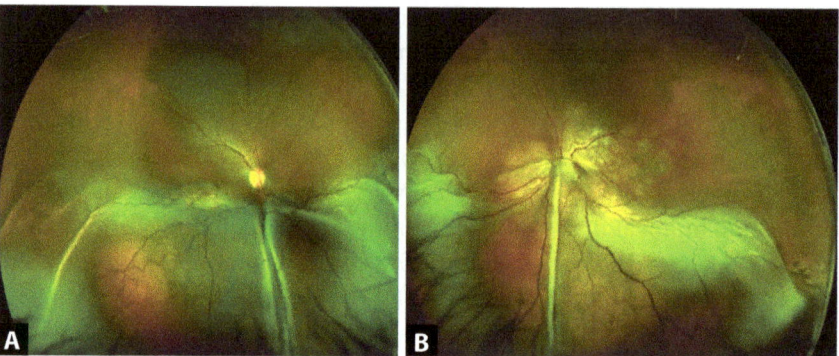

**Figs. 1A and B:** Fundus photographs of right and left eyes, respectively, showing a diffuse ill-defined creamy-yellow subretinal mass lesion with overlying exudative retinal detachment. Note that the detachment is out of proportion to the size of lesions in both eyes.

---

**BOX 1:** Differential diagnosis of choroidal metastasis.

- Choroidal melanoma
- Choroidal nevus
- Circumscribed choroidal hemangioma
- Choroidal osteoma
- Choroidal granuloma
- Subretinal abscess
- Nodular posterior scleritis
- Choroidal neovascularization with disciform scar
- Congenital hypertrophy of RPE
- Organized subretinal hemorrhage
- Vogt–Koyanagi–Harada disease
- Central serous chorioretinopathy
- Posterior uveal effusion syndrome
- Solitary idiopathic choroiditis
- Choroidal detachment

(RPE: retinal pigment epithelium)

---

posterior scleritis, and other rare lesions **(Box 1)**. Choroidal metastases are distinguished from other choroidal lesions by distinctive characteristics on ophthalmoscopy and using different imaging modalities.

The assessment starts with a proper systemic history since the majority of patients present with an established primary cancer diagnosis. Ophthalmic evaluation, particularly dilated fundus examination, is essential. A patient with an obvious lesion in one eye should be carefully looked for any lesion in the other eye as the disease is bilateral in 20–40% of patients. These lesions should be documented with fundus photographs to compare

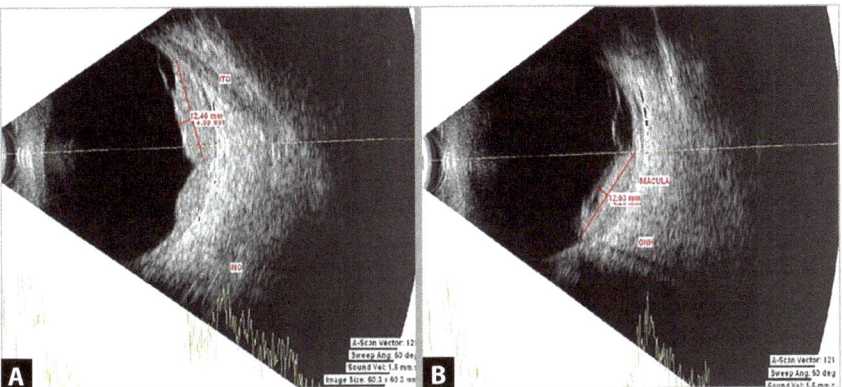

**Figs. 2A and B:** Ultrasonography of right and left eyes showing irregular mass lesions with moderate internal reflectivity with a lower height-to-base ratio. Overlying retinal detachment can be seen. (INO: internuclear ophthalmoplegia; ONH: optic nerve hypoplasia).

with subsequent examinations to assess growth and treatment response. Following investigations are commonly performed that help establish the diagnosis of choroidal metastases.

## Ultrasonography

Ultrasonography remains one of the most important ancillary investigations for diagnosis and differentiation of choroidal metastases from other choroidal lesions, particularly melanoma. Tumor size and echogenicity are assessed using ultrasound technology. A broad, ill-defined echogenic choroidal mass with a characteristically lower height-to-base ratio is characteristic on a B-scan ultrasonography **(Figs. 2A and B)**. Acoustic hollowing as in choroidal melanoma is typically absent in metastatic lesions. Moderate-to-high internal reflectivity, solid consistency, and little to no internal vascularity are all visible on an A-scan ultrasonography. In rare circumstances, choroidal detachment may be seen in addition to the more typical overlying retinal detachment. Ultrasonography can be used to measure the height of a metastatic tumor so that the lesion's reduction can be observed after treatment.

## Fundus Autofluorescence

Fundus autofluorescence, a noninvasive diagnostic technique, can identify the intrinsic autofluorescence of ocular tissue. Lipofuscin, which is composed of digested photoreceptor outer segments and found in the retinal pigment epithelium (RPE), is the molecule responsible for autofluorescence. Choroidal metastases with underlying subretinal fluid and lipofuscin appear hyperautofluorescent **(Figs. 3A and B)**, which aids in distinguishing them

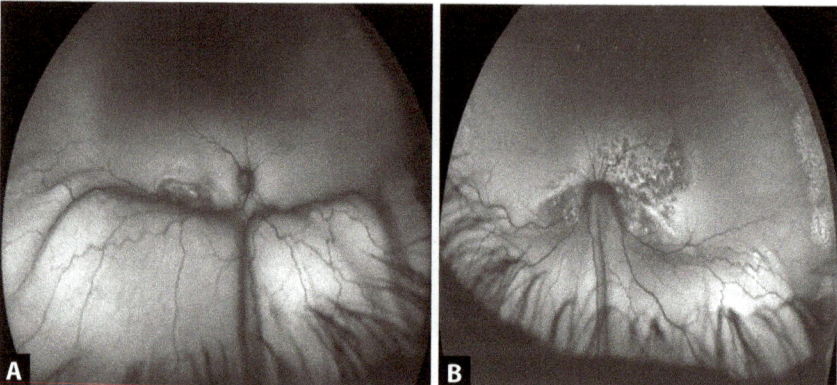

**Figs. 3A and B:** Fundus autofluorescence of both eyes of the same patient as in **Figures 1A and B**.

from other lesions.[6] These observations can be used to determine tumor surface characteristics as well as progressing tumor margins.[6-9]

## Fluorescein Angiography and Indocyanine Green Angiography

Fundus fluorescein angiography can help to differentiate choroidal metastases and choroidal melanoma or hemangiomas. Fluorescein angiography typically shows a hypofluorescent pattern in early arterial phases, with hyperfluorescence in the late venous phases **(Figs. 4A and B)**.[3,5,6] Choroidal metastases also can have dilated retinal capillaries with a pinpoint leakage at the tumor border in 73% of cases compared to 16% in melanoma.[10,11] Indocyanine green angiography (ICGA) is a more sensitive tool that shows a blockage of the background staining and a patchy staining of the tumor surface **(Figs. 4C and D)**. No intratumoral vessels could be detected using ICGA.[11]

## Optical Coherence Tomography

Optical coherence tomography (OCT) with enhanced depth imaging of these lesions usually reveals a characteristic "lumpy bumpy" choroidal surface with compression of the choriocapillaris and irregularities of the outer retinal layers **(Fig. 5)**. Micrometastases can also be detected using OCT, which is typically not possible with fundoscopy.[12]

## Magnetic Resonance Imaging

Magnetic resonance imaging often shows a well-demarcated choroidal mass which appears isointense on T1-weighted images and hypointense on T2-weighted images. It can also detect metastatic lesions in the brain.

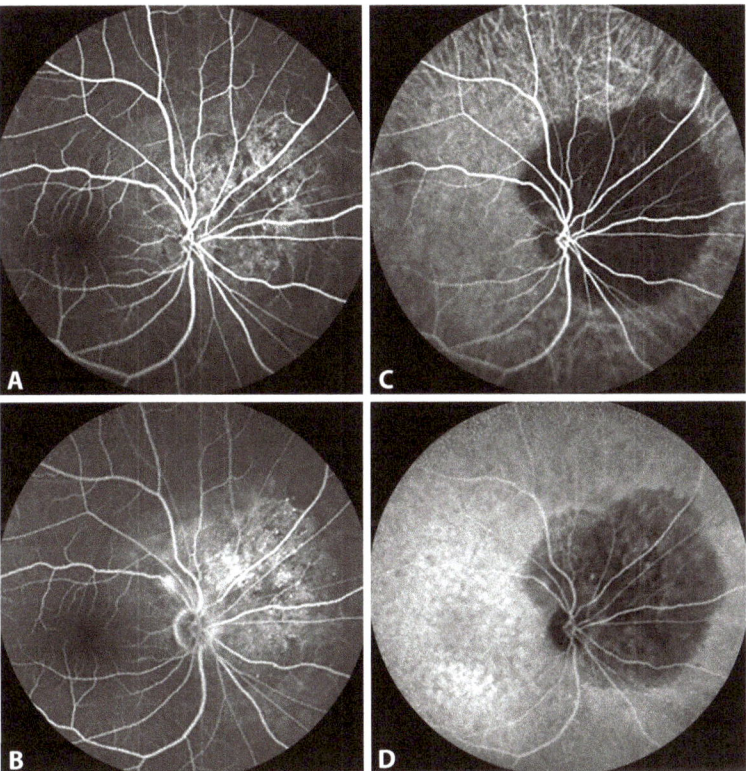

**Figs. 4A to D:** (A and B) Fundus fluorescein angiography of patient with choroidal metastasis demonstrating a typical hypofluorescent pattern in the early arterial phase with hyperfluorescence in the venous phase; (C and D) Indocyanine green angiography of the same patient showing blockage of background staining and a patchy staining of the tumor surface.

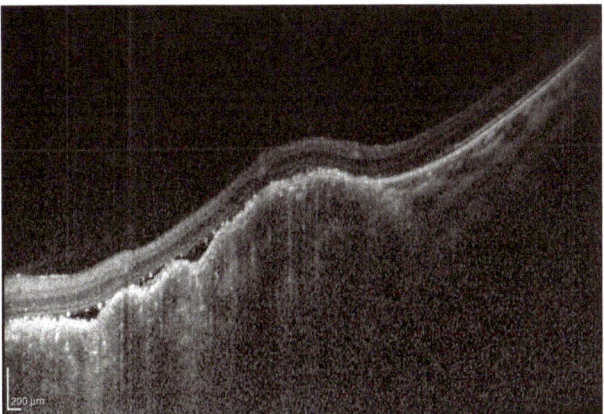

**Fig. 5:** Optical coherence tomography passing through a choroidal metastatic lesion showing a classic lumpy-bumpy appearance of the choroid with subretinal fluid.

### Whole-body Positron Emission Tomography-Computed Tomography

Whole-body F18-fluorodeoxyglucose, positron emission tomography-computed tomography (FDG, PET-CT) is a sensitive method to localize choroidal lesions, especially in known cases of systemic carcinoma with multiorgan involvement.

### Fine-needle Aspiration Biopsy

When the primary source is unknown and diagnostic findings indeterminate, fine-needle aspiration biopsy can be helpful to have a cytological evidence of metastasis or primary occurrence.[3] For posterior segment lesions with no retinal detachment, biopsy is obtained through pars plana and transvitreal approach, whereas cases of overlying retinal detachment require a trans-scleral equatorial approach.[13]

## ■ TREATMENT

The treatment of choroidal metastasis depends on the patient's general health and systemic status, number of choroidal tumors, location, and laterality. For patients with multifocal or bilateral metastases, systemic chemotherapy, immunotherapy, hormone therapy, or whole eye radiotherapy may be tried; for solitary metastases, plaque radiotherapy, transpupillary radiotherapy, or photodynamic therapy (PDT) are the treatment options; and for painful, blind eyes, enucleation may be necessary. Observation is recommended for patients with poor systemic status.

External beam radiotherapy (EBRT), at a dose of 40–60 Gy, can help tumor regression in 85–93% of patients while improving or stabilizing vision in 56% of eyes.[14] Cataract (7%), radiation retinopathy (3%), exposure keratopathy (3%), optic neuropathy (2%), and neovascularization of the iris (2%) are EBRT-related side effects.[15]

Gamma knife radiosurgery (GKR) has also been used to treat both choroidal metastases and uveal melanomas.[3] This method uses several gamma rays to target the lesion and requires an average dose of 30 Gy over 10 days.

Proton beam radiotherapy (PBT) enables more focused irradiation since protons are supplied through a beam and penetrate tissues at varying depths depending on their energy, with less scatter to the neighboring tissues.[16] The average dosage is 28 Gy divided over two treatments.[16] Complications reported are madarosis (28%), lid burns (17%), iris neovascularization and neovascular glaucoma (8%), cataract (11%), radiation maculopathy (19%), and radiation papillopathy (22%).[15,16]

In comparison to EBRT, plaque radiation offers more focused, targeted radiotherapy, which leads to improved tumor control and fewer complications. Shields et al. used plaque irradiation to treat 36 patients with choroidal metastases and saw prompt remission in 100% of cases and long-lasting remission in 94% over an average follow-up of 11 months.[17] In three patients (8%), radiation retinopathy and/or papillopathy developed. Optic nerve atrophy (40%) and radiation retinopathy (20%) were late radiation side effects.

Transpupillary thermotherapy (TTT) uses diode laser and works by heating the choroid and RPE, causing tumor necrosis.[18] In a trial of 59 eyes with choroidal metastasis treated with TTT as the main mode of therapy, 71% of the eyes displayed regression or growth inhibition, whereas 7% manifested progression over a 15-month follow-up period.[18]

Photodynamic treatment results in tumor necrosis through the formation of reactive singlet oxygen as well as verteporfin-induced intravascular thrombosis and subsequent tumor infarction. PDT has been used to treat a number of ocular disorders, including age-related macular degeneration, melanomas, choroidal hemangiomas, and retinal astrocytic hamartomas. PDT has been utilized successfully for the management of choroidal metastases as a main or secondary treatment option.[19]

Intravitreal antivascular growth factor (anti-VEGF) has also been used in the management for ocular tumors, including metastases. The use of intravitreal bevacizumab and ranibizumab to block angiogenesis is a useful therapy option since metastases depend on neovascularization for growth.[20] Primary or adjunct eye therapy with anti-VEGF injections has been shown to be effective in managing metastases from breast, lung, and colorectal carcinomas. Injections are repeated every 1–3 months, depending on the tumor response. Regression is observed after a follow-up period of 4–22 months.[20]

## ■ CONCLUSION

Choroidal metastases are the most common intraocular malignancy in adults. More number of population with cancer can present with metastases as more effective treatment options become accessible and cancer patients live longer. It is crucial to effectively control these lesions. In certain circumstances, systemic chemotherapy is able to manage the tumor; however, targeted therapy is indicated when the tumor is causing vision loss or when the patient is not responding to systemic therapy.

## ■ ACKNOWLEDGMENT

We would like to thank Dr Pukhraj Rishi for his help and contributions.

## ■ REFERENCES

1. Cohen VML. Ocular metastases. Eye (Lond). 2013;27(2):137-41.
2. Ferry AP, Font RL. Carcinoma metastatic to the eye and orbit. I. A clinicopathologic study of 227 cases. Arch Ophthalmol. 1974;92:276-86.

3. Avram AM, Gielczyk R, Su L, Vine AK, Sisson JC. Choroidal and skin metastases from papillary thyroid cancer: case and a review of the literature. J Clin Endocrinol Metab. 2004;89:5303-7.
4. Shields CL, Shields JA, Gross NE, Schwartz GP, Lally SE. Survey of 520 eyes with uveal metastases. Ophthalmology. 1997;104:1265-76.
5. Harbour JW, De Potter P, Shields CL, Shields JA. Uveal metastasis from carcinoid tumor. Clinical observations in nine cases. Ophthalmology. 1994;101:1084-90.
6. Ishida T, Ohno-Matsui K, Kaneko Y, Tobita H, Hayashi K, Shimada N, et al. Autofluorescence of metastatic choroidal tumor. Int Ophthalmol. 2009;29:309-13.
7. Collet LC, Pulido JS, Gündüz K, Diago T, McCannel C, Blodi C, et al. Fundus autofluorescence in choroidal metastatic lesions: a pilot study. Retina. 2008;28:1251-6.
8. Natesh S, Chin KJ, Finger PT. Choroidal metastases fundus autofluorescence imaging: correlation to clinical, OCT, and fluorescein angiographic findings. Ophthalmic Surg Lasers Imaging. 2010;41:406-12.
9. Almeida A, Kaliki S, Shields CL. Autofluorescence of intraocular tumours. Curr Opin Ophthalmol. 2013;24:222-32.
10. Li L, Wang WJ, Chen RJ, Qian J, Luo CQ, Zhang YJ, et al. Fundus fluorescein angiography in metastatic choroidal carcinomas and differentiating metastatic choroidal carcinomas from primary choroidal melanomas. Zhonghua Yan Ke Za Zhi. 2011;47:27-34.
11. Shah SU, Mashayekhi A, Shields CL, Walia HS, Hubbard 3rd GB, Zhang J, et al. Uveal metastasis from lung cancer: clinical features, treatment, and outcome in 194 patients. Ophthalmology. 2014;121:352-7.
12. Al-Dahmash SA, Shields CL, Kaliki S, Johnson T, Shields JA. Enhanced depth imaging optical coherence tomography of choroidal metastasis in 14 eyes. Retina. 2014;34:1588-93.
13. Shields JA, Shields CL, Ehya H, Eagle Jr RC, De Potter P. Fine-needle aspiration biopsy of suspected intraocular tumors. The 1992 Urwick Lecture. Ophthalmology. 1993;100:1677-84.
14. Fernandez-Perez S, Ruiz-Moreno O, Pueyo V, de la Mata G, Pablo L. Bilateral choroidal metastases as presentation of dissemination of cutaneous malignant melanoma. Case Rep Ophthalmol Med. 2012;2012:486167.
15. Rudoler SB, Corn BW, Shields CL, De Potter P, Hyslop T, Shields JA, et al. External beam irradiation for choroid metastases: identification of factors predisposing to long-term sequelae. Int J Radiat Oncol Biol Phys. 1997;38:251-6.
16. Tsina EK, Lane AM, Zacks DN, Munzenrider JE, Collier JM, Gragoudas ES. Treatment of metastatic tumors of the choroid with proton beam irradiation. Ophthalmology. 2005;112:337-43.
17. Shields CL, Shields JA, De Potter P, Quaranta M, Freire J, Brady LW, et al. Plaque radiotherapy for the management of uveal metastasis. Arch Ophthalmol. 1997;115:203-9.
18. Romanowska-Dixon B, Kowal J, Pogrzebielski A, Markiewicz A. Transpupillary thermotherapy (TTT) for intraocular metastases in choroid. Klin Oczna. 2011;113:132-5.
19. Mauget-Faysse M, Gambrelle J, Quaranta-El Maftouhi M, Moullet I. Photodynamic therapy for choroidal metastasis from lung adenocarcinoma. Acta Ophthalmol Scand. 2006;84:552-4.
20. Tolentino M. Systemic and ocular safety of intravitreal anti-VEGF therapies for ocular neovascular disease. Surv Ophthalmol. 2011;56:95-113.

# CHAPTER 16

# Artificial Intelligence in Neuro-ophthalmology

*Hima Pendharkar, Rishabh Rathi*

## ABSTRACT

Advances in technology have aided human intelligence and quest for solving problems in several ways. The application of artificial intelligence (AI) in medicine has been of help in several fields, especially in image-based areas. Ophthalmology is one such field where images of the fundus can be obtained and reviewed by specialists either via telemedicine or these images can be used to develop AI algorithms which may be implemented at various medical establishments. Further, these AI algorithms aid in identifying emergency situations of neuro-ophthalmology correctly even in the absence of a trained specialist. This chapter briefly addresses the clinical use of AI in neuro-ophthalmology.

***Keywords:*** Artificial intelligence; machine learning; papilledema; optic neuritis; anterior ischemic optic neuropathy; optical coherence tomography; pituitary tumor.

## ◼ INTRODUCTION

Eyes are a reflection of several things from emotions to disease. Just as a photographer captures the emotions reflected in the eyes beautifully, the ophthalmologist precisely captures the features in the eyes that express the underlying pathology. And we thus know that the eye reflects a wide spectrum of abnormalities that point toward a certain diagnosis. At times the findings are specific for a given condition; at times they direct further workup. Neuro-ophthalmology is, hence, an important direction in identifying systemic diseases.

Technological advances have aided tremendously in enhancing healthcare. Artificial intelligence (AI), which may be defined as any computer method that performs tasks normally requiring human intelligence currently, is the basis for many advances in medicine.[1] The progress in AI has shown benefits in several fields of modern medicine.

Humans have always intended to replicate knowledge into machines. Computers that could handle textual data and arithmetic were the first step in this process. Computing involves feeding data and problem methodology into a computer using structured "computer languages." These programs could be run on computers and answers provided back to the user. Large problems hitherto deemed unsolvable by humans could thus be run on computers. Even these computers with high computing power did not attempt to replicate human cognition. The search for computers that could mimic human cognition, hence, developed parallel to the development of faster computers. An area of work in this regard was to develop computing techniques that mimic the human nervous system.

As a first step, the function of the neuron was implemented and simple neural networks were created. The "neurons" created were known as *perceptrons*. Of all the properties of neurons, the presence of a threshold potential and the fact that neurons communicate and transfer messages downstream were used to create rudimentary neural networks. Learning as a concept was introduced into these networks using a principle called *backpropagation*. Backpropagation involves a method using differential equations to change the neural parameters. This is done repeatedly and systematically "back from the result." There is, therefore, a training set that is used to change the neuronal parameters and achieve learning. Once learning is completed, a test object is recognized by the neural net. The major success of neural networks was in image processing. Image processing refers to the identification of parts or whole of an image. Two important paradigms are worthy of mention. One is the labeling of individual images. Thus, a network learns on a training set and accurately "labels" a new image. Another is called image segmentation, where individual objects on an image are recognized and labeled.

From very primitive multilayered neural networks, more sophisticated networks evolved. These are called convolutional neural networks (CNNs). More sophisticated methods, such as generative adversarial network (GAN) and long short-term memory (LSTM), are now common in the AI workplace. These networks are complex iterations of the smaller neural networks.

Artificial intelligence enables a technical system of human-like behavior that consists of receiving, interpreting, and learning from data before achieving a particular goal.[2] AI has two subsets to it—machine learning (ML) and deep learning (DL). The term machine learning was coined 50 years ago by Arthur Samuel, who stated that machines could have the ability to learn without being programmed.[3] ML is a subset of AI in which a model "learns" to solve a particular task by encountering multiple example inputs for that task. DL is an approach that utilizes multiple neural networks to learn the representation of data using multiple levels of abstraction.[4] It involves the process of training a multilayer network of neurons containing millions of parameters to perform a given task. Training involves "showing" the network a large set of images as pixels (training data) and programming it to produce an output. A detailed discussion of the technical aspects of ML/DL is beyond the scope of this chapter; interested readers may refer to the studies that discuss these techniques.[5-7]

Few specialties in medicine, with imaging being the foremost as dermatology and pathology, have immensely benefited from AI. Ophthalmology, too, has been utilizing the data from multiple diagnostic procedures such as automated perimetry, optical coherence tomography (OCT), and fundus photography to develop AI algorithms that would help identify various ocular pathologies.[8]

## NEED FOR ARTIFICIAL INTELLIGENCE IN OPHTHALMOLOGY

The evaluation of ocular fundus gives invaluable clues to identifying the underlying etiology which at times may be an emergency. However, when a patient comes to an acute care setup or a general hospital, pediatric hospital, and so on, a trained ophthalmologist or neuro-ophthalmologist may not always be available for fundus evaluation. Though reporting of fundus photographs through telemedicine has addressed this issue to a certain extent, it may not always be feasible, especially in developing countries. AI offers the next best solution to overcome this limitation.

However, it must be borne in mind that the limited data available in various neuro-ophthalmic conditions makes it a little difficult to apply AI on a basis as wide as in certain other specialties. With more data collection and analysis and also advances in ML/DL, this issue would definitely be addressed in coming years.

## ARTIFICIAL INTELLIGENCE IN OPHTHALMOLOGY

Major ophthalmic diseases in which DL techniques have been used include diabetic retinopathy (DR), glaucoma, age-related macular degeneration (AMD), and retinopathy of prematurity (ROP). Several other eye diseases are also being studied with progress and evolution in AI technology.

### Diabetic Retinopathy

Patients with diabetes suffer many life-limiting and life-threatening complications, including macrovascular-related stroke, ischemic heart disease, peripheral artery disease, and/or microvascular-related retinopathy, neuropathy, and nephropathy. DR is the most common microvascular complication of diabetes and currently affects almost 100 million people worldwide, and expected to become an ever-increasing health burden.[9,10]

*Clinically, DR is divided into two types:* Nonproliferative diabetic retinopathy (NPDR) and proliferative diabetic retinopathy (PDR). NPDR represents the early stage of DR, wherein increased vascular permeability and capillary occlusion are two main observations in the retinal vasculature. During this stage, retinal pathologies, including microaneurysms, hemorrhages, and hard exudates, can be detected by fundus photography although the patients may be asymptomatic. PDR, a more advanced stage of DR, is characterized by neovascularization. During this stage, the patients may experience severe visual impairment when the new abnormal vessels bleed into the vitreous (vitreous hemorrhage) or when tractional retinal detachment is present.[11] The presence and severity of peripheral DR lesions are predictive of future rates of DR worsening.[12]

Of the various techniques used to visualize the retina, retinal photographs utilize adaptive optics technology and have greatly expanded the ability to visualize it on a cellular level. OCT is a widely utilized option for imaging the diabetic neural retina that uses light interferometry to create cross-sectional images of the retina in which individual retinal layers can be distinguished.[13,14]

Having obtained the fundus photographs, interpretation still remains a challenge. On similar lines to that of teleradiology, in ophthalmology, images that are captured by fundus cameras can be sent over to ophthalmologists elsewhere across the globe for their opinion. Telemedicine, however, is limited by the inherent requirements. To cite an example, The Singapore Integrated Diabetic Retinopathy Program (SiDRP) obtains fundus images remotely and gets them evaluated by ophthalmologic professionals.[15] However, traditional telemedicine still relies on human resources to grade the fundus images of patients.

In 2018, for the first time in medicine, the Food and Drug Administration (FDA) authorized the marketing of a commercially available, autonomous artificial intelligence-based diagnostic system for the detection of DR: IDx-DR (Digital Diagnostics Inc., Coralville, USA). It uses Topcon NW400 to capture fundus images, following which the doctor uploads the images to the cloud server. The software provides results according to the images. If the image quality is high enough and either mild or severe DR is detected, the doctor will be prompted to refer the patient to an ophthalmologist; if the severity is not higher than mild DR, it will prompt the patient to retest in 12 months.[16] The FDA-approved autonomous AI system became a highly effective system for DR detection.

Once DR is detected, its grading is also necessary for further management. Compared with manual work, AI systems are more sensitive and less specific for the diagnosis of DR and can greatly reduce the workload of manual grading of DR. Instead of going to specialized hospitals with ophthalmologists, AI systems enable patients to collect fundus photographs or OCT images at a relatively close primary health care clinic, which can be used to directly perform grading and receive further suggestions for follow-up or referral. This characteristic makes it more convenient and efficient for diabetic patients to undergo fundus screening and greatly reduces the workload of ophthalmologists as well as improves the compliance of diabetic patients for screening.[17] EyeArt was the first AI system to detect DR on smartphone, thus conveying that it is feasible for the system on a mobile device to perform remote DR detection.[18]

In the past few decades, a large number of fundus photographs have been collated in the screening network for pathologies such as DR and papilledema that have helped to develop AI algorithms.[19] Though DL is used to train automatic systems to detect DR, however, challenging cases such as ischemic optic neuropathy still have some limitations with the use of these automatic detection systems.[20]

## Glaucoma

Glaucoma is a group of optic neuropathies associated with characteristic structural changes at the optic nerve head (ONH) (increased cup/disk ratio, notching) that may lead to visual field (VF) loss and, ultimately, irreversible vision loss. It affects 3.5% of individuals between the age of 40 and 80 years worldwide.[21] Given the high prevalence of undiagnosed yet treatable glaucoma patients, AI and, more specifically, DL neural network algorithms have attempted to automatically detect the disease on digital fundus images and thus aid in treatment.[22]

Glaucoma typically presents with ONH cupping. However, it is critical to appropriately identify a compressive optic neuropathy that can, at times, mimic glaucoma. Yang et al. utilized DL to differentiate glaucomatous optic neuropathy (GON), defined as enlarged cupping of the ONH with corresponding VF defect, from nonglaucomatous optic neuropathy (NGON) due to compression, hereditary diseases, chronic ischemia, inflammation, trauma, or toxin through analyzing ONH fundus photographs with the use of AI.[23] With appropriate application of AI to distinguish GON from NGON, understandably, the referral of patients who need treatment can be addressed and attended to on a priority.

Glaucoma is considered to be one of the diseases ideal for screening because it is a chronic disease that progresses slowly and, if treated early, the irreversible visual decline can be prevented. Though AI can screen for glaucoma, the priority presently should be focused on automated identification of moderate glaucoma when patients begin to experience functional changes or VF abnormalities and are more likely to experience visual disability over their lifetime.

### Age-related Macular Degeneration

The global prevalence of AMD is 8.69%, being higher among Europeans than among Asians or Africans.[24] AMD is classified as either dry or wet AMD. Dry AMD is characterized by multiple drusen deposits which rarely affect vision. Dry AMD can progress not only to geographic atrophy (GA) but also to wet AMD, which is characterized by active choroidal neovascularization (CNV) and leads to significant vision impairment.[25] Intravitreal injection of antivascular endothelial growth factor (anti-VEGF) drugs is considered to be the optimal treatment for CNV. However, any improvement is accompanied by long-term monthly intravitreal injections and uncertainty concerning the treatment duration and possible recurrence of CNV.[26] Screening and early detection of active CNV are, therefore, crucial.

In AMD, AI has been deployed to estimate the number of anti-VEGF injections needed and to predict GA progression.[27,28] Hwang et al. integrated the concepts of cloud computing and telemedicine with AI in diagnosing AMD and providing treatment recommendations. This underscores the fact that smart health practices lead to accurate diagnostic tools, more effective patient care, and devices that improve quality of life.[25]

## ■ ARTIFICIAL INTELLIGENCE IN NEURO-OPHTHALMOLOGY

Truly said, "eyes are the gateway to the brain." The eye can voice out many neurological manifestations. This has made a big shift in the management of neurological conditions by an early catch in the diagnosis, progression, and prognosis. This advent of knowledge has allowed a great scope in the development of neuro-ophthalmology. In the current scenario, the expertise of a neuro-ophthalmologist cannot be fulfilled in every tertiary care center. The need of expert opinion and their availability in the current time has become a strong catalyst for the development of AI in the field of neuro-ophthalmology. The present era of fifth generation internet and telecommunication has assisted AI to expand its platform.[29,30]

There is a whole paradigm shift in the management and monitoring of neurological diseases by AI-driven algorithms, especially using DL. Today, most of the available research done using DL and ML rely on fundus images to rule out changes in ONH abnormalities. Recent studies are using other imaging modalities, such as OCT, to evaluate and differentiate optic disk abnormalities. The combination of deep learning systems (DLSs) along with new innovative hardware solutions could bring revolution in early diagnosis and monitoring of neuro-ophthalmic conditions and healthcare.[31] AI-based DL algorithms for detecting optic disk abnormalities showed reasonable performance in differentiating neuropathies. A study has recently looked into the possibility of discriminating between normal disks, swollen disks due to various optic neuropathies, and pseudopapilledema.[32] ML techniques have been applied to OCT data in neuro-ophthalmology, allowing differentiation between controls and patients with multiple sclerosis (MS) even in the absence of optic neuritis attack.[23]

Applications of AI in common neuro-ophthalmic conditions are described below.

## Papilledema

Papilledema is defined as bilateral swelling of the ONH from raised intracranial pressure. Understandably, the diagnosis and management of the patient with papilledema depend on the fundus findings. On one hand, a false diagnosis of papilledema can lead to unnecessary, expensive, and invasive investigations and, on the other hand, failure to detect papilledema and its cause may lead to irreversible neurologic dysfunction, permanent vision loss, and even death.[33] Availability of ophthalmologist/neuro-ophthalmologist is one of the limiting factors in many healthcare setups and, hence, use of ML/AI in the field of neuro-ophthalmology is of utmost importance.

Machine learning algorithms require visual evaluation of optic disk for diagnosing and monitoring of the underlying disease in papilledema. Physical appearance of the ONH is dependent on its structural integrity. The ONH pathologies and their appearance are based on axonal loss, which can give a variable clinical picture depending upon the underlying neuro-ophthalmic disorders. They are usually differentiated by three characteristic ONH findings: (1) Pallor, which suggests atrophy; (2) cupping suggestive of glaucomatous changes; and (3) swelling seen in various neuropathies, such as ischemic, inflammatory, infiltrative, infective, toxic, and compressive.[34]

The availability of fundus photography has allowed the development of computer-aided detection (CAD). ML algorithms offer a solution for fast, automated, and accurate interpretation of ONH appearance and the potential underlying diagnosis. Colored fundus photographs with proper segmentation can be trained to develop an automated system to recognize features and classify ONH conditions by DL algorithms. These algorithms require large training datasets with robust ground reality that can even outperform ML algorithms for the classification and categorization of images.

In fundus photography, correct placement with simultaneous positioning and proper segmentation of the optic nerve is one basic necessity for the detection of a lesion. There are three methods for locating optic disk in traditional ML: (1) Based on the characteristics of the optic disk, (2) based on vascular structure, and (3) combination of the two methods.[35] "Characteristics-based methodology" relies on identification of an approximate circular shape, an area with high brightness, and large internal gray contrast to locate the optic disk. As this method is completely based on the "characteristics of optic disk" changes in fundus photography images may, therefore, affect the accuracy. Although the method for locating the optic disk based on the vascular structure relies on locating the optic disk and the blood vessels converging on the optic disk, as well as the characteristics of blood vessels, this method of understanding vascular changes has shown good robustness for fundus changes. However, there is a drawback with this processing too as vascular segmentation in associated pathologies, where the vasculature is irregular or damaged, will not be accurate and may lead to misdiagnosis.

Data from prior studies done to differentiate papilledema from normal ONH had shown promising results and also marked the severity gradings using fundus photographs when used retrospectively.[36] In these studies, ONH was classified on the basis of four classical features (textural, color, disk obscuration, and vascular), and processing was done with support vector machine classifier and radial basis function kernel. The yield from this system showed high accuracies of 92.9 and 97.9% for the detection and grading of papilledema, respectively. There have been few other studies using data augmentation and classical CNN with tensor flow and transfer learning to differentiate true ONH swelling from pseudo-swelling with high accuracy (~95%).[32] Studies using different combinations of ONH feature extraction and ML algorithms have shown good agreement for papilledema grading when compared to an expert neuro-ophthalmologist.[37]

In the post-COVID era, the development in the field of AI had been on a fast track. During this period, an ML system was designed wherein a new model was compared with the three most commonly used ML classifiers, GoogleNet Inception v3, 19 layers of super deep convolutional network from visual geometry group, and 50 layers of deep residual learning network (ResNet). The accuracy and area under the receiver operating characteristic (AUROC) curve were analyzed. Results from this new model study concluded that ML technology could distinguish between pseudopapilledema and an edematous optic disk of optic neuropathy.[32]

The Brain and Optic Nerve Study with Artificial Intelligence (BONSAI) consortium was a large collaborative effort made across 24 ophthalmology centers in 15 countries for the development of a DLS. The DLS, enabled segmentation (U-Net), and classification (DensNet) networks were trained to classify ONHs into three classes: Normal, papilledema, and other ONH abnormalities. They have been able to classify papilledema and other ONH abnormalities.[38] In a follow-up study from the BONSAI consortium, a DLS was developed and trained to "classify" papilledema severity. The DLS was trained to differentiate different grades of papilledema. The DLS yielded an accuracy of 87.9%, a sensitivity of 91.8%, and a specificity of 82.6% in classifying papilledema.[39]

Using AI with collation of large medical datasets has stimulated great interest in the development of DL algorithms. Today, DL algorithms can figure out pathology related to ONH not only faster but also accurately when compared to subjective and traditional-DL driven AI.[40] There are two types of research presented in DLSs for optic disk: (1) Detection of the optic disk in the image and (2) classification of ONH in cropped image.[41,42] There might be some limitations in DL for optic disk pathologies as most advanced object detection algorithms are still lacking, and also, the influence of comorbid pathologies on the function of these algorithms is still unclear because the algorithms have been trained and tested on datasets that exclude other eye conditions such as retinal diseases and high myopia.[43] To overcome this limitation, Rogers et al. used different sets of CNN, each responsible for different tasks in spotting optic disk, macula, and other pathological lesions.[44] It is basically a cloud-based AI system, "Pegasus," to evaluate fundus photography. CNN is used to recognize and extract, and then a standardized format is used as an input into another CNN to classify it. Another study by Milea et al. also trained, validated, and externally tested a DLS to classify the optic disk as normal, with papilledema or with other abnormalities, and also to accurately classify the severity of papilledema.[38]

A new and different learning system is proposed to diagnose uncommon optic disk disorders, which uses a small sample learning framework based on a visualization tool.[45] The framework extends the CNN to detect rare cases in fundus images, such as optic disk edema, by learning with only a small number of samples. Experiments showed AUC to be >0.8 which was achieved in around 90% of cases. Therefore, this framework can be considered superior to other frameworks in detecting rare cases. These richer predictions may facilitate quicker adoption of automatic ophthalmic pathological screening and can change the clinical practice of ophthalmology in the future. Another recent study evaluated the results from DLS-based AI for the classification of optic disk appearance.[46] The evaluation was done by randomly presented fundus images without clinical information, and the performance of DLS was at par with two expert professional neuro-ophthalmologists in classifying optic disk abnormalities.

Fully automated detection of papilledema and its distinction from normal optic disks has been reported with CAD systems using complex hybrid feature extraction methods.[36,47] But these studies have only differentiated papilledema from normal disks, which is a binary (normal or papilledema) and not a real-life situation. In real life, understandably, there are more than just two alternatives related to the optic disk appearance, identification of which gives the direction toward a possible diagnosis.[38] Therefore, before the liberal application of AI technology into clinical practice as the standard of care, further prospective studies on real-world datasets are required to validate the utility of DL algorithms as decision-making support tools.

## Optic Neuritis

Optic nerve is the exit pathway carrying all the impulses generated within the layers of the retina to the brain. Optic neuropathy is a broad term used to describe a variety of conditions affecting the optic nerve due to a wide range of causes, such as infections, trauma, vascular insufficiency, metastases, toxins, and nutritional deficiencies.

Optic neuritis is the inflammation of the optic nerve. It can lead to irreversible vision loss if not diagnosed and managed timely. It is classified into three types on the basis of morphology: (1) Papillitis, (2) retrobulbar neuritis, and (3) neuroretinitis. The diagnosis of papillitis is made on the appearance of a fiery-red optic disk often associated with peripapillary splinter hemorrhages. In contrast, in retrobulbar neuritis, the changes over the disk are subtle or may not be present at all and, therefore, can often be easily missed. A classic example of retrobulbar neuritis is demyelinating optic neuropathy due to MS. There has always been an open gateway for the use of AI with the help of fundus photography. Researchers are constantly trying to study the various methods to derive early and better ways of diagnosis using AI.[48]

Multiple sclerosis is the most common chronic autoimmune demyelinating disorder of the central nervous system. It causes pathophysiological changes in the optic nerve, which include demyelination and atrophy. In MS, a DL-based disease classification of prior optic neuritis is feasible and has the potential to outperform "peripapillary retinal nerve fiber layer (pRNFL) thickness-based classification" of eyes with and without a history of prior optic neuritis. In the acute stage, the RNFL swells in the area surrounding the ONH. It is then followed by persistent thinning of this layer due to compensatory response. These changes can be studied using OCT imaging which captures high-resolution measurements of structural retinal thickness that reflect the integrity of the optic nerve.[49] pRNFL thickness as measured by OCT distinguishes eyes with a prior history of optic neuritis and may provide evidence to support a demyelinating attack. These measurements have been suggested as diagnostic biomarkers in MS that not only reflect structural but also functional visual outcomes in patients of MS.[50-52] As such, the pRNFL thickness is reduced within weeks to months after optic neuritis, and increased magnitude of thickness reduction is associated with worsening of visual function.[53] However, the large individual ranges of normal OCT measurements render absolute thickness measurements of pRNFL alone less useful for detecting optic neuritis.[54,55]

Artificial intelligence, using DL and CNN, allows image classification based on raw imaging data. ML-based classification of eyes with previous episodes of optic neuritis in MS utilizing standard OCT parameters has been promising.[56] However, optic neuritis will not always lead to measurable neuroaxonal damage, and this is one of its limitations. Alternatively, optic nerve magnetic resonance imaging (MRI) or visual evoked potentials (VEPs) may provide valuable biomarkers to determine the diagnosis of MS in these cases.[57,58]

## Anterior Ischemic Optic Neuropathy

Anterior ischemic optic neuropathy (AION) is caused by compromised blood supply to the optic nerve. AION is generally categorized into two types: (1) Arteritic AION (AAION), which is due to inflammation, and (2) nonarteritic AION (NAION), which can be due to noninflammatory causes.[59,60] Only few studies have documented the use of AI automatic detection systems in AION. This is because the standard DLS requires many examples of both AAION and NAION for fetching the correct diagnosis.[20]

Optical coherence tomography has increasingly been used to measure pRNFL thickness in NAION and demyelinating optic neuritis.[61-63] It has become an indispensable tool in the management of ischemic optic neuropathy as accurate RNFL thickness measurement data is necessary for both diagnosis and follow-up of these patients.[64] DL approach with accurate segmentation of the retinal layers would allow accurate estimation of the thickness of RNFL, which is comparable to manual segmentation. However, studies are lacking about the use of DL for RNFL segmentation in NAION cases.

A study reported that the neural network can detect AION 94.7% of the time as compared to clinicians, with the capability of distinguishing AION from optic neuritis in the presence of overlapping features.[65] Another study described the ability of a computerized classification system to characterize NAION severity based on Humphrey VF testing. However, this study lacked clinical applicability.[66]

Recently, Liu et al. presented their research on high-performance DLS for semantic labeling of neuro-ophthalmic images using small datasets.[67] The system modified the Residual Network-152 (ResNet-152) deep CNN that was pretrained on ImageNet, which can distinguish between normal and abnormal optic disks and can also detect laterality. The system could detect a variety of neuro-ophthalmic disorders, including AION, optic disk hypoplasia and atrophy, and papilledema, which offers a ray of hope for the clinical use of AI in the field of neuro-ophthalmology.

## Neuro-ophthalmic Tumors

The most common cause of chiasmal compression is pituitary tumors. They compress structures in the vicinity of pituitary gland, predominantly optic chiasma, leading to visual disturbances and VF defects classically manifesting as bitemporal hemianopia.[68] These tumors can be nonsecreting, which present initially with vision loss and subsequently can reach large size without causing much symptoms. However, hormonally active tumors are detected before they cause significant loss of vision due to accompanying systemic features. Acute hemorrhage or infarction in the pituitary tumor, known as *pituitary apoplexy*, causes diplopia, visual loss, and VF defects. The role of ophthalmologists is, therefore, crucial in the diagnosis and management of pituitary tumors.

Lesions of the visual pathway are accompanied by characteristic VF defects.[69] There may be typical changes in VF which help in reaching to a diagnosis; however, at times, challenging cases present with atypical VF defects or with multiple pathologies.[70,71] Sometimes, it is also important, yet difficult, to distinguish between an undiagnosed compressive pituitary mass and glaucomatous progression in a patient presenting with worsening temporal VF loss.[72,73]

Artificial intelligence has been applied to detect neuro-ophthalmic tumors by harnessing the power of DL to classify patterns of VF defects by a trained feedforward backpropagation artificial neuronal network (ANN).[74] The trained ANN was evaluated in two ways: (1) Trained on 70% of the total available bilateral VF representations and (2) using a "needle in a haystack" algorithm where pituitary visual defects with confirmed pituitary lesions on neuroimaging were withheld from the training dataset and the trained DLS was evaluated for its detection with glaucomatous damage. The model was programmed to rank the probability of VF presented from the most likely bitemporal hemianopia defect to the least likely. However, such an algorithm, if used in clinical practice, could trigger a high false-positive result leading to unnecessary and expensive neuroimaging for patients.

Alternatively, exploration through visual electrophysiology diagnostic tests such as VEP is a future possibility. Although studies with small sample sizes utilizing ML and ANN have shown high accuracy for the detection of optic nerve abnormalities on VEPs, most VEP tests are still interpreted correctly by trained experts only.[75,76] Furthermore, a study suggests that VEP responses during intracranial surgery, for sellar region tumors, such as pituitary adenoma, can be automatically interpreted by neural network algorithms (DL models), thereby potentially assisting real-time VEP monitoring during the surgical resection.[77]

## CONCERNS WITH ARTIFICIAL INTELLIGENCE IN NEURO-OPHTHALMOLOGY

As a relatively new technology trying to match human intelligence, AI is often looked at with several concerns and doubts. The availability of adequately large datasets to gather precise information from the datasets that represent various geographical regions of differing socioeconomic strata, the sensitivity and specificity of AI for the given entity, etc., are some of the major concerns. The quality control for obtaining these datasets is also an issue of worry. Given these limitations, presently, a well-trained ophthalmologist is often necessary for quality control in automated or semiautomated AI systems.[2] The ethical concerns include individual privacy in data sharing and deidentification and reidentification of data which are important for retinal photographs because of the unique retinal vascular patterns that remain unchanged throughout a patient's life.[78-80] As we understand more and more about these systems and as new technology improves the outcomes of AI, these issues will be ably addressed.

# FUTURE OF ARTIFICIAL INTELLIGENCE IN OPHTHALMOLOGY

In the coming years, AI will aid in diagnosis and guiding treatment of several ophthalmological disorders. AI is likely to play not only a larger role in detecting ophthalmological diseases but also will help in providing information on whether there is a common link to systemic diseases such as hypertension, stroke, dementia, cardiovascular diseases, and neurological disorders. The utility of AI and OCT in screening for anemia and distinguishing patients with Alzheimer's disease from healthy control has been demonstrated.[81,82] Lee et al. noted that DL algorithms help in creating a strong association between neurofibrillary tangles and development of dementia in patients with significant amyloid plaques from neuropathology specimens.[83] Retinal biomarkers may eventually be able to even screen and monitor the progression of Alzheimer's disease.[84] To develop AI further, it is important that the ophthalmologists work closely with the multidisciplinary AI team to work on the present and future, which will benefit the patient eventually.

# CONCLUSION

The importance of neuro-ophthalmological assessment in patients is evident more so in emergency situations. Similarly, different conditions which are preventable and/or treatable, if identified early and correctly, can direct medical/surgical management to the patient on time and help salvage eyesight. Here, AI has the potential to play a big role in the future. Also, given the technological advances and the extensive research in the field of AI, it is understandable that AI will very soon be clinically applied in multiple neuro-ophthalmological disorders. Moreover, the ophthalmological conditions where these AI algorithms can be applicable will increase with time. The requirement of human supervision might decrease eventually. What seemingly continues to be a challenge is the ability to implement AI technology in remote areas in developing countries where the needy underprivileged patients can also get access and benefit.

## ACKNOWLEDGMENTS

We acknowledge the encouragement, trust, and support of Late Professor Hari Nema to contribute toward the "Recent Advances in Ophthalmology" series. Moreover, we thank Dr Vikas V, Professor of Neurosurgery, NIMHANS, Bangalore, for his guidance and valuable inputs on the technical aspect of AI. Further, we feel grateful to Dr Anthony Vipin Das, LV Prasad Eye Institute, Hyderabad, for meticulously reviewing our chapter.

## REFERENCES

1. Zaharchuk G, Gong E, Wintermark M, Rubin D, Langlotz CP. Deep learning in neuroradiology. AJNR Am J Neuroradiol. 2018;39(10):1776-84.
2. Leong YY, Vasseneix C, Finkelstein MT, Milea D, Najjar RP. Artificial intelligence meets neuro-ophthalmology. Asia Pac J Ophthalmol (Phila). 2022;11(2):111-25.
3. Samuel AL. Some studies in machine learning using the game of checkers. In: Computer Games. New York: Springer; 1988. pp. 335-65.
4. LeCun Y, Bengio Y, Hinton G. Deep learning. Nature. 2015;521(7553):436-44.
5. Rajkomar A, Dean J, Kohane I. Machine learning in medicine. N Engl J Med. 2019;380(14):1347-58.
6. Kapoor R, Walters SP, Al-Aswad LA. The current state of artificial intelligence in ophthalmology. Surv Ophthalmol. 2019;64(2):233-40.
7. Ongole P. Artificial intelligence, machine learning and deep learning. In: 2017 15th International Conference on ICT and Knowledge Engineering (ICT KE); 2017. pp. 1-6.
8. Mortensen PW, Wong TY, Milea D, Lee AG. The eye is a window to systemic and neuro-ophthalmic diseases. Asia Pac J Ophthalmol (Phila). 2022;11(2):91-3.
9. Antonetti DA, Klein R, Gardner TW. Diabetic retinopathy. N Engl J Med. 2012;366(13):1227-39.
10. Leasher JL, Bourne RRA, Flaxman SR, Jonas JB, Keeffe J, Naidoo K, et al. Global estimates on the number of people blind or visually impaired by diabetic retinopathy: a meta-analysis from 1990 to 2010. Diabetes Care. 2016;39(9):1643-9.
11. Wang W, Lo ACY. Diabetic retinopathy: pathophysiology and treatments. Int J Mol Sci. 2018;19(6):1816.
12. Silva PS, Cavallerano JD, Haddad NMN, Kwak H, Dyer KH, Omar AF, et al. Peripheral lesions identified on ultrawide field imaging predict increased risk of diabetic retinopathy progression over 4 years. Ophthalmology. 2015;122(5):949-56.
13. Shin HJ, Lee SH, Chung H, Kim HC. Association between photoreceptor integrity and visual outcome in diabetic macular edema. Graefes Arch Clin Exp Ophthalmol. 2012;250(1):61-70.
14. Sun JK, Lin MM, Lammer J, Prager S, Sarangi R, Silva PS, et al. Disorganization of the retinal inner layers as a predictor of visual acuity in eyes with center-involved diabetic macular edema. JAMA Ophthalmol. 2014;132(11):1309-16.
15. Nguyen HV, Tan GS, Tapp RJ, Mital S, Ting DS, Wong HT, et al. Cost-effectiveness of a national telemedicine diabetic retinopathy screening program in Singapore. Ophthalmology. 2016;123(12):2571-80.

16. US Food and Drug Administration. (2018). US-FDA permits marketing of artificial intelligence-based device to detect certain diabetes-related eye problems. [online] Available from: https://www.fda.gov/news-events/press-announcements/fda-permits-marketing-artificial-intelligence-based-device-detect-certain-diabetes-related-eye. [Last accessed February, 2023].
17. Fenner BJ, Wong RLM, Lam WC, Tan GSW, Cheung GCM. Advances in retinal imaging and applications in diabetic retinopathy screening: a review. Ophthalmol Ther. 2018;7(2):333-46.
18. Rajalakshmi R, Subashini R, Anjana RM, Mohan V. Automated diabetic retinopathy detection in smartphone-based fundus photography using artificial intelligence. Eye (Lond). 2018;32(6):1138-44.
19. Cao P, Ren F, Wan C, Yang J, Zaiane O. Efficient multi-kernel multi-instance learning using weakly supervised and imbalanced data for diabetic retinopathy diagnosis. Comput Med Imaging Graph. 2018;69:112-24.
20. Gulshan V, Peng L, Coram M, Stumpe MC, Wu D, Narayanaswamy A, et al. Development and validation of a deep learning algorithm for detection of diabetic retinopathy in retinal fundus photographs. JAMA. 2016;316:2402-10.
21. Tham YC, Li X, Wong TY, Quigley HA, Aung T, Cheng CY. Global prevalence of glaucoma and projections of glaucoma burden through 2040: a systematic review and meta-analysis. Ophthalmology. 2014;121(11):2081-90.
22. Devalla SK, Liang Z, Pham TH, Boote C, Strouthidis NG, Thiery AH, et al. Glaucoma management in the era of artificial intelligence. Br J Ophthalmol. 2020;104(3):301-11.
23. Yang HK, Kim YJ, Sung JY, Kim DH, Kim KG, Hwang JM. Efficacy for differentiating nonglaucomatous versus glaucomatous optic neuropathy using deep learning systems. Am J Ophthalmol. 2020;216:140-6.
24. Wong WL, Su X, Li X, Cheung CMG, Klein R, Cheng CY, et al. Global prevalence of age-related macular degeneration and disease burden projection for 2020 and 2040: a systematic review and meta-analysis. Lancet Glob Health. 2014;2(2):e106-16.
25. Hwang DK, Hsu CC, Chang KJ, Chao D, Sun CH, Jheng YC, et al. Artificial intelligence-based decision-making for age-related macular degeneration. Theranostics. 2019;9(1):232-45.
26. Mitchell P, Korobelnik JF, Lanzetta P, Holz FG, Prünte C, Schmidt-Erfurth U, et al. Ranibizumab (Lucentis) in neovascular age-related macular degeneration: evidence from clinical trials. Br J Ophthalmol. 2010;94(1):2-13.
27. Bogunovic H, Waldstein SM, Schlegl T, Langs G, Sadeghipour A, Liu X, et al. Prediction of anti-VEGF treatment requirements in neovascular AMD using a machine learning approach. Invest Ophthalmol Vis Sci. 2017;58(7):3240-8.
28. Pfau M, Möller PT, Künzel SH, von der Emde L, Lindner M, Thiele S, et al. Type 1 choroidal neovascularization is associated with reduced localized progression of atrophy in age-related macular degeneration. Ophthalmol Retina. 2020;4(3):238-48.
29. Niwas SI, Lin W, Bai X, Kwoh CK, Jay Kuo CC, Sng CC, et al. Automated anterior segment OCT image analysis for angle closure glaucoma mechanisms classification. Comput Methods Programs Biomed. 2016;130:65-75.
30. Li Z, He Y, Keel S, Meng W, Chang RT, He M. Efficacy of a deep learning system for detecting glaucomatous optic neuropathy based on color fundus photographs. Ophthalmology. 2018;125:1199-206.

31. Girard MJA, Panda SK, Tun TA, Wibroe EA, Najjar RP, Tin A, et al. (2021). 3D structural analysis of the optic nerve head to robustly discriminate between papilledema and optic disc drusen. [online] Available from: http://arxiv.org/abs/2112.09970. [Last accessed February, 2023].
32. Ahn JM, Kim S, Ahn KS, Cho SH, Kim US. Accuracy of machine learning for differentiation between optic neuropathies and pseudopapilledema. BMC Ophthalmol. 2019;19:178.
33. Poostchi A, Awad M, Wilde C, Dineen RA, Gruener AM. Spike in neuroimaging requests following the conviction of the optometrist Honey Rose. Eye (Lond). 2018;32(3):489-90.
34. Bruce BB, Thulasi P, Fraser CL, Keadey MT, Ward A, Heilpern KL, et al. Diagnostic accuracy and use of nonmydriatic ocular fundus photography by emergency physicians: phase II of the FOTO-ED study. Ann Emerg Med. 2013;62(1): 28-33.e1.
35. Balasubramanian K, Ananthamoorthy NP. State-of-the-art techniques in optic cup and disc localization for glaucoma diagnosis: research results and issues. Crit Rev Biomed Eng. 2020;48:63-83.
36. Akbar S, Akram MU, Sharif M, Tariq A, Yasin UU. Decision support system for detection of papilledema through fundus retinal images. J Med Syst. 2017;41(4):66.
37. Agne J, Wang JK, Kardon RH, Garvin MK. Determining degree of optic nerve edema from color fundus photography. In: Hadjiiski LM, Tourassi GD (Eds). Proc. SPIE 9414, Medical Imaging 2015: Computer-Aided Diagnosis. Orlando, Florida: SPIE Medical Imaging; 2015. p. 94140F.
38. Milea D, Najjar RP, Zhubo J, Ting D, Vasseneix C, Xu X, et al. Artificial intelligence to detect papilledema from ocular fundus photographs. N Engl J Med. 2020;382:1687-95.
39. Frisén L. Swelling of the optic nerve head: a staging scheme. J Neurol Neurosurg Psychiatry. 1982;45:13-8.
40. Liu H, Li L, Wormstone IM, Qiao C, Zhang C, Liu P, et al. Development and validation of a deep learning system to detect glaucomatous optic neuropathy using fundus photographs. JAMA Ophthalmol. 2019;137:1353-60.
41. Mvoulana A, Kachouri R, Akil M. Fully automated method for glaucoma screening using robust optic nerve head detection and unsupervised segmentation based cup-to-disc ratio computation in retinal fundus images. Comput Med Imaging Graph. 2019;77:101643.
42. Martins J, Cardoso JS, Soares F. Offline computer-aided diagnosis for Glaucoma detection using fundus images targeted at mobile devices. Comput Methods Programs Biomed. 2020;192:105341.
43. Hirota M, Mizota A, Mimura T, Hayashi T, Kotoku J, Sawa T, et al. Effect of color information on the diagnostic performance of glaucoma in deep learning using few fundus images. Int Ophthalmol. 2020;40:3013-22.
44. Rogers TW, Jaccard N, Carbonaro F, Lemij HG, Vermeer KA, Reus NJ, et al. Evaluation of an AI system for the automated detection of glaucoma from stereoscopic optic disc photographs: the European Optic Disc Assessment Study. Eye (Lond). 2019;33:1791-7.
45. Quellec G, Lamard M, Conze PH, Massin P, Cochener B. Automatic detection of rare pathologies in fundus photographs using few-shot learning. Med Image Anal. 2020;61:101660.

46. Vasseneix C, Najjar RP, Xu X, Tang Z, Loo JL, Singhal S, et al. Accuracy of a deep learning system for classification of papilledema severity on ocular fundus photographs. Neurology. 2021;97:e369-77.
47. Fatima KN, Hassan T, Akram MU, Akhtar M, Butt WH. Fully automated diagnosis of papilledema through robust extraction of vascular patterns and ocular pathology from fundus photographs. Biomed Opt Express. 2017;8(2):1005-24.
48. Carelli V, Ross-Cisneros FN, Sadun AA. Mitochondrial dysfunction as a cause of optic neuropathies. Prog Retin Eye Res. 2004;23(1):53-89.
49. Jurkute N, Yu-Wai-Man P. Leber hereditary optic neuropathy: bridging the translational gap. Curr Opin Ophthalmol. 2017;28:403-9.
50. Brandt AU, Martinez-Lapiscina EH, Nolan R, Saidha S. Monitoring the course of MS with optical coherence tomography. Curr Treat Options Neurol. 2017; 19(4):15.
51. Petzold A, de Boer JF, Schippling S, Vermersch P, Kardon R, Green A, et al. Optical coherence tomography in multiple sclerosis: a systematic review and meta-analysis. Lancet Neurol 2010;9(9):921-32.
52. Petzold A, Balcer LJ, Calabresi PA, Costello F, Frohman TC, Frohman EM, et al. Retinal layer segmentation in multiple sclerosis: a systematic review and meta-analysis. Lancet Neurol. 2017;16(10):797-812.
53. Costello F, Coupland S, Hodge W, Lorello GR, Koroluk J, Pan YI, et al. Quantifying axonal loss after optic neuritis with optical coherence tomography. Ann Neurol. 2006;59(6):963-9.
54. Bock M, Brandt AU, Dörr J, Kraft H, Weinges-Evers N, Gaede G, et al. Patterns of retinal nerve fiber layer loss in multiple sclerosis patients with or without optic neuritis and glaucoma patients. Clin Neurol Neurosurg. 2010;112(8):647-52.
55. Motamedi S, Gawlik K, Ayadi N, Zimmermann HG, Asseyer S, Bereuter C, et al. Normative data and minimally detectable change for inner retinal layer thicknesses using a semi-automated OCT image segmentation pipeline. Front Neurol. 2019;10:1117.
56. Brandt AU, Specovius S, Oberwahrenbrock T, Zimmermann HG, Paul F, Costello F. Frequent retinal ganglion cell damage after acute optic neuritis. Mult Scler Relat Disord. 2018;22:141-7.
57. Outteryck O, Lopes R, Drumez É, Labreuche J, Lannoy J, Hadhoum N, et al. Optical coherence tomography for detection of asymptomatic optic nerve lesions in clinically isolated syndrome. Neurology. 2020;95(6):e733-44.
58. Vidal-Jordana A, Rovira A, Arrambide G, Otero-Romero S, Río J, Comabella M, et al. Optic nerve topography in multiple sclerosis diagnosis: the utility of visual evoked potentials. Neurology. 2021;96(4):e482-90.
59. Saxena R, Singh D, Sharma M, James M, Sharma P, Menon V. Steroids versus no steroids in nonarteritic anterior ischemic optic neuropathy: a randomized controlled trial. Ophthalmology. 2018;125(10):1623-7.
60. Atkins EJ, Bruce BB, Newman NJ, Biousse V. Treatment of nonarteritic anterior ischemic optic neuropathy. Surv Ophthalmol. 2010;55(1):47-63.
61. Fard MA, Afzali M, Abdi P, Chen R, Yaseri M, Azaripour E, et al. Optic nerve head morphology in nonarteritic anterior ischemic optic neuropathy compared to open-angle glaucoma. Invest Ophthalmol Vis Sci. 2016;57(11):4632-40.
62. Fard MA, Ghahvehchian H, Subramanian PS. Optical coherence tomography in ischemic optic neuropathy. Ann Eye Sci. 2020;5:6.

63. Yadegari S, Gholizade A, Ghahvehchian H, Aghsaei Fard M. Effect of phenytoin on retinal ganglion cells in acute isolated optic neuritis. Neurol Sci. 2020;41:2477-83.
64. Mayro EL, Wang M, Elze T, Pasquale LR. The impact of artificial intelligence in the diagnosis and management of glaucoma. Eye (Lond). 2020;34:1-11.
65. Levin LA, Rizzo 3rd JF, Lessell S. Neural network differentiation of optic neuritis and anterior ischaemic optic neuropathy. Br J Ophthalmol. 1996;80(9):835-9.
66. Feldon SE, Levin L, Scherer RW, Arnold A, Chung SM, Johnson LN, et al. Development and validation of a computerized expert system for evaluation of automated visual fields from the Ischemic Optic Neuropathy Decompression Trial. BMC Ophthalmol. 2006;6:34.
67. Liu TYA, Ting DSW, Yi PH, Wei J, Zhu H, Subramanian PS, et al. Deep learning and transfer learning for optic disc laterality detection: implications for machine learning in neuro-ophthalmology. J Neuroophthalmol. 2020;40:178-84.
68. Danesh-Meyer HV, Yoon JJ, Lawlor M, Savino PJ. Visual loss and recovery in chiasmal compression. Prog Retin Eye Res. 2019;73:100765.
69. Bhatti MT. (2021). American Academy of Ophthalmology. Neuro-ophthalmology. [online] Available from: https://search.ebscohost.com. [Last accessed February, 2023].
70. Lee IH, Miller NR, Zan E, Tavares F, Blitz AM, Sung H, et al. Visual defects in patients with pituitary adenomas: the myth of bitemporal hemianopsia. AJR Am J Roentgenol. 2015;205(5):W512-8.
71. Ogra S, Nichols AD, Stylli S, Kaye AH, Savino PJ, Danesh-Meyer HV. Visual acuity and pattern of visual field loss at presentation in pituitary adenoma. J Clin Neurosci. 2014;21(5):735-40.
72. Drummond SR, Weir C. Chiasmal compression misdiagnosed as normal-tension glaucoma: can we avoid the pitfalls? Int Ophthalmol. 2010;30:215-9.
73. Greenfield DS, Siatkowski RM, Glaser JS, Schatz NJ, Parrish 2nd RK. The cupped disc. Who needs neuroimaging? Ophthalmology. 1998;105(10):1866-74.
74. Thomas PBM, Chan T, Nixon T, Muthusamy B, White A. Feasibility of simple machine learning approaches to support detection of non-glaucomatous visual fields in future automated glaucoma clinics. Eye (Lond). 2019;33(7):1133-9.
75. Kara S, Güven A. Neural network-based diagnosing for optic nerve disease from visual-evoked potential. J Med Syst. 2007;31:391-6.
76. Güven A, Polat K, Kara S, Güneş S. The effect of generalized discriminate analysis (GDA) to the classification of optic nerve disease from VEP signals. Comput Biol Med. 2008;38(1):62-8.
77. Qiao N, Song M, Ye Z, He W, Ma Z, Wang Y, et al. Deep learning for automatically visual evoked potential classification during surgical decompression of sellar region tumors. Transl Vis Sci Technol. 2019;8(6):21.
78. World Health Organization. (2021). Ethics and governance of artificial intelligence for health: WHO guidance. [online] Available from: https://apps.who.int/iris/bitstream/handle/10665/341996/9789240029200-eng.pdf. [Last accessed February, 2023].
79. Batlle JC, Dreyer K, Allen B, Cook T, Roth CJ, Kitts AB, et al. Data sharing of imaging in an evolving health care world: report of the ACR Data Sharing Workgroup, part 1: data ethics of privacy, consent, and anonymization. J Am Coll Radiol. 2021;18(12):1646-54.

80. Akram MU, Abdul Salam A, Khawaja SG, Naqvi SGH, Khan SA. RIDB: a dataset of fundus images for retina based person identification. Data Brief. 2020;33:106433.
81. Chen Z, Mo Y, Ouyang P, Shen H, Li D, Zhao R. Retinal vessel optical coherence tomography images for anemia screening. Med Biol Eng Comput. 2019;57(4):953-66.
82. Tian J, Smith G, Guo H, Liu B, Pan Z, Wang Z, et al. Modular machine learning for Alzheimer's disease classification from retinal vasculature. Sci Rep. 2021;11(1):238.
83. Lee CS, Latimer CS, Henriksen JC, Blazes M, Larson EB, Crane PK, et al. Application of deep learning to understand resilience to Alzheimer's disease pathology. Brain Pathol. 2021;31(6):e12974.
84. Yuan A, Lee CS. Retinal biomarkers for Alzheimer disease: the facts and the future. Asia Pac J Ophthalmol (Phila). 2022;11(2):140-8.

CHAPTER 17

# Updates in Artificial Intelligence in Ophthalmology

*Ng Yu Ci Faye, Dinesh Visva Gunasekeran, Rupesh Agrawal, Gangadhara Sundar*

## ABSTRACT

Artificial intelligence (AI) is a branch of computer science that aims to create intelligent machines that can independently perform cognitive functions such as learning, reasoning, and solving problems, as humans do, being dubbed as the "fourth industrial revolution" of mankind. With the continued and rapidly progressive development of computational technologies, big data acquisition, and advanced clinical imaging methods, the application of AI in medicine is constantly expanding. Ophthalmology is at the forefront of the development and deployment of AI technology, and already in use in the clinical diagnosis, reading of diagnostic imaging such as automated perimetry and optical coherence tomography (OCT), and in the implementation of cutting-edge technology such as surgical robotics. We herein provide an introduction and update to AI and related concepts, its current applications in the field of ophthalmology, and explain the judicious and fruitful utilization of AI, with an eye on future opportunities and challenges.

***Keywords:*** Artificial intelligence; machine learning; big data; virtual reality; augmented reality; robotic surgery.

## ■ INTRODUCTION

Artificial intelligence (AI) is the fourth industrial revolution in the history of mankind.[1] AI was first conceived in the 1940s by pioneers such as Alan Turing and John von Neumann from the field of computing, who hypothesized that machines could "think." The technology has since expanded and been integrated into fields as diverse as finance, transportation, education, and healthcare. Today, AI is a branch of computer science that aims to create intelligent machines that can independently perform cognitive functions as humans do. These may include learning, reasoning, and solving problems. AI algorithms can be trained to identify patterns and make inferences and decisions based on given data. Through each iteration of data processing, learning AI systems update predictive capabilities and enhance result accuracy based on their prior performance during training and validation.

Artificial intelligence is transforming the way we live, work, and play by enabling new technologies, such as self-driving cars, and improving old ones, such as search engines' algorithms. Increasingly, AI permeates the various aspects of our daily lives. It can recognize faces in photographs on Apple's photo application, has triumphed over the world champions in chess and "Go," and may process speech instructions on digital devices via Siri and Alexa. More recently, AI is being employed in Amazon's latest experiment: A surveillance-powered, no-checkout convenience store known as "Go," where consumers simply grab their groceries and walk out of the store and are charged an accurate receipt of their purchases afterward. This is enabled by an advanced system of cameras and computer vision algorithms that seamlessly track and estimate the intention of every person in the store.

With the continuous development of computational technologies, big data acquisition, and advanced clinical imaging methods, the application of AI in medicine is constantly expanding. Today, AI-driven solutions are being used to solve real-world complex problems in healthcare. The aspiration for AI is for it to augment the ability of humans to provide healthcare, giving both physicians and patients greater quality assurance, efficiency, and convenience. As a specialty, ophthalmology is at the forefront of AI technology development and deployment in clinical practice. In ophthalmology, there are numerous examples of AI applications across the care continuum, from diagnosis and prognosis to management and treatment of patients.[2] Clinical applications of AI have made tremendous progress in the field of ophthalmology, matching human experts in the detection of eye diseases on ophthalmic imaging, and even providing additional insights such as differentiating gender based on retinal photographs or optical coherence tomography (OCT) images.[3] The burgeoning global burden of eye diseases provides an urgent impetus for the continued relevance and potential for AI in the field.

## ■ PRINCIPLES AND CONCEPTS

Artificial intelligence refers to computer systems that simulate or display a specific aspect of human intelligence and can be programmed to perform tasks commonly associated with a human mind, such as learning, reasoning, or problem solving. Rather than a single technology, AI is a range of intelligent processes and behaviors driven by computational models and algorithms. Real-world applications of AI to date include machine learning (ML), natural language processing (NLP), and intelligent robots, among others **(Fig. 1)**.

### Machine Learning

Machine learning is a general-purpose method of AI that gains knowledge about relationships from existing data without the need to define them a priori.[4] It uses large datasets to identify interaction patterns among variables,

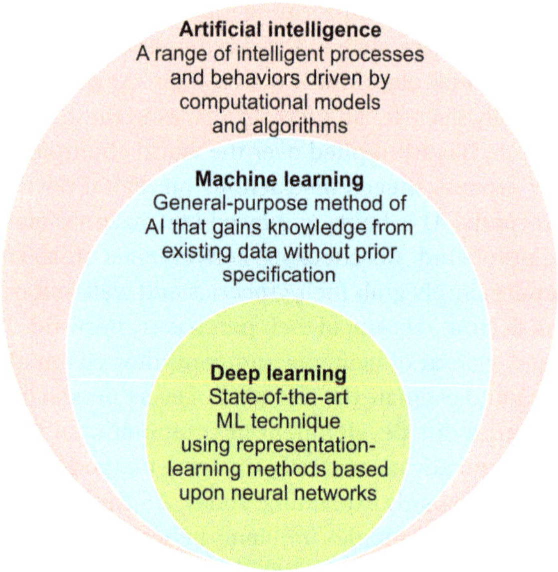

**Fig. 1:** Relationship between artificial intelligence and its subtypes. (ML: machine learning)

**Artificial intelligence**
A range of intelligent processes and behaviors driven by computational models and algorithms

**Machine learning**
General-purpose method of AI that gains knowledge from existing data without prior specification

**Deep learning**
State-of-the-art ML technique using representation-learning methods based upon neural networks

discover previously unknown associations, and generate novel insights for further evaluation. It is especially useful when predictive models need to be derived without established explanations about underlying mechanisms, which may be unknown or insufficiently defined.[5] ML utilizes intelligent algorithms to mimic human learning, allowing machines to improve and refine their functions over time, becoming increasingly accurate when making predictions or classifications.

Machine learning approaches can be categorized into supervised methods, unsupervised methods, and reinforcement learning. Supervised methods are used for classification and regression and require large labeled datasets for training. Examples include detection of lung nodules from chest X-rays,[6] risk estimation of anticoagulation therapy,[7] and prediction of in-hospital mortality of sepsis patients in the intensive care unit (ICU).[8] On the other hand, unsupervised learning does not require labeled datasets but instead aims to identify hidden patterns present within data to generate novel hypotheses through data exploration.[6] For example, drug repurposing methods utilize data from failed clinical trials with different drugs for heart failure patients to identify subclasses of patients who might benefit from specific therapies.[9] Finally, reinforcement learning is a combination of supervised learning and unsupervised learning.[10] The algorithm maximizes accuracy of results through trial and error, learning by interacting with its environment and getting either a positive or a negative reward. Common algorithms in reinforcement learning include temporal difference, deep adversarial networks, and Q-learning.[11]

## Deep Learning

Deep learning (DL) is a state-of-the-art ML technique with widespread applications. DL uses representation-learning methods composed of multiple processing layers based upon neural networks with multiple levels of abstraction to sort through input data.[12] This removes the need for manual feature engineering by recognizing features that contribute to accurate classification from high dimensions through projection onto data in lower dimensions. Every subsequent layer of a DL system produces a representation of observed logic derived from the data it obtains as inputs from the layer prior. There are no limitations in terms of its number of layers, connections, or its capacity to make additional abstractions.[13] There is no need for a local supervised criterion unlike traditional ML models, and layers of features are learned from data using a general-purpose learning procedure. DL uses complete images and associates the entire image with a diagnostic output, eliminating the use of "hand-drawn" image features.[14]

## Natural Language Processing

Natural language processing utilizes computational methods to automatically analyze and represent human languages and can be applied in speech recognition, question answering, sentiment analysis, and text classification, among others.[15] NLP can be readily applied in healthcare, since most forms of healthcare data, such as doctors' notes, test results, laboratory reports, medication orders, and discharge instructions, are unstructured textual data. NLP can be used to extract important information about patients from the above sources of descriptive data, synthesizing large amounts of data to generate insights to improve diagnosis and treatment recommendations. For example, adverse events in healthcare are often collated in incident reports which contain unstructured free text, and NLP can help reduce human workload associated with its analysis and generate meaningful insights.[16] NLP can also be deployed in categorization of electronic dialog data of patients to better engage with and educate them, such as in the development of a chatbot interacting with patients with inflammatory bowel disease.[17]

## Intelligent Robots

Medical robots have been used to assist surgical operations, facilitate rehabilitation and assisted living, and engage patients in social interaction. In particular, intelligent robots have made tremendous headway in the surgical realm. Robotic anastomosis of porcine intestine performed using an AI-driven surgical robot has been demonstrated to outperform results by expert surgeons,[18] while various other semiautonomous robots have been utilized in orthopedic, neurologic, and ophthalmologic procedures.[16] Compared to traditional surgery, AI robot-assisted surgery is minimally invasive and portends better patient outcomes such as reduced hospital stay duration, complication rates, and errors. Apart from conducting surgical interventions, AI can also be applied to clinical decision support system (CDSS). It is able to recommend the best timing of surgery and surgical approach by analyzing medical records and clinical imaging, tailoring treatment plans for each individual patient. It can also provide data-driven insight into the potential risks and benefits of surgery and predict postoperative outcomes depending on each patient's risk profile.

## CURRENT APPLICATIONS OF ARTIFICIAL INTELLIGENCE IN OPHTHALMOLOGY

Artificial intelligence technologies can be wielded as powerful tools and assistants to enhance, extend, and expand human capabilities to deliver care to patients and enhance clinical effectiveness through the domains of quality, safety, and efficiency. Through automated clinical decision-making systems and workflows, AI extends access to ophthalmologic care and increases the affordability of services provided.

### Patient Experience

Artificial intelligence can provide convenience to patients, offering the possibility of screening for eye diseases from the comfort of the patient's home at any time of the day. The prevalence of smartphones, coupled with the availability of affordable, easy-to-use adapters for retinal photographs with AI evaluation algorithms, enable eye screening services to be conducted by nonspecialists through analyses of fundus photographs captured by technicians that can be sited in out-of-hospital settings or even in the community.[19] In-home, app-based testing for diseases such as age-related macular degeneration (AMD) and diabetic retinopathy (DR) could be the future, improving ease of screening for patients and enabling more patients to have access to basic eye care.[20] Models built on AI have been shown to improve the cost-effectiveness of screening[21] and further benefit patients by being personalized and predictive.[22]

This has major implications on public and preventive health, especially in middle to low-income countries where large segments of the population may not have access to the healthcare system but are connected to the network through their smartphones. It is both feasible and effective as it leverages on the resources patients already have to augment their interaction with regional or global healthcare ssytems, thus lowering the barrier of entry, for clinical case presentations, seeking early medical attention and thus encouraging positive health-seeking behavior. Apart from retinal diseases, AI applications have also been developed to screen for strabismus through objective classification of ocular versions[23] as well as perform eyelid measurements.[24]

Additionally, AI can be deployed clinically to relieve the workload in the office by acting as a support tool for diagnostic and triaging purposes, freeing up a physician's time for patient care and interaction. For example, retinal photograph-based AI algorithms have been developed to help classify referral cases from primary care settings into urgent and nonurgent cases, relieving the overwhelming patient load often experienced at tertiary eye clinics.[25] Patients can also rely on app-based AI-powered chatbots to obtain preliminary medical advice about eye symptoms and signs, or undertake AI-driven questionnaires that serve as a first-line triage for eye diseases.[26] In follow-up care, patients can self-monitor and report their progress through an AI-based app without physical visits to the clinics, which flags up dangerous symptoms prompting early follow-up at clinics. This improves allocation of healthcare resources, whereby ophthalmologists are thereby able to identify patients with either critical or serious eye conditions and dedicate more time and attention to each individual patient.[27] As most AI-driven tools are able to give feedback to instantaneous results, these also encourage more timely referrals and earlier detection of cases. Consequently, this reduces delays in sight-preserving interventions and alleviates the growing burden of preventable vision loss.[28]

Finally, the integration of AI with other digital health solutions such as mobile applications or extended reality can help patients better navigate the healthcare system.[29] AI-enabled mobile applications offer patients insights to queue lengths and waiting times, allow patients to schedule their appointments online, and remind patients to pick up their medications at the pharmacy once ready, letting patients better plan and organize their visits to the clinic.[30] AI-powered technologies can also allow staff at eye centers to better predict and respond to patient volumes as well as streamline workflows for operational efficiency and redirect personnel to meet evolving manpower needs.[31] All these contribute to more efficient work processes in the healthcare system and result in improvements of eye care delivery.

## Clinical Imaging

Digital images provide millions of anatomical and morphological datapoints that can be analyzed using AI in a fast and comprehensive manner. Given AI's ability to build automated prediction models large amounts of data, and the discipline of Ophthalmology's extensive and long standing expertise in high-resolution imaging such as fundus photography, OCT and digital data, AI is perfectly suited for advanced screening and diagnostic grading aiding early and better management of ophthalmic disorders.

Methods based on ML, and in particular DL, can identify, localize, and quantify pathological features in eye diseases, with automated detection of disease activity, recurrences, quantification of therapeutic effects, and identification of relevant targets for novel therapeutic approaches. Incredible progress has already been made in landmark innovations, including Google's validated detection algorithms for referable DR[32] as well as an AI system to detect referable DR from retinal photographs, the first autonomous dialogistic system to be approved in any field of medicine by the United States Food and Drug Administration (USFDA).[33]

Deep learning has been shown to be highly effective in discovering intricate structures in high-dimensional data and obtaining incredible accuracy at object detection in images, advancing medical imaging analysis.[34] Within ophthalmology, DL has shown robust diagnostic performance in ocular imaging for DR,[35] glaucoma,[36] AMD,[37] and retinopathy of prematurity (ROP),[38] in fundus photographs and OCT. Additionally, DL is able to estimate refractive errors and cardiovascular risk factors from retinal fundus photographs as well.[39,40]

These applications have been demonstrated by many academic and research groups internationally for applications ranging from screening, prediction, and even CDS for driving management decisions in eye diseases such as DR.[21] Of note, technology industry players have recently entered these spaces, including Google and Ping An Smart Healthcare.[41] For example, experts from Ping An have expanded into the AI space by creating technologies related to the diagnosis of eye diseases, including quality control, screening, lesion detection, segmentation, and quantization of retinal structure or lesion areas. In an OCT screening system developed by the group, the accuracy rate of the image quality control model, the pathological changes screening model, and the lesions-detection model were 99, 96.8, and 97.5%, respectively. The imaging model's smart enhancements resulted in an average of 46% in time savings from clinical encounters. Ping An Smart Healthcare has since rolled out smart ophthalmic imaging technology to >100 hospitals in 15 provinces and cities, including Beijing, Shanghai, Shenzhen, and Gansu. By deploying the AI model on its platform, Ping An Cloud receives de-identified OCT images from hospitals, processes the results, and feeds them back to end users through the network.

## Risk Prediction and Stratification

Unsupervised models and DL networks are able to self-learn predictive features from input data without being explicitly programmed to detect specific features. Hence, AI is able to determine disease risk and progression using a variety of factors in a more holistic and comprehensive way.[21] The predictive capabilities of AI are not biased by a physician's existing knowledge of disease or patient, providing a more accurate analysis of patient outcomes based on objective measures and indicators.[13] The AI may even be able to pool datapoints together to uncover new associations regarding risk and disease that was previously unknown.

Many ophthalmologic conditions are sight threatening, and it is crucial to catch patients at an early juncture in their condition to avoid permanent vision loss. AI prioritizes resource allocation and promotes timely intervention by identifying patients most in need of treatment through well-defined criteria and standards. For example, not all diabetic patients will develop DR, and not all patients with DR will eventually require treatment in tertiary centers for severe DR with proliferative changes. Existing methods of basing the risk of DR on blood glycemic indices are imprecise and only explain 11% in variation of the risk, as evidenced in the Diabetes Control and Complications trial.[42] AI circumvents this problem by deriving insight from a broader, more complex range of data to predict and stratify risk, and focuses on analyzing imaging modalities that have been shown to yield more accurate findings. AI has been shown to be effective in detecting disease progression between consecutive retinal images for DR[43] as well as visual fields in glaucoma in consecutive functional screenings. Its algorithms have also been designed to prognosticate disease progression in high-risk patients with glaucoma and AMD.[44] With advances in the technology, prediction and prognostic findings by AI could potentially be used to guide targeted and personalized eye care for patients in the future, such as the recommendation for early referral for assessment or shorter screening intervals.

## Surgical Robotics

A lesser-known but equally exciting application of AI in ophthalmology is its role in surgical care. AI offers an additional edge when integrated into preoperative, intraoperative, and postoperative tools and decision-making algorithms by providing surgeons with insights gathered from clinical data. Preoperatively, inputting patients' OCT and visual acuity data into an ML algorithm can guide the surgeon on the rate of progression of an epiretinal membrane to determine the optimal timing of surgery.[45] AI tools can also be utilized to guide surgeons in choosing the correct intraocular lens (IOL) power and have contributed to refinements of existing IOL formulas for refractive surgery.[46] An IOL "super formula" that incorporates postoperative outcomes was able to continuously improve the model using an AI-hybrid approach.[47]

Ophthalmic microsurgery is technically demanding due to the small surgical field requiring a high level of precision and the nature of operating on awake and nonparalyzed patients. Intraoperatively, AI-programmed surgical robots can analyze data from preoperative scans and findings to guide a surgeon's instrument in real time during a procedure.[45] AI assistance can range from intraoperative image guidance to full automation via autonomous robotic surgery, with robotic models with various levels of autonomy being developed.[18] Given that most ophthalmologic surgeries are performed using operating microscopes with near-fixed surgical fields, large amounts of surgical video data can also be generated to train ML algorithms to provide intraoperative guidance and program future robotic eye surgery.[45] With the convergence of DL and ophthalmic robotic microsurgery, AI will also have an increasing role in enhancing the safety, efficacy, and reliability of robotic platforms, such as the development of an active interventional control framework (AICF) to predict surgeon movements and prevent the exertion of excessive force to the sclera.[48]

## Medical Education

In medical and ophthalmic education, novel AI-based and virtual reality (VR) technologies can allow trainees to improve and hone their skillsets by facilitating surgical training prior to the operating theatre as well as enhancing feedback received from the actual procedure. One example of a VR-based simulator is the Eyesi˙ Surgical platform, software that offers a controlled environment for novice surgeons to "operate" in and provides timely, objective, and detailed feedback of the learner's performance afterward for review.

Artificial intelligence can also provide real-time surgical guidance by incorporating augmented reality (AR) into "smart" operating microscopes to provide step-by-step direction. Taking the example of cataract surgery, convolutional neural network (CNN) models can be developed to accurately recognize the phase of cataract surgery in real time and overlay a respecified capsulorrhexis size indicator on the anterior capsule. Meanwhile, instrument tracking, alongside intraoperative imaging such as microscope-integrated OCT, can help estimate the depth of microinstrumentation within the cataract nucleus during phacoemulsification. The same technology may also enable to ascertain forceps distance from the retinal surface during macular membrane or posterior hyaloid maneuvers. Warnings of possible errors or complications can be triggered as a part of real-time vibrotactile or other forms of feedback to the novice surgeon. OCT AI-enhanced technologies can be integrated into the instrument tip to assist in retinal surface detection and tremor compensation as well (cf. image stabilization in digital cameras).[49]

An overview of various applications of AI in ophthalmology is shown in **Figure 2**.

## ■ THE FUTURE

The current applications of AI in ophthalmic practice are described in this chapter. Latest research has demonstrated how it can improve the accuracy

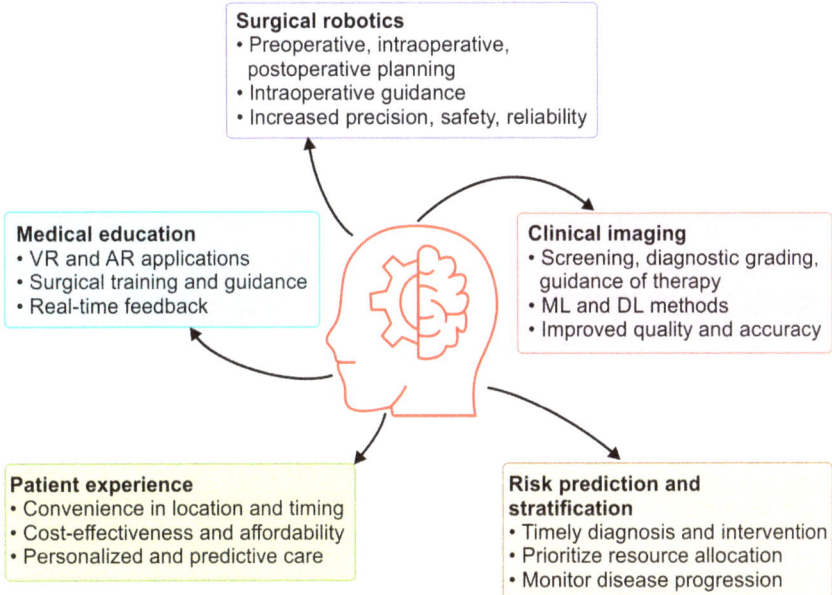

**Fig. 2:** Artificial intelligence (AI) applications and use cases in ophthalmology. (AR: augmented reality; DL: deep learning; ML: machine learning; VR: virtual reality)

of OCT imaging by serving as an aid to clinicians, optimizing patients' experience in the clinic, home, and throughout the healthcare system, hence increasing work efficiency and enhancing the quality and efficiency of care. It also has the potential to alleviate the problem of insufficient medical resources and expertise in ophthalmology and, when combined with clinical validation to fulfill early screening and standardized treatment of common diseases, may alleviate the risk of permanent eye damage and blindness for the individual and the society at large.

Although AI has created unprecedented opportunities for ophthalmology to adapt new models of care supported by digital innovations, there remain several clinical and technical challenges in implementation which need to be addressed. Firstly, it is important to note that AI models are highly dependent upon the datasets they are trained on, and learn only what they are presented with. If an AI tool is given insufficient datasets to train on, or the datasets provided are not representative of the entire population, the algorithm is unlikely to generate accurate or reliable outcomes. Most AI studies in the initial stages train on limited datasets from a specific population resulting in a homogenous patient demographic,[32] which might not be applicable or relevant to the larger population and thus may limit generalizability in application. In addition, retinal images, which form the current mainstay of training datasets in ophthalmology, are often subject to technical and imaging factors, including width of field, field of view, image magnification, and image quality, thereby biasing results.[50] Diversifying the dataset in terms of ethnicity and standardizing the image-capture hardware could help mitigate this challenge.

Secondly, the robustness of an AI model is dependent on the volume of information fed. It is thus difficult to train algorithms on rare ophthalmic diseases, such as orbital and ocular tumors and retinitis pigmentosa, due to the limited availability of patient data. To overcome the rarity of such diseases, there is a need for wide-ranging and organized collaboration between tertiary care centers and research laboratories involved in the treatment of rare eye diseases on an international level. Researchers have to collaborate between different research centers and across geographies to enroll patients and aggregate sufficient datasets over time. Effective recruitment of patients can also be achieved through partnership with patient organizations, rare disease registries, and centers of expertise. In the process, full patient consent and data anonymity must be respected.

Thirdly, AI models may not work as well for diseases where there has historically been disagreement and interobserver variability in definition of disease phenotype and labeling of fundal images such as glaucoma, ROP, orbital and orbitofacial fractures, or even thyroid eye disease. More evidence to support clinical decision-making and establish high-quality ground-truth labels are thus required to establish the validity of these algorithms. Adjudication grades by ophthalmic subspecialists have been shown to be a more rigorous reference standard than majority decision in diagnosis of DR, and usage of such high-quality datasets can improve algorithm performance.[51] A similar process could potentially benefit diseases with high disagreement and interobserver variability.

A final barrier to the widespread adoption of AI in healthcare lies in its unknown nature and "black box" characteristic. Even though AI has been shown to outperform humans in certain aspects of clinical diagnosis and decision-making, the lack of explainability for its output is a barrier for adoption as providers may not fully trust the recommendations from clinical AI.[52] For example, the use of DL architecture has been shown to improve performance for image pattern recognition and classification tasks in the diagnosis of multiple ophthalmologic diseases. However, the ability to observe "cause and effect" from automated systems decreases with the use of DL methods.[53] By virtue of their scientific training and the rigorous, rational nature of medicine, trained physicians gravitate toward solutions with clear explanations and known mechanisms. Physicians need to know not only the quantitative performance metrics but also the logic and methods by which the algorithm arrives at its conclusions.

To promote greater physician acceptance of AI algorithms, developers are working on solution-based strategies such as visualization of hidden layers in a neural network to improve the explainability of algorithms.[54] They have also generated heat maps highlighting the regions of interest in an image contributing to the algorithm's analysis, such as the DL system developed by the Moorfields Eye Hospital and DeepMind, where a segmentation network model is used to quantify relevant areas of retinal pathology in an intermediate tissue representation.[55]

Ongoing research is critical to investigate how AI can be integrated into current clinical workflows as well as evaluate the clinical benefit and cost-effectiveness of such technologies to patients. To this end, AI algorithms need to continue to be designed with the highest standards and transparency, with rigorous guidelines guiding their development to ensure clinical efficacy and patient safety. Core ethical and professional principles, regulatory frameworks, and protocols need to be established to allow AI to be utilized in clinical practice in a safe and responsible manner. Legal and regulatory uncertainties as well as the liability concerns are issues that will need to be continually discussed by medical, ethical, legal, and regulatory experts to allow these novel technologies to benefit patient and population health.

Timely reporting of new findings by the AI community is also essential to enable communication and collaboration in the space and allow optimization of algorithms toward patient care. The standardization of vocabulary involving AI documentation and sharing of data across platforms are imperative for future growth, while taking into consideration user privacy and anonymity in the collection and usage of data. As the scope, application, and the sophistication of AI continue to grow exponentially, the fundamentals of AI in ophthalmic imaging will also need to be included in the training of ophthalmologists to encourage understanding of both the technical basis and the clinical implications of the technology. Future ophthalmologists will also need to work in tandem with AI computer scientists and researchers to develop algorithms in line with established guidelines.

## ■ CONCLUSION

Artificial intelligence has immense potential to further revolutionize the field of ophthalmology. It is poised to further impact and transform the practice of healthcare in the imminent future. It has already demonstrated great promise in detecting multiple eye diseases, with clinically acceptable diagnostic performance, and continues to extend its influence in the realms of screening, diagnosis, prognosis, and management. The key to integrating AI into the practice of ophthalmology is to foster a mutually reinforcing human–machine partnership. This has to maintain the fine balance between the personal human care and interaction that stakeholders value in healthcare and the levels of automation that AI technologies present. Despite evidence that AI models may outperform expert ophthalmologists in specific aspects of clinical care such as evaluating risk stratification from retinal fundus photos, patients will ultimately want to receive care and reassurance from their "human" physicians instead of relying on a machine to explain their results. The need for better integration of human understanding, empathy, and personalization to meet the varying needs, wishes, and demands of patients provides food for thought for the future generations and applications of AI technology.

## ■ REFERENCES

1. Forum WE. (2016). The fourth industrial revolution: what it means, how to respond. [online] Available from https://www.weforum.org/agenda/2016/01/the-fourth-industrial-revolution-what-it-means-and-how-to-respond. [Last accessed February, 2023].
2. Sundar G. Surgical audits, big data, professionalism, and patient-centric care. TNOA J Ophthalmic Sci Res. 2020;58:145-7.
3. Korot E, Pontikos N, Liu X, Wagner SK, Faes L, Huemer J, et al. Predicting sex from retinal fundus photographs using automated deep learning. Sci Rep. 2021;11(1):10286.
4. Murphy KP. Machine Learning: A Probabilistic Perspective. London, England: The MIT Press; 2012.
5. Bishop CM. Pattern Recognition and Machine Learning (Information Science and Statistics). New York, United States: Springer; 2007.
6. Deo RC. Machine learning in medicine. Circulation. 2015;132(20):1920-30.
7. Lip GY, Nieuwlaat R, Pisters R, Lane DA, Crijns HJ. Refining clinical risk stratification for predicting stroke and thromboembolism in atrial fibrillation using a novel risk factor-based approach: the euro heart survey on atrial fibrillation. Chest. 2010;137(2):263-72.
8. Kong G, Lin K, Hu Y. Using machine learning methods to predict in-hospital mortality of sepsis patients in the ICU. BMC Med Inform Decis Mak. 2020;20(1):251.
9. Noorbakhsh-Sabet N, Zand R, Zhang Y, Abedi V. Artificial intelligence transforms the future of health care. Am J Med. 2019;132(7):795-801.
10. Botvinick M, Ritter S, Wang JX, Kurth-Nelson Z, Blundell C, Hassabis D. Reinforcement learning, fast and slow. Trends Cogn Sci. 2019;23(5):408-22.
11. Mahesh B. Machine learning algorithms—a review. Int J Sci Res (IJSR). 2020;9:381-6.
12. LeCun Y, Bengio Y, Hinton G. Deep learning. Nature. 2015;521(7553):436-44.
13. Miotto R, Wang F, Wang S, Jiang X, Dudley JT. Deep learning for healthcare: review, opportunities and challenges. Brief Bioinform. 2018;19(6):1236-46.
14. Ting DSW, Peng L, Varadarajan AV, Keane PA, Burlina PM, Chiang MF, et al. Deep learning in ophthalmology: the technical and clinical considerations. Prog Retin Eye Res. 2019;72:100759.
15. Chen M, Decary M. Artificial intelligence in healthcare: an essential guide for health leaders. Healthc Manage Forum. 2020;33(1):10-8.
16. Young IJB, Luz S, Lone N. A systematic review of natural language processing for classification tasks in the field of incident reporting and adverse event analysis. Int J Med Inform. 2019;132:103971.

17. Zand A, Sharma A, Stokes Z, Reynolds C, Montilla A, Sauk J, et al. An exploration into the use of a chatbot for patients with inflammatory bowel diseases: retrospective cohort study. J Med Internet Res. 2020;22(5):e15589.
18. Panesar S, Cagle Y, Chander D, Morey J, Fernandez-Miranda J, Kliot M. Artificial intelligence and the future of surgical robotics. Ann Surg. 2019;270(2):223-6.
19. Pieczynski J, Kuklo P, Grzybowski A. The role of telemedicine, in-home testing and artificial intelligence to alleviate an increasingly burdened healthcare system: diabetic retinopathy. Ophthalmol Ther. 2021;10(3):445-64.
20. Schmid MK, Thiel MA, Lienhard K, Schlingemann RO, Faes L, Bachmann LM. Reliability and diagnostic performance of a novel mobile app for hyperacuity self-monitoring in patients with age-related macular degeneration. Eye (Lond). 2019;33(10):1584-9.
21. Gunasekeran DV, Ting DSW, Tan GSW, Wong TY. Artificial intelligence for diabetic retinopathy screening, prediction and management. Curr Opin Ophthalmol. 2020;31(5):357-65.
22. Schmidt-Erfurth U, Sadeghipour A, Gerendas BS, Waldstein SM, Bogunović H. Artificial intelligence in retina. Prog Retin Eye Res. 2018;67:1-29.
23. de Figueiredo LA, Dias JVP, Polati M, Carricondo PC, Debert I. Strabismus and artificial intelligence app: optimizing diagnostic and accuracy. Transl Vis Sci Technol. 2021;10(7):22.
24. Chen HC, Tzeng SS, Hsiao YC, Chen RF, Hung EC, Lee OK. Smartphone-based artificial intelligence-assisted prediction for eyelid measurements: Algorithm Development and Observational Validation study. JMIR Mhealth Uhealth. 2021;9(10):e32444.
25. Tham YC, Husain R, Teo KYC, Tan ACS, Chew ACY, Ting DS, et al. New digital models of care in ophthalmology, during and beyond the COVID-19 pandemic. Br J Ophthalmol. 2022;106(4):452-7.
26. Lee JH, Jeong MS, Cho JU, Jeon HK, Park JH, Shin KD, et al. Developing an Ophthalmic Chatbot System. Presented at: Proceedings of 15th International Conference on Ubiquitous Information Management and Communication. 2021; 1-7.
27. Gunasekeran DV, Tham YC, Ting DSW, Tan GSW, Wong TY. Digital health during COVID-19: lessons from operationalising new models of care in ophthalmology. Lancet Digit Health. 2021;3(2):e124-34.
28. Foot B, MacEwen C. Surveillance of sight loss due to delay in ophthalmic treatment or review: frequency, cause and outcome. Eye (Lond). 2017;31(5):771-5.
29. Ong CW, Tan MCJ, Lam M, Koh VTC. Applications of extended reality in ophthalmology: systematic review. J Med Internet Res. 2021;23(8):e24152.
30. Li X, Tian D, Li W, Dong B, Wang H, Yuan J, et al. Artificial intelligence-assisted reduction in patients' waiting time for outpatient process: a retrospective cohort study. BMC Health Serv Res. 2021;21(1):237.
31. Li JO, Liu H, Ting DSJ, Jeon S, Chan RVP, Kim JE, et al. Digital technology, telemedicine and artificial intelligence in ophthalmology: a global perspective. Prog Retin Eye Res. 2021;82:100900.
32. Gulshan V, Peng L, Coram M, Stumpe MC, Wu D, Narayanaswamy A, et al. Development and validation of a deep learning algorithm for detection of diabetic retinopathy in retinal fundus photographs. JAMA. 2016;316(22):2402-10.

33. Abràmoff MD, Lavin PT, Birch M, Shah N, Folk JC. Pivotal trial of an autonomous AI-based diagnostic system for detection of diabetic retinopathy in primary care offices. NPJ Digit Med. 2018;1(1):39.
34. Zhang X, Zou J, He K, Sun J. Accelerating very deep convolutional networks for classification and detection. IEEE Trans Pattern Anal Mach Intell. 2016;38(10):1943-55.
35. Ting DSW, Cheung CY, Lim G, Tan GSW, Quang ND, Gan A, et al. Development and validation of a deep learning system for diabetic retinopathy and related eye diseases using retinal images from multiethnic populations with diabetes. JAMA. 2017;318(22):2211-23.
36. Li Z, He Y, Keel S, Meng W, Chang RT, He M. Efficacy of a deep learning system for detecting glaucomatous optic neuropathy based on color fundus photographs. Ophthalmology. 2018;125(8):1199-206.
37. Burlina PM, Joshi N, Pekala M, Pacheco KD, Freund DE, Bressler NM. Automated grading of age-related macular degeneration from color fundus images using deep convolutional neural networks. JAMA Ophthalmol. 2017;135(11):1170-6.
38. Brown JM, Campbell JP, Beers A, Chang K, Ostmo S, Chan RVP, et al. Automated diagnosis of plus disease in retinopathy of prematurity using deep convolutional neural networks. JAMA Ophthalmol. 2018;136(7):803-10.
39. Varadarajan AV, Poplin R, Blumer K, Angermueller C, Ledsam J, Chopra R, et al. Deep learning for predicting refractive error from retinal fundus images. Invest Ophthalmol Vis Sci. 2018;59(7):2861-8.
40. Poplin R, Varadarajan AV, Blumer K, Liu Y, McConnell MV, Corrado GS, et al. Prediction of cardiovascular risk factors from retinal fundus photographs via deep learning. Nat Biomed Eng. 2018;2(3):158-64.
41. Liu X, Zhao C, Wang L, Wang G, Lv B, Lv C, et al. Evaluation of an OCT-AI-based telemedicine platform for retinal disease screening and referral in a primary care setting. Transl Vis Sci Technol. 2022;11(3):4.
42. Lachin JM, Genuth S, Nathan DM, Zinman B, Rutledge BN, DCCT/EDIC Research Group. Effect of glycemic exposure on the risk of microvascular complications in the diabetes control and complications trial—revisited. Diabetes. 2008;57(4):995-1001.
43. Ribeiro L, Oliveira CM, Neves C, Ramos JD, Ferreira H, Cunha-Vaz J. Screening for diabetic retinopathy in the central region of Portugal. Added value of automated 'disease/no disease' grading. Ophthalmologica. 2015;233:96-103.
44. Yousefi S, Elze T, Pasquale LR, Saeedi O, Wang M, Shen LQ, et al. Monitoring glaucomatous functional loss using an artificial intelligence-enabled dashboard. Ophthalmology. 2020;127(9):1170-8.
45. Mishra K, Leng T. Artificial intelligence and ophthalmic surgery. Curr Opin Ophthalmol. 2021;32(5):425-30.
46. Ladas J, Ladas D, Lin SR, Devgan U, Siddiqui AA, Jun AS. Improvement of multiple generations of intraocular lens calculation formulae with a novel approach using artificial intelligence. Transl Vis Sci Technol. 2021;10(3):7.
47. Ladas JG, Siddiqui AA, Devgan U, Jun AS. A 3-D "super surface" combining modern intraocular lens formulas to generate a "super formula" and maximize accuracy. JAMA Ophthalmol. 2015;133(12):1431-6.

48. He C, Patel N, Shahbazi M, Yang Y, Gehlbach P, Kobilarov M, et al. Toward safe retinal microsurgery: development and evaluation of an RNN-based active interventional control framework. IEEE Trans Biomed Eng. 2020;67(4):966-77.
49. Cheon GW, Huang Y, Cha J, Gehlbach PL, Kang JU. Accurate real-time depth control for CP-SSOCT distal sensor based handheld microsurgery tools. Biomed Opt Express. 2015;6(5):1942-53.
50. Yip MYT, Lim G, Lim ZW, Nguyen QD, Chong CCY, Yu M, et al. Technical and imaging factors influencing performance of deep learning systems for diabetic retinopathy. NPJ Digit Med. 2020;3:40.
51. Krause J, Gulshan V, Rahimy E, Karth P, Widner K, Corrado GS, et al. Grader variability and the importance of reference standards for evaluating machine learning models for diabetic retinopathy. Ophthalmology. 2018;125(8):1264-72.
52. Beede E, Baylor E, Hersch F, Iurchenko A, Wilcox L, Ruamviboonsuk P, et al. A human-centered evaluation of a deep learning system deployed in clinics for the detection of diabetic retinopathy. Presented at: Proceedings of the 2020 CHI Conference on Human Factors in Computing Systems; 2020; Honolulu, HI, USA.
53. Varghese J. Artificial intelligence in medicine: chances and challenges for wide clinical adoption. Visc Med. 2020;36(6):443-9.
54. Dreiseitl S, Ohno-Machado L. Logistic regression and artificial neural network classification models: a methodology review. J Biomed Inform. 2002;35(5-6):352-9.
55. De Fauw J, Ledsam JR, Romera-Paredes B, Nikolov S, Tomasev N, Blackwell S, et al. Clinically applicable deep learning for diagnosis and referral in retinal disease. Nat Med. 2018;24(9):1342-50.

# Index

Page numbers followed by *b* refer to box, *f* refer to figure, *fc* refer to flowchart, and *t* refer to table.

## A

Aberration correction 58
Ablation profiles, types of 45
Accurate refraction methods 22
Acquired vitelliform lesion 215
Active interventional control
 framework 280
Advanced clinical imaging methods 273
Advanced machine learning 35
Advanced refractive correction 66, 68
 systems 68
Age-related macular degeneration 11, 21, 34, 95, 98, 175, 182, 184, 185*t*, 187, 196, 203, 217*f*, 255, 258, 276
 detection of 189
 diagnosis of 184, 186*t*
 dry 187*t*
 initial detection of 184
 management 184*fc*
 neovascular 203
 non-neovascular 207, 216
 progression of 187, 188*t*
 sign of 1
 subtypes of non-neovascular 207
Alzheimer's disease 265
Amazon's latest experiment 273
Amyotrophic lateral sclerosis 152
Anaplastic astrocytoma 228
Anesthesia, topical 59
Angiography, dye-based 195
Anterior chamber
 angle 94
 depth 38
Anterior lenticule
 cut 60*f*
 surface 60
Anti-inflammatory agents 118
Antivascular endothelial growth factor 188*t*
 intravitreal injection of 258
 treatment 187
Aphakic refractive error 110
Apple's photo application 273
Aqueous humor 111
Area under receiver operating
 characteristic curve 260

Artificial intelligence 1, 6, 11, 20, 22, 29, 30*t*, 33, 37, 40, 97-99, 99*f*, 100, 133, 135*fc*, 137, 140, 142*fc*, 142*t*, 143, 145, 151, 152, 155, 168, 174, 175, 182, 183, 185*t*-188*t*, 253, 262, 264, 272, 273, 274*f*, 276, 281*f*
 algorithms 98
  types of 34, 34*fc*
 application of 167, 183
 background of 183
 challenges with 188
 contribution of 184*fc*
 current applications of 276
 development of 175, 189
 enigma of 102
 future of 1, 265
 implementing 99*t*
 integration, monitor with 141*f*
 limitations of 38
 model 101, 136, 139*t*
 need for 255
 pitfalls of 145
 role of 144*f*, 184
 subclasses 134*f*
 subsets 21*f*
 system, functioning of 175
 unexplainable 103*fc*
 updates in 272
 use of 103, 179
 utility of 157
 work 136
Artificial neural network 90, 153, 183
 backpropagation 264
Artiphakia 70
Asphericity asymmetry index, posterior 38
Asteroid hyalosis 179*f*
Astigmatism 51
 lower-order 57
Astrocytes 223
Astrocytic hamartoma 240
Atrophy meetings, classification of 212
Attention model 23*fc*
Attention technique 23
Augmented reality 272
Autofluorescence, significantly
 decreased 200

Autoimmune demyelinating disorder, chronic 262
Automated detection methods 132
Automated perimetry 255, 272
Automatic ophthalmic pathological screening 261
Axial length measurement 108, 112

# B

Basal laminar drusen 213*f*, 214*f*
Behçet's disease 119, 124
Best vitelliform macular dystrophy 203
Biconvex lens 113
Big data 272
   acquisition 273
Bioptics 75
   treatment for 76
Black box 169
   phenomenon 135
Blindness, cause of 182
Blood
   glycemic indices 279
   pressure 34
Blood-borne 236
   metastasis
      cases of 239
      invasion 236
Body mass index 34
Both eyes, fundus autofluorescence of 248*f*
Brain and optic nerve study 260
Branching vascular network 203
Breast cancer 244, 245
Bruch's membrane opening 87
B-scan ultrasonography 233*f*

# C

Calcified psammoma bodies 230*f*
Cancer
   risk of secondary 227
   treatment of primary source of 239
Cap opening incision 64*f*
Capillary hemangioma 240
Cascaded deep learning system, framework of 176
Cataract 95, 111, 118, 124, 178, 183
   causes 118
   complicated 118, 119, 120*f*
   dense brown 122
   diagnosis 12
   extraction 122
      extracapsular 122
   hard 108
   haze 179*f*
   incidence of 119, 119*t*
   surgery 68, 107, 110, 118, 121
      indications for 120
      phase of 280
      total 120*f*
Cavernous hemangioma 240
Central cornea 57
Central nervous system 227, 262
Central retinal
   thickness 144
   vascular trunk 26
Central serous chorioretinopathy 196, 200*f*, 201, 203, 204*f*, 205*f*, 207*f*
   acute 197*f*, 198, 201
   chronic 198*f*, 201
   episodes of 200
   masquerades of 201
Chiasmal compression, cause of 263
Choriocapillaris
   loss 212
   nonperfusion 201
Choroid 196
   detachment 128
   granuloma 245
   hemangioma 245
   melanoma 223, 238*f*, 245
   metastatic lesion 249*f*
   neovascularization 187, 206, 245
   nevus 235
   osteoma 245
   structure of 86*f*
   vessels 212
Choroidal metastasis 244, 248, 249*f*
   clinical features 245
   diagnosis 245
   differential diagnosis of 246*b*
   treatment 250
   ultrasonography 247
Choroidal neovascularization, active 258
Ciliary body medulloepithelioma 237
Ciliary dysfunction 127
Classic lumpy-bumpy appearance 249*f*
Clectronic medical record 9
Clinical decision support system 8, 276
Collagen fibers, peripheral 61
Color fundus photograph 139*t*, 194
Common macular diseases, multimodal imaging in 196
Communication
   human 13
   system 8
Compound annual growth rate 4*f*
Computational technology, development of 273

Index

Computer languages 254
Computer systems 33
Computer vision 134
Computer-aided detection, development of 259
Computer-based image analysis 151
Contact interface, application of 55*f*
Contact lens 50
  sensor 12
Contoura
  vision 43
  workstation 56*f*
Contralateral choroid 245
Conventional ablation 46
Conventional dissection 64*f*
Convolution neural network 11, 36, 135, 138*f*, 153, 178*fc*, 182, 183, 185-188, 254, 280
  basic structure of 175*f*
Cornea
  clear 127*f*
  contact interface 59*f*
  demonstrates, anterior 45
  ectasias 11
  edema 128
  endothelial cell 71
  lenticule extraction 66, 68
  nerves, lower number of 62
  side cut 60*f*
  thinner 50
  tissue 52
  tomographic technologies 38
  topography 33
  transplantation 68
  treatment in thinner 50
  visualization scheimpflug technology 37
  volume 38
Corneal lenticule extraction 64
  different 68
Corneal stroma 67
  edema 122
Corneal thickness, half 73
Corticosteroids 118
COVID-19, pandemic of 145
Cryoretinopexy, adjunctive 112
Crystalline lens 74*f*
  normal 70
Current femtosecond lasers 65*t*
Cuticular drusen 211
Cyclitic membrane 128, 129
Cycloplegic refraction 71
Cyclotorsion compensation 47

Cystoid macular edema 118, 122, 125, 127, 128, 128*f*
Cysts, predominantly 128*f*

## D

Data 2
  augmentation 153
  collection, method of 29*f*
  generated 5
  lack of integration of 39
  training set 134
  types of 23
Data-driven decisions, era of 15
Deep convolutional neural networks, working of 135*f*
Deep learning 20, 36, 97, 134, 151, 153, 182, 184, 186, 254, 275
  based image analysis, future of 168
  system 12
    combination of 258
Deep neural network 23, 160
  architecture 24*fc*
Deep residual learning network, layers of 260
Diabetes, burden of 132
Diabetic macular edema 111, 132, 141, 142*t*, 144, 175, 182
  diagnosis of 140
  identifying 140
Diabetic retinopathy 9, 12, 21, 34, 132, 136, 143, 144, 144*f*, 175, 183, 255, 276
  annotation of 138*f*
  detection 145
  diagnose 182
  identifying 137, 143
  management of 156
  nonproliferative 144, 256
  proliferative 132, 256
  screening for 132, 133
    evolution of 133
  sign of 1
Digital devices via Siri and Alexa 273
Digital technologies 2
Diopters 28
Dipping sign 201
Disciform scar 245
Disease
  identification of stage of 160
  progression 50
Doppler optical coherence tomography 94
Double-layer sign 208, 217
Drusen 210

Drusenoid pigment epithelial detachment 212, 215*f*, 216, 216*f*
Dry eye disease 67

# E

Eccentric photorefraction
   method, advantages of 28
      prediction with 27*fc*
Ectasia 70
Electronic medical records 8
Emmetropia 113
Emmetropic refraction 113
En face scan 84
Endoscopic endonasal techniques 231
Endothelial growth factor 182
Enucleated eyeball, cut section of 226*f*
Epi-laser-assisted in situ keratomileusis, steps of 49*f*
Epiretinal membrane 111
Epithelial flap 49*f*
Excimer laser 44
   ablation 49*f*
      stromal 55*f*
   flying spot placement of 45*f*
   types of 45, 45*b*
External beam radiotherapy 250
External validation, lack of 38
Extracellular signal-regulated kinase 227
Exudative retinal detachment 128, 244
Eye 35, 107, 112
   asymptomatic fellow 200
   care professional 98
   disease, diabetic 9
   enucleated 230*f*, 237, 238*f*
   keratoconic 50
   left 233*f*, 246*f*, 247*f*
   leukemic 237*f*
   movement 47
      intraoperative 47
   right 202*f*, 205*f*, 214*f*, 246*f*, 247*f*
   tracking in excimer laser 46
   unaffected 35
   vitrectomized 111, 114
Eyeball, enucleated 226*f*
Eyelashes 179*f*
Eyelid speculum 47

# F

Femtosecond laser 61*b*, 66
   assisted small incision lenticule extraction, surgical steps of 62*f*

Femtosecond laser in situ keratomileusis 52
   advantages of 54
   performing 67
Femtosecond lenticule extraction 61
Fibrin
   central serous chorioretinopathy 202*f*
   composed of 201
   membrane 118, 127*f*
      post-uveitic cataract extraction 127*f*
Fibrovascular pigment epithelial detachment 208
Fiery-red optic disk, appearance of 262
Fine-needle aspiration biopsy 250
Flap creation, laser settings for 54, 54*b*
Flapless procedure 48
Fluorescein
   angiogram 140, 143, 144
   angiography 248
Focal external limiting membrane 196
Foveal cone photoreceptors 25
Foveomacular vitelliform dystrophy, adult-onset 218*f*
Fuchs heterochromic iridocyclitis 119
Fuchs iridocyclitis 125
Fundus
   autofluorescence 156, 193, 195, 197, 197*f*, 247
   camera, quality of 166
   color photographs 132, 137
   fluorescein angiography 128*f*, 193, 196, 208, 233*f*, 249*f*
   images
      cases in 261
      evaluation of 159
   pathology, treatment of 120

# G

Galilei analyzer 37
Gamma knife radiosurgery 250
Ganglion cell
   analysis 85
   complex 85, 91
   inner plexiform layer 86
   layer 80, 82, 86
Gas tamponade 112
   effect of 112
Gastrointestinal tract carcinoma 245
Gene therapy 227
Geographic atrophy 187, 212, 258
Glaucoma 11, 12, 21, 34, 80, 85, 89*t*, 93, 94, 97, 98, 104, 121, 126, 129, 151, 182, 183, 255, 257

assessment of 98
care 97
case of 100
diagnosis of 80, 90, 97-99, 99*t*, 100
    model in 99*f*
early 93
management of 97, 104
mild 85
neovascular 126
normal tension 94
prediction 90
preperimetric 93
progression analysis 88, 89*t*
progression of 95, 99
screening 91, 98
secondary angle-closure 73
sign of 1
suspicious for 92
Glaucomatous optic neuropathy 100, 257
Glioma, malignant 228
Granulomatous iridocyclitis, anterior 121

## H

Hand-drawn image features, use of 275
Harnessing information 168
Health Insurance and Portability and
    Accountability Act 5
Healthcare
    data 3
    providers 8, 15
    research 5*f*
Hemorrhage
    preretinal 132
    splinter 236, 237*f*
    vitreous 178, 179*f*
Human brain, function of 35
Human leukocyte antigen 125
Hyalinized connective tissues 227*f*
Hyaloid traction, posterior 142
Hyperautofluorescence 200
Hyperechoic small dome-shaped
    lesion 233*f*
Hyperfluorescence, zones of 201
Hypermetropia 26
Hyperopia 51, 71
    correction of 67
Hyperopic small incision lenticule
    extraction 67
    treatment 68*f*
Hyphema 71, 122
Hypoautofluorescence, patches of 216
Hypotony 118, 121, 127
    chronic 128

## I

Ideal opaque bubble layer 53*f*
Images captured, quality of 166
Implant, pupillary capture of 128
Implantable collamer lens 70
Indocyanine green 196
    angiography 193, 208, 248
Infections 262
Inflammation 263
    before surgery, control of 118
    management of 122
    postoperative 125
    preoperative control of 121
Inflammatory cytokines 119
Infrared cameras 46
Inner plexiform layer 82, 86
Intelligent robots 273, 275
Intensive care unit 274
Internal limiting membrane 168
Internal reflectivity, moderate 216
Internuclear ophthalmoplegia 247
Intracorneal implants 43
Intraocular gas 113
Intraocular lens 33, 43, 112, 125, 179*f*
    calculation of 108
    contraindication of 119
    correct 279
    estimation of 107
    formula, accuracy of 114
    placement 118
    power, adjusting 113
Intraocular malignancy 244
Intraocular pressure 12, 52, 66, 125
    elevated 126
    lower 121
Intraocular tumors 236
    cases of 237
Intraretinal fluid 142, 208
Intraretinal neovascularization 206
Intrastromal lenticule 67
    refractive correction 64
Intravitreal antivascular growth factor 251
Intrinsic noise interference 88
Iridotomy, peripheral 73
Iris
    mid-peripheral 70
    registration of 46, 48*f*
    spatula 123
Ischemic index 144
Ischemic optic neuropathy,
    anterior 253, 263

# Index

## J

Juvenile idiopathic arthritis 118, 119
Juvenile rheumatoid arthritis 125
Juxtapapillary choroidal melanoma 235

## K

Keratectasia 50
Keratitis, infective 33
Keratoconus 33, 38, 50
    diagnosis 37*t*
    management of 33
    topography-guided treatment for 50
Keratometric flattening 50
Keratometry, paracentral mean 38
Keratopathy, band-shaped 120*f*, 121, 129
Keratorefractive procedures 75, 76
Kidney cancer 245
K-nearest neighbors 35

## L

Lamellar keratitis, diffuse 54
Laser epithelial keratomileusis 48
Laser in situ keratomileusis 43, 51
    flaps, used for 69
    microkeratome 52
    steps of microkeratome 52*f*
    surgical steps of 54
    topography-guided 56, 57
Laser system's optical aperture 58
Laser vision correction 76
    advantages of 76
Laser-assisted in situ keratomileusis 66
    thin flap 62
Late-phase hyperfluorescence, evidence of 232
Learning
    transfer 154
    unsupervised 35
Left eye 233*f*, 246*f*, 247*f*
    fundus photograph of 232*f*
Lens
    position, effective 111
    proteins, oxidation of 107
    thickness 112
    vault 73
Lens-iris diaphragm 113
Lenticule extraction, performing manual 60
Lenticule side cut 60*f*, 64*f*
Lenticuloschisis 63, 64*f*
Linear discriminant analysis 90
Lipofuscin 247
Lung cancer 244, 245

## M

Machine learning 9, 21, 97, 98, 133, 134, 151, 152, 182, 184, 186, 188, 253, 254, 272-274
    algorithms, types of 20
    application of 6
    supervised 35
    techniques 168
    utilizing, types of 37*t*
Macula 128*f*
    thickness of 88
Macular diseases
    multimodal imaging in 193
    variety of 194
    vitrectomy for 111
Macular disorders, common 193
Macular edema, identifying 140
Macular ganglion cell 91*f*
    complex analysis 91
Macular holes 111
Macular neovascularization 208*t*
    type 1 203, 205*f*, 206*f*
Macular pathology 111
Macular retinal pigment epithelium lesions 213*f*
Magnetic resonance imaging 248
Malignancy, primary systemic 245
Medical device 10
Medical education 280
Melanocytoma 231
    histopathology of 234*f*
Melanoma cells 238*f*
    malignant 234
    positive 237
Memory, long short-term 22, 254
Meningeal tumors 236
Meningioma 223
Meningoepithelial cells, proliferation of 228
Meniscus lenses 113
Metastasis 223, 244, 262
Methyl methacrylate 123
Microkeratome 52
Micrometastases 248
Microplasma
    bubbles, small 54
    formation 53
Mitomycin C 49*f*
Mobile application 142*f*
Modern refractive corneal lenticule extraction 65*t*
Morphology, types on basis of 262
Multifocal visual-evoked potential 229

Index

Multiple sclerosis 259
Multiscale analysis, retinal image 158
Munnerlyn equation 44
Myopia 26, 27, 29, 48, 156
    correct 51
    high 261
Myopic correction 44

# N

National Health Service 4
National Indigenous Eye Health Survey 140
Natural language processing 10, 21, 273, 275
Near vision, correction for 20
Near-infrared
    band 29$f$
    reflectance 193, 194
Neodymium-doped yttrium aluminum garnet 127
Neovascular membrane, types of 203
Neovascular ocular conditions 182
Neovascularization, types of 206
Nerve tissue, sampling of 90
Neural network 36, 182
Neurofibromatosis-1 224
Neurons 254
Neuro-ophthalmic
    conditions 255
    disorders, variety of 263
    tumors 263
Neuro-ophthalmology 253, 258, 259, 264
    field of 258, 263
Neuroretinitis 262
Neuroscientific theory 153
Neurosensory detachment 202$f$
Nongovernmental organizations 7
Noninflammatory causes 263
Nonlinear anisotropic filters 88
Nonmydriatic fundus camera 176
Nonsteroidal anti-inflammatory drugs 122
Nutritional deficiencies 262

# O

Occlusive retinal vasculopathies 238
Ocular examination, repeated 156
Ocular hypertension 118
Ocular hypotony 127
Ocular oncology 244
Ocular pathologies 95, 255
Ocular surface disorders 33
Ocular tissue, intrinsic autofluorescence of 247
Ocular tumors 11
Ocular wavefront 51
Opaque bubble layer 54
    pattern of 53
Ophthalmic diseases 282
Ophthalmic disorders 14
Ophthalmology
    clinical practice of 261
    disorders, treatment of 265
Ophthalmoscopy 133
Optic chiasma 228
Optic disk 82$f$, 86$f$, 100, 261
    appearance 261
    characteristics of 259
    cube 82$f$, 85$f$, 87$f$
    detection of 261
    disorders 261
    edema 235, 261
        bilateral 238
    metastasis, diagnosis of 239
    metastatic melanoma to 235
    pathologies 261
    photographs 12
    surface 232$f$
    visual evaluation of 259
Optic disk melanocytoma 231, 232$f$
    complications 235
    differential diagnosis 235
    histopathology 233
    investigations 232
    management 234
    pathogenesis 231
    transformation of 234
Optic nerve 237$f$, 238$f$
    cut section of 238$f$
    edges of 232$f$
    hypoplasia 247$f$
    inflammation of 262
    kinking of 225$f$
    magnetic resonance imaging 263
    melanocytoma 223
    meningioma, morphology of 230$f$
    parenchyma 226$f$
    right 229$f$
    secondary metastasis of 239$f$
Optic nerve glioma 223, 224
    investigations 225
    management 226
    pathogenesis 224
    right-sided 225$f$
Optic nerve head 25, 82, 87$f$, 98, 257
    classification of 261
Optic nerve sheath meningioma 223, 228
    investigations 229

## Index

management 229
  specimen of 231*f*
Optic nerve tumors
  primary 223, 224
  recent advances in 223
  secondary 223, 235
Optic neuritis 253, 262, 263
Optic neuropathy, demyelinating 262
Optic pathway glioma, part of 224
Optic zone, larger effective 74
Optical biometry 107, 109
Optical coherence tomography 27, 30, 37, 66, 80, 87*f*, 89*f*, 93, 98, 128*f*, 140, 141, 142*t*, 144*f*, 156, 193, 195, 248, 253, 255, 272, 273
  adaptive optics 93
  angiography 143, 193, 208
  anterior segment 74*f*
  common spectral domain 81*t*
  devices 81
  home-based 141*f*
  image
    posterior segment 27
    preprocessing 88
    segmentation 88
  intraoperative 66, 69
  method
    advantages of posterior segment 27
    disadvantages of posterior segment 27
  polarization-sensitive 94
  spectral domain 93, 185-188, 193, 208, 216
Optimizing intraocular lens power calculation 107
Orbital fractures 282
Orbitofacial fractures 282
Otago Diabetic Eye Monitoring Service 140

## P

Palpebral fissure 60
Papilledema 253, 259
  different grades of 260
  severity of 261
Papillitis 262
  diagnosis of 262
Paraneoplastic optic neuropathy 239
Pediatric uveitic cataract 118
  cause of 128
  surgery 128
Pegasus 261
PentaCam 36, 37
Perceptrons 254

Peripapillary retinal nerve fiber layer 80, 82
  thickness 262
Peripapillary splinter hemorrhages 262
Peripapillary staphylomas 95
Peripapillary vitreous hemorrhage 235
Peripheral retinal lesions 177
Peripupillary membranectomy 123
Phacovitrectomy 112
  combined 114
  procedures 112
Phakic intraocular implants 43
Phakic intraocular lens 70
  demonstrating 74*f*
  implantation 70
  indications of 71
  iris-supported 70
  types of 70
Phakic technology, posterior chamber 75
Photoablation 44
Photodynamic therapy 244, 250
Photodynamic treatment 251
Photorefraction, theory of 28
Photorefractive keratectomy 44, 48
  advantages of 48
Phototherapeutic keratectomy 49*f*, 51
  topography-assisted 51
Phthisis bulbi 128
Pigment dispersion 122, 232
Pigment epithelial detachment 208
Pituitary apoplexy 264
Pituitary gland, vicinity of 263
Pituitary tumor 253, 263
Plaque radiotherapy 244, 250
Plus disease 155
  automated diagnosis of 162
  conundrum 158
  detection of 163
  diagnostic accuracy of 159
  identification of 162
Polychromatic luster 119
Polymethyl methacrylate 114
Polypoidal choroidal vasculopathy 201, 204*f*, 217, 219*f*
Positron emission tomography 239
Post-cataract surgery 128*f*
Post-COVID era 260
Posterior capsular
  opacification 127, 128
  opacity 178
  rupture 123
Posterior chamber phakic intraocular lens, advantages of 74
Posterior lenticule
  cut 60*f*
  surface 60

# Index

Postuveitic cataract extraction  126
Postvitrectomy cataract  107, 108
Power, calculation of  71
Presbyopia  26
Presbyopic correction  43
Presbyopic phakic intraocular lens  75, 75$f$
Prior optic neuritis, history of  262
Procarbazine  227
Prostate cancer  245
Protected health information  6
Proton beam radiotherapy  250
Pseudohypopyon  203
Pseudophakia  70
Psychophysical methods  25
Pterygia  72
Pterygium excision  68
Pupil  29
    centroid  46, 47
        shift  47
    management  123
    small  123

## Q

Quality of life, vision-related  67

## R

Racemose hemangioma  240
Radial scan  83
Radiation therapy  230
Raster scan  84
Real-life scenarios, translation to  101
Rectified linear unit  135
Recurrent chronic serous
        chorioretinopathy  198$f$
Recurrent neural network  22, 36, 188
Red blood cells  126
Refametinib  227
Refraction  22
Refractive corneal lenticule extraction,
        advantages of  66
Refractive error  11, 20, 22, 29, 33, 112
    degree of  24
    detection network  22
        visualization in  28$f c$
    diagnosis of  30$t$
    postoperative  110
    predicting  22, 27
    range of  26
Refractive lenticule extraction  58
Refractive surgery  33, 43, 76
    advances in  43
    formulas for  279

Regression tree  90
Reinforcement learning  36
Relex smile  61
Reticular pseudodrusen  211, 213$f$, 214$f$
Retina
    computer-assisted image
        analysis of  159
    glial tumor of  240
    hamartoma of  235
    multiple layers of  237$f$
    normal  176$f$
    specialists  12, 186
    stability of  113
    vascular tumors of  240
Retinal angiomatous proliferation  206,
        208, 211$f$
Retinal atrophy, outer  216, 217$f$
Retinal blood flow  94
Retinal detachment  11, 132, 174, 175, 177$f$,
        178
    detection  175
    diagnosis of  174
    stages of  164
Retinal disease  174
    single  193
Retinal edema  235
Retinal exudation  235
Retinal fundus
    image method, disadvantages of  26
    images  22, 25, 26, 163
    photograph  23
Retinal hemorrhage  235
Retinal imaging, field of  193
Retinal landmark  25, 26
Retinal nerve fiber  92
    layer  80, 82, 84, 87$f$, 98
Retinal photographs  265, 273
Retinal pigment epithelial
    detachment  196
    progression of  217$f$
Retinal pigment epithelium  109, 196, 199$f$,
        216, 235, 247
    adenoma of  235
    hyperplasia of  235
Retinal surface detection  280
Retinal thickness  142
    structural  262
Retinal vascular occlusion  11
Retinal vein occlusion  182, 235
Retinitis  238
Retinoblastoma  237
Retinopathy of prematurity  11, 12, 34, 98,
        151, 154, 157, 167, 182, 255, 278
    automated analysis of  161

automated identification of 161
deep learning in 160
developing 167
diagnosis of 161
    stage in 162
evaluation of infants for 155
learning-derived 165
management of 121, 155
screening 167
telemedical 162
teleophthalmology for 157
threatening stages of 168
treatment-requiring 155
Retinopathy, exudative 238
Retrobulbar neuritis 262
    classic example of 262
Rhegmatogenous retinal detachment 176$f$
Ribonucleic acid 152
Rigid gas permeable 50
Robotic surgery 272
Rosenthal fibers 223, 227$f$
Rubeosis 129

## S

Sagging sign 201
Sarcoidosis 119, 125
Sawtooth pattern 211
Scanning laser ophthalmoscopy 196
Scleral buckling procedure 112
Serous
    chorioretinopathy, chronic 199$f$
    macular detachment 197$f$, 198$f$
Silicone oil 107, 110$t$, 111
    filled eye 108, 109, 113
    incomplete 109
    refractive index of 113
Simple automated detectors 35
Simulate human
    behavior 11
    conversation 13
Simulate intuitive human behavior 11
Singapore Integrated Diabetic Retinopathy Program 140, 256
Skin cancer 245
Small incision lenticule extraction 58, 60$f$, 61, 61$b$, 62, 63$f$, 66
    advantages of 61
Smoking status 34
Smooth stromal interface 69
Soft drusen, multimodal imaging of 212$f$
Solitary metastasis 244, 250
Spectral domain optical coherence tomography, limitations of 95

Spherical aberrations 62
Spherical equivalent 22
Sphincter tissue 123
Standard management protocols 226
Steeper central corneal configuration 67
Stereotactic radiotherapy 230
Steroid treatment, aggressive 127$f$
Strabismus 11
Stretch pupilloplasty 123, 124$f$
Striate keratopathy post-cataract extraction 127$f$
Subcapsular cataract, posterior 118, 120$f$
Subfoveal choroidal thickness, reduced 216
Submandibular gland 245
Subretinal fluid 201, 208
    localized 235
Subretinal hyperreflective material 201
Subretinal mass, yellow-white 245
Subretinal neovascularization 206
Subretinal polypoidal lesions 217
Suction peak pressure 69
Supervised learning, workflow of 102$fc$
Support vector machine 14
Surgery, posterior segment 107
Surgical robotics 279
Synechiolysis, posterior 123
Systemic immunosuppressive drugs 125

## T

Telemedicine
    application in 174
    role in 180
Teleophthalmology 155
Temozolomide 227
Thioguanine 227
Three-dimensional scan 82
Topography measurement machines 38
Topo-guided
    ablation profile 46
    approach 50
Tortuosity index 159
Toxoplasmosis, reactivation of 122
Trabeculectomy 126
Traction retinal detachment 142
Train neural networks 11
Tram track sign 229
Trametinib 227
Transepithelial photorefractive keratectomy 49$f$, 50
Transpupillary radiotherapy 244, 250
Transpupillary thermotherapy 244, 251
Tumors 245
Typical ophthalmoscopic features 245

# Index

## U

Ultrasound biometry 107
Ultrawide field fundus color
 photographs 140
Ultrawide field image 176$f$
Unique retinal vascular patterns 265
Unsupervised learning, workflow of 103$fc$
Uveal metastasis 238
Uveitic cataract 118, 119, 127
 extraction 125
 management of 118, 129
 surgery 121, 122, 124, 128
  complication of 127
Uveitic entities 119$t$, 125$t$
Uveitis 119, 126$f$, 128$f$
 cataract surgery 119
 flare-up of 128
 herpetic 119
 HLA-B27 125
 intermediate 119
 pediatric 129
 phacoantigenic 120
 type of 125

## V

Validation sets 134
Vascular endothelial growth factor 184
Vascular insufficiency 262
Vascular severity score 163, 164, 169
Videokeratoscope 36, 37
Virtual reality technologies 280
Viscoelastic cannula 123
Viscosities 110$t$
Vision
 and eye health surveillance system 7
 decreased 33
 impairment, treatment for 1

Vision loss 97, 228, 235
 irreversible 262
 severe 182
Vision-threatening
 diabetic retinopathy, identifying 140
 late, developing 189
Visual acuity 126$f$, 232
 best-corrected 144
 uncorrected distance 56
Visual debility, permanent 175
Visual evoked potentials 263
Visual field, lead to 257
Visual loss
 moderate 235
 severe progressive 239
Visual morbidity 180
Visual pathway, lesions of 264
Visual quality, degradation of 50
Visualization tool 261
VisuMax laser system 69
 femtosecond 59$f$
Vitelliform macular dystrophy 207$f$
Vitrectomy
 complications of 107
 posterior 122
Vitreomacular traction 111
Vitreoretinal pathologies 107
Vitreous
 detachment, posterior 84
 replacement of 111
 seeds 235
Vitritis 178
Vulnerable cohorts, identification of 4

## W

Wavefront-guided ablation 46
Wavefront-optimized ablation 46
White-to-white diameter, measurement
 of 71, 72$f$

Milton Keynes UK
Ingram Content Group UK Ltd.
UKHW050739090724
445259UK00003B/17